Vascular Surgery and Endovascular Therapy

Editor

GIRMA TEFERA

SURGICAL CLINICS
OF NORTH AMERICA

www.surgical.theclinics.com

Consulting Editor
RONALD F. MARTIN

August 2013 • Volume 93 • Number 4

ELSEVIER

1600 John F. Kennedy Boulevard • Suite 1800 • Philadelphia, Pennsylvania, 19103-2899
http://www.surgical.theclinics.com

SURGICAL CLINICS OF NORTH AMERICA Volume 93, Number 4
August 2013 ISSN 0039–6109, ISBN-13: 978-0-323-18616-2

Editor: John Vassallo, j.vassallo@elsevier.com
Developmental Editor: Susan Showalter

Surgical Clinics of North America (ISSN 0039–6109) is published bimonthly by Elsevier Inc., 360 Park Avenue South, New York, NY 10010-1710. Months of publication are February, April, June, August, October, and December. Business and Editorial Offices: 1600 John F. Kennedy Blvd., Suite 1800, Philadelphia, PA 19103-2899. Periodicals postage paid at New York, NY and additional mailing offices. Subscription prices are $353.00 per year for US individuals, $598.00 per year for US institutions, $173.00 per year for US students and residents, $432.00 per year for Canadian individuals, $741.00 per year for Canadian institutions, $487.00 for international individuals, $741.00 per year for international institutions and $238.00 per year for Canadian and foreign students/residents. To receive student/resident rate, orders must be accompanied by name of affiliated institution, date of term, and the *signature* of program/residency coordinator on institution letterhead. Orders will be billed at individual rate until proof of status is received. Foreign air speed delivery is included in all *Clinics* subscription prices. All prices are subject to change without notice. POSTMASTER: Send address changes to *Surgical Clinics*, Elsevier Health Sciences Division, Subscription Customer Service, 3251 Riverport Lane, Maryland Heights, MO 63043. **Customer Service (orders, claims, online, change of address): Telephone: 1-800-654-2452 (U.S. and Canada); 314-447-8871 (outside U.S. and Canada). Fax: 314-447-8029. E-mail: journalscustomerservice-usa@elsevier.com (for print support); journalsonline support-usa@elsevier.com (for online support).**

Reprints. For copies of 100 or more, of articles in this publication, please contact the Commercial Reprints Department, Elsevier Inc., 360 Park Avenue South, New York, New York 10010-1710. Tel. (212) 633-3812, Fax: (212) 462-1935, e-mail: reprints@elsevier.com.

The Surgical Clinics of North America is also published in Spanish by McGraw-Hill Interamericana Editores S.A., P.O. Box 5-237 06500 Mexico D.F. Mexico; and in Portuguese by Interlivros Edicoes Ltda., Rua Comandante Coelho 1085, CEP 21250, Rio de Janeiro, Brazil; and in Greek by Paschalidis Medical Publications, Athens Greece.

The Surgical Clinics of North America is covered in *MEDLINE/PubMed (Index Medicus), EMBASE/Excerpta Medica, Current Contents/Clinical Medicine, Current Contents/Life Sciences, Science Citation Index*, and *ISI/BIOMED.*

Printed and bound by CPI Group (UK) Ltd, Croydon, CR0 4YY

Transferred to digital print 2012

Contributors

CONSULTING EDITOR

RONALD F. MARTIN, MD, FACS
Staff Surgeon, Department of Surgery, Marshfield Clinic, Marshfield, Wisconsin; Clinical Associate Professor, University of Wisconsin School of Medicine and Public Health, Madison, Wisconsin; Colonel, Medical Corps, United States Army Reserve

EDITOR

GIRMA TEFERA, MD
Vice Chair, Division of Vascular Surgery, Department of Surgery, University of Wisconsin School of Medicine and Public Health, Chief of Vascular Surgery at William S. Middleton VA Hospital, Madison, Wisconsin

AUTHORS

TRISSA BABROWSKI, MD
Fellow, Section of Vascular Surgery and Endovascular Therapy, The University of Chicago Medical Center, Chicago, Illinois

MATTHEW J. BLECHA, MD
Section of Vascular Surgery and Endovascular Therapy, The University of Chicago Medical Center; St. Joseph Hospital, Chicago, Illinois

JOSEPH L. BOBADILLA, MD
Assistant Professor, Vascular & Endovascular Surgery, Department of Surgery, University of Kentucky, Lexington, Kentucky

KELLIE R. BROWN, MD
Associate Professor of Surgery and Radiology, Division of Vascular Surgery, The Medical College of Wisconsin, Milwaukee, Wisconsin

RACHAEL A. CALLCUT, MD, MSPH
Assistant Professor, Department of Surgery, San Francisco General Hospital, University of California-San Francisco (UCSF), San Francisco, California

RABIH A. CHAER, MD
Associate Professor of Surgery, Division of Vascular Surgery, University of Pittsburgh Medical Center, Pittsburgh, Pennsylvania

COURTNEY DALY, MD
Vascular Surgery Resident, Division of Vascular Surgery, Feinberg School of Medicine, Northwestern University, Chicago, Illinois

CHRISTOPHER J. FRANÇOIS, MD
Associate Professor, Department of Radiology, University of Wisconsin School of Medicine and Public Health, Madison, Wisconsin

HEATHER A. HALL, MD
Clinical Associate, Section of Vascular Surgery and Endovascular Therapy, The University of Chicago Medical Center, Chicago, Illinois

PETER K. HENKE, MD
Professor, Section of Vascular Surgery, University of Michigan, Ann Arbor, Michigan

JOHN R. HOCH, MD
Professor of Surgery, Division of Vascular Surgery, Department of Surgery, University of Wisconsin School of Medicine and Public Health, Madison, Wisconsin

ANDREW W. HOEL, MD
Assistant Professor, Division of Vascular Surgery, Feinberg School of Medicine, Northwestern University, Chicago, Illinois

KAKRA HUGHES, MD, FACS
Assistant Professor of Surgery, Director of Endovascular Surgery, Department of Surgery, Howard University Hospital, Howard University College of Medicine, Washington, DC

HEATHER M. JOHNSON, MD
Division of Cardiovascular Medicine, University of Wisconsin School of Medicine and Public Health, Madison, Wisconsin

JORDAN P. KNEPPER, MD
Section of Vascular Surgery, University of Michigan, Ann Arbor, Michigan

PETER J. MASON, MD, MPH
Division of Cardiovascular Medicine, University of Wisconsin School of Medicine and Public Health, Madison, Wisconsin

MATTHEW W. MELL, MD, MS
Assistant Professor, Division of Vascular Surgery, Department of Surgery, Stanford University School of Medicine, Stanford, California

SAMANTHA MINC, MD
Fellow, Section of Vascular Surgery and Endovascular Therapy, The University of Chicago Medical Center, Chicago, Illinois

HERON E. RODRIGUEZ, MD
Associate Professor of Vascular Surgery and Radiology, Division of Vascular Surgery, Feinberg School of Medicine, Northwestern University, Chicago, Illinois

DAVID A. ROSE, MD, FACS
Associate Professor, Chief of Vascular Surgery, Department of Surgery, Howard University Hospital, Howard University College of Medicine, Washington, DC

PETER J. ROSSI, MD
Assistant Professor of Surgery and Radiology, Division of Vascular Surgery, The Medical College of Wisconsin, Milwaukee, Wisconsin

EMMANUEL SONAIKE, MD
Surgical Resident, Department of Surgery, Howard University Hospital, Howard University College of Medicine, Washington, DC

PASITHORN A. SUWANABOL, MD
Surgical Resident, Department of Surgery, University of Wisconsin School of Medicine and Public Health, Madison, Wisconsin

TOSHIO TAKAYAMA, MD, PhD
Division of Vascular Surgery, Department of Surgery, University of Wisconsin School of Medicine and Public Health, Madison, Wisconsin

MATTHEW C. TATTERSALL, DO
Division of Cardiovascular Medicine, University of Wisconsin School of Medicine and Public Health, Madison, Wisconsin

WILLIAM WU, MD
Division of Vascular Surgery, University of Pittsburgh Medical Center, Pittsburgh, Pennsylvania

DAI YAMANOUCHI, MD, PhD
Assistant Professor, Division of Vascular Surgery, Department of Surgery, University of Wisconsin School of Medicine and Public Health, Madison, Wisconsin

Contents

Foreword: Vascular Surgery and Endovascular Therapy   xiii

Ronald F. Martin

Preface: Vascular Surgery and Endovascular Therapy   xvii

Girma Tefera

Noninvasive Imaging Workup of Patients with Vascular Disease   741

Christopher J. François

> The diagnostic workup of patients with cardiovascular disease is frequently challenging, and requires a multimodality approach to appropriately determine management. Depending on the presenting symptoms and their acuity, noninvasive diagnostic imaging strategies can include radiography, ultrasonography, computed tomography, and magnetic resonance imaging. This article provides an introduction to the use of these imaging modalities for commonly encountered diseases of the aorta, mesenteric arteries, and renal arteries, focusing on how the acuity of presentation and likelihood of disease affects the workup of patients with known or suspected vascular disease.

Contemporary and Optimal Medical Management of Peripheral Arterial Disease   761

Matthew C. Tattersall, Heather M. Johnson, and Peter J. Mason

> Atherosclerotic lower extremity peripheral arterial disease (PAD) is a highly prevalent condition associated with a significant increase in risk of all-cause mortality and cardiovascular morbidity and mortality. PAD is underdiagnosed and undertreated. Treatment is focused on (1) lowering cardiovascular risk and cardiovascular disease event rates and (2) improvement in symptoms and quality of life. Multidisciplinary and intersociety guidelines guide optimal medical therapy. Substantial evidence supports implementation of tobacco cessation counseling and pharmacotherapy to help achieve tobacco abstinence, antiplatelet therapy, HMG-CoA reductase inhibitors (statins) therapy, and antihypertensive therapy for the purpose of lowering cardiovascular event rates and improving survival.

Diagnosis, Prevention, and Treatment of Claudication   779

Jordan P. Knepper and Peter K. Henke

> Lower extremity chronic ischemia due to atherosclerosis represents the continuum of peripheral arterial disease, encompassing intermittent claudication, rest pain, and tissue loss. Traditionally, the indication for invasive intervention has been critical limb ischemia as a means to prevent amputation. This article highlights claudication and reviews its diagnosis, available treatment modalities, and preventative measures.

Critical Limb Ischemia

789

Matthew J. Blecha

Critical limb ischemia refers to the clinical state of advanced arterial occlusive disease, placing an extremity at risk for gangrene and limb loss. Critical limb ischemia has 2 broad clinical subcategories that are vital to differentiate: acute limb ischemia and chronic arterial occlusive disease. This article reviews the etiologies, diagnosis, and treatment of critical limb ischemia.

Carotid Artery Occlusive Disease

813

Courtney Daly and Heron E. Rodriguez

Carotid disease is a major contributor to stroke, one of the leading causes of death and disability in the United States. Clinically significant stenosis can be detected by duplex ultrasound using well-established criteria. In addition to optimal medical management, surgical and endovascular revascularizations of carotid disease have been demonstrated to be effective interventions that reduce the risk of stroke in properly selected patients.

Nonarteriosclerotic Vascular Disease

833

William Wu and Rabih A. Chaer

Thromboangiitis obliterans, or Buerger disease, is a chronic nonatherosclerotic endarteritis manifesting as inflammation and thrombosis of distal extremity small and medium-sized arteries resulting in relapsing episodes of distal extremity ischemia. Takayasu arteritis is a rare syndrome characterized by inflammation of the aortic arch, pulmonary, coronary, and cerebral vessels, presenting with cerebrovascular symptoms, myocardial ischemia, or upper extremity claudication in young, often female, patients. Kawasaki disease is a small- and medium-vessel acute systemic vasculitis of young children, with morbidity and mortality stemming from coronary artery aneurysms. Microscopic polyangiitis, Churg-Strauss syndrome, and Wegener granulomatosis are systemic small-vessel vasculitides, affecting arterioles, capillary beds and venules, and each presenting with variable effects on the pulmonary, renal and gastrointestinal systems.

Aneurysmal Disease: The Abdominal Aorta

877

Toshio Takayama and Dai Yamanouchi

Abdominal aortic aneurysm (AAA) is one of the leading causes of death in the United States. Approximately 80% of AAAs occur in the infrarenal abdominal aorta. Most are caused by a degenerative process in the aortic wall, and smoking is the risk factor most strongly associated with AAA. Contrast-enhanced computed tomography is the most reliable imaging modality. Open repair is more invasive initially but more durable, whereas endovascular aneurysm repair is less invasive but less durable. Since degradation of the aorta progresses with age, continuous follow-up after aneurysmal repair improves the long-term outcome.

Aneurysmal Disease: Thoracic Aorta   893

Andrew W. Hoel

Thoracic aortic aneurysms are clinically significant for their high mortality risk in the face of rupture. This article reviews the natural history and pathophysiology of thoracic and thoracoabdominal aortic aneurysms, discusses the evaluation of these patients, and details the treatment options. Specifically discussed are treatment advances arising from the development of endovascular technology.

Peripheral Artery Aneurysm   911

Heather A. Hall, Samantha Minc, and Trissa Babrowski

Peripheral aneurysms typically present as asymptomatic incidental findings or may present with symptoms when there is local compression of other structures, such as nerves or veins, with ischemia, or rarely with rupture. Larger and symptomatic aneurysms should be repaired. Ultrasonography, computed tomography angiography, and magnetic resonance angiography can be used to define inflow and outflow and better characterize the aneurysm, particularly size and thrombus. Repair of peripheral aneurysms typically involves resection with interposition grafting, although certain anatomic sites may be amenable to endovascular approaches. Femoral pseudoaneurysms can be managed with observation, surgical repair, ultrasound-guided compression, or ultrasound-guided thrombin injection.

Mesenteric Ischemia   925

Joseph L. Bobadilla

This article reviews the presentation, diagnosis, evaluation, and treatment of the various forms of mesenteric ischemia, including acute and chronic ischemia. In addition, nonocclusive mesenteric ischemia and median arcuate ligament compressive syndrome are covered. The goals are to provide a structured and evidence-based framework for the evaluation and management of patients with these intestinal ischemia syndromes. Special attention is given to avoiding typical pitfalls in the diagnostic and treatment pathways. Operative techniques are also briefly discussed, including an evidence-based review of newer endovascular techniques.

Modern Advances in Vascular Trauma   941

Rachael A. Callcut and Matthew W. Mell

Early diagnosis and intervention are paramount for improving the likelihood of a favorable outcome for traumatic vascular injuries. As technology has rapidly diversified, the diagnostic and therapeutic approaches available for vascular injuries have evolved. Mortality and morbidity from vascular injury have declined over the last decade. The use of vascular shunts and tourniquets has become standard of care in military medicine.

Superficial Venous Disease   963

Kellie R. Brown and Peter J. Rossi

Superficial venous disease is a common clinical problem. The concerning disease states of the superficial venous system are venous reflux, varicose veins, and superficial venous thrombosis. Superficial venous reflux can be a significant contributor to chronic venous stasis wounds of the lower extremity, the treatment of which can be costly both in terms of overall health care expenditure and lost working days for affected patients. Although commonly thought of as a benign process, superficial venous thrombosis is associated with several underlying pathologic processes, including malignancy and deep venous thrombosis.

Venous Thromboembolic Disease   983

Pasithorn A. Suwanabol and John R. Hoch

Venous thromboembolic disease is extremely common. Conventional treatment with anticoagulation alone aims to impede the progression of thrombus, and prevent recurrence and the development of pulmonary embolism. This is appropriate for most patients. However, in certain patient populations, this alone does not address the long-term complications of venous thromboembolic disease. Surgeons should be familiar with the surgical techniques that have been demonstrated to improve outcomes with low risk. Recent studies of catheter-directed thrombolysis have demonstrated its safety, efficacy, and possibly the superiority over standard treatment alone.

Hemodialysis Access   997

David A. Rose, Emmanuel Sonaike, and Kakra Hughes

The number of patients requiring dialysis is increasing, in particular those patients over the age of 75. The arteriovenous fistula is the preferred access for hemodialysis due to fewer complications and decreased mortality. Access complications are common and require early recognition and treatment. Postoperative access surveillance is important to ensure timely diagnosis and treatment of access-related complications. There is a continued need for high-quality data to assist in determining the best access for each patient.

Index   1013

SURGICAL CLINICS OF NORTH AMERICA

FORTHCOMING ISSUES

October 2013
Abdominal Wall Reconstruction
Michael Rosen, MD, *Editor*

December 2013
Current Topics in Transplantation
A. Osama Gaber, MD, *Editor*

February 2014
Acute Care Surgery
George Velmahos, MD, *Editor*

RECENT ISSUES

June 2013
Modern Concepts in Pancreatic Surgery
Stephen W. Behrman, MD, FACS, and
Ronald F. Martin, MD, FACS, *Editors*

April 2013
Multidisciplinary Breast Management
George M. Fuhrman, MD, and
Tari A. King, MD, *Editors*

February 2013
**Complications, Considerations and
Consequences of Colorectal Surgery**
Scott R. Steele, MD, *Editor*

December 2012
Surgical Critical Care
John A. Weigelt, MD, *Editor*

ISSUE OF RELATED INTEREST

Clinics in Plastic Surgery January 2011 (Vol. 38, Issue 1)
Vascular Anomalies
Arin K. Greene, MD, MMSc, and Chad A. Perlyn, MD, PhD, *Editors*

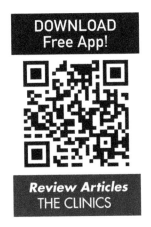

NOW AVAILABLE FOR YOUR iPhone and iPad

Foreword

Vascular Surgery and Endovascular Therapy

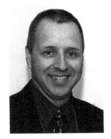

Ronald F. Martin, MD, FACS
Consulting Editor

DEFINITION OF AUTONOMY

1. The quality or state of being self-governing; *especially*: the right of self-government
2. Self-directing freedom and especially moral independence
3. A self-governing state

MEDICAL DEFINITION OF AUTONOMY

1. The quality or state of being independent, free, and self-directing
2. Independence from the organism as a whole in the capacity of a part for growth, reactivity, or responsiveness

—Merriam-Webster Dictionary

Some of us choose a path in our careers and follow it without wavering. Some of us make considerable course changes along the way. I began my surgical career fairly convinced I would become a vascular surgeon. When I look back on things, it still seems like it would have been a good idea, or at least a satisfying career. I was never one of those people who had an epiphany as to what to do, as it appears many of the applicants who apply to our training program report in their personal statements on the residency application. I suppose I followed a philosophy of wanting to work with people whose talents and work ethic I admired. During my medical school days, I was fortunate to spend time with a very capable group of vascular surgeons. They were brilliant, confident, and demanding as could be. I would find it hard to believe that the level of demand they placed on residents and students—though never more than on themselves from what I could see—would be tolerated in most institutions

Surg Clin N Am 93 (2013) xiii–xv
http://dx.doi.org/10.1016/j.suc.2013.06.008
0039-6109/13/$ – see front matter © 2013 Published by Elsevier Inc.

anymore. Still it wasn't just that rigor that I found intriguing. What drew me in was that they always had a plan and they could *always* articulate that plan. It didn't matter what complex problem came up because there were fundamental principles that led to actions that when combined properly got us through complex challenges. One of the absolute requirements of successful participation on this service was adherence to strict precision of language. One was simply not allowed to be sloppy or cavalier in how one described anything. I believe some of my colleagues (ie, medical students) felt that the rigidity and precision were somehow meant to be punitive. Some of us though preferred to think of the requirement as liberating because it improved our odds of success for and with the patient. Those of us who believed in this approach felt fairly confident that the need for precision was because our professors realized something we only guessed at—the whole situation can pivot dramatically on one significant detail.

I recently attended the Association of Program Directors in Surgery meeting in Florida. As always, it is a meeting equally filled with happiness from connecting with old and new friends and with trepidation as we listen to the changes that are likely to come as we try to manage the overall process of self-replication of the profession. Most years, there seems to be a buzzword that appears a bit overrepresented in discussions and in the program. This year that buzzword seemed to be "Autonomy." Lamentations of how we have lost autonomy, how residents no longer develop autonomy, ways in which we can simulate autonomy (maybe through group activity), and perhaps, even ways to test autonomy.

To me, the constant cry for "autonomy" is akin to the plaintive wail of an overtired 4-year-old who insists that she doesn't want help getting buckled into her car seat before the drive home. She informs me that she "can do it herself." It is possible that some of you are more patient than I and could wait to see this buckle get latched by less than nimble small fingers. I confess, at that point, my reaction is that getting home is a team project and autonomy is a minor consideration.

I would submit that we as surgeons lose perspective when we suggest we are autonomous or that our goal is to train someone to be autonomous. I will go so far to say it is a ludicrous concept in some regards because at the bare minimum there is the surgeon and the patient—and without the patient there is no need whatsoever for the surgeon. Even if it just boils down to the patient and the surgeon, I won't speak for you, but I am pretty much useless at the things I generally do without anesthesiologists, nurses, surgical technicians, other surgeons, etc. As a matter of fact, I am about the least autonomous person I know of from a professional standpoint.

Despite this desired romantic notion of the lone surgeon fearlessly facing down death and disease, the reality is we mostly play parts on teams. That is not our weakness—that is our strength. Good surgical teams are fluid and match the best resources to achieve the best results for those whom we serve. And as I have said before, it is remarkable what you can accomplish when you don't care who gets the credit.

I suggest we dispense with this professed fondness of autonomy for a bit and shift our focus. What is perhaps more important is that we train people to be leaders: leaders of not just other surgeons but of all kinds of teams. To do that, we have to train people to understand the roles of all, or at least most, of the members of the team. In many instances, we have to train people to play multiple variations of their own positions on the team (that is what residency does well). We need to teach people how to manage teams (something I think residency does less well since the work hour restrictions were put in place). Learning new responsibilities continues throughout practice independent of where one works. We should embrace that. If you are reading this text, you have tacitly recognized that you wish to learn from others; you are not alone.

It doesn't take a doctorate in linguistics to realize that what most people are referring to when they invoke "autonomy" is that they want the resident to have greater independence of thought and greater capacity to play a substantial leadership role that will hopefully lead to a greater sense of ownership of the patient's problems, thereby developing a more useful surgeon. Who shouldn't want that? Still, if that is what we desire, then that goal is what we must clearly and precisely articulate. Only then can we test our tactics at developing these traits against something of merit. Surgeons are not meant to stand alone; we are meant to stand among and to lead.

I miss the world of vascular surgery, or my remembrance of it, in many ways. Mostly I miss the rigor and dedication that it takes to be a good vascular surgeon. I would like to think that the field I eventually concentrated on had the same discipline but, alas, I spend most of my clinical time working on an organ whose main fluid flows from distal to proximal—sigh, we can't compete linguistically or anatomically. Still, we can all learn from our vascular colleagues. The principles by which they live are useful to every surgeon at some time. There are few people who so readily prove their dedication as the vascular surgeon, who spends many hours restoring blood flow to a limb only to go to the recovery room to give one last pulse check, sadly realizing it is time to go back to the OR—something is amiss.

Dr Tefera and his colleagues have compiled a wealth of information for us. I commend it to you no matter what you do. We all learn from one another. That is what makes this fun.

Ronald F. Martin, MD, FACS
Department of Surgery
Marshfield Clinic
1000 North Oak Avenue
Marshfield, WI 54449, USA

E-mail address:
martin.ronald@marshfieldclinic.org

Preface

Vascular Surgery and Endovascular Therapy

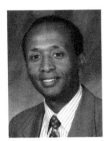

Girma Tefera, MD
Editor

Over the past couple of decades, vascular surgery has undergone transformative changes in all aspects of vascular care. These changes occurred primarily because of major innovative technical advances in both the diagnostic area and the area of therapeutic choices. The scope of work of the vascular surgeon has changed significantly. We provide comprehensive vascular care that includes medical management, minimally invasive percutaneous endovascular therapy, and standard open surgical interventions. Most importantly, the multidisciplinary approach to vascular patients has become indispensable and standard of care in most institutions. This issue *of Surgical Clinics of North America* will provide the reader with a comprehensive review of the current status in the diagnosis and treatment of peripheral vascular, aneurysmal arterial disease, venous diseases, and management of dialysis access.

The first article by Dr François covers the current advances in imaging modalities used for vascular diagnosis in acute and chronic conditions. The advantages and limitations of these studies are clearly outlined. Dr Mason and coworkers from the University of Wisconsin School of Medicine and Public Health discuss the optimal medical therapy in the vascular patient. Understanding cardiovascular event rates and identifying risk factors are critical steps in the comprehensive care of the vascular patient. The authors of this article emphasize identification of risk factors and the multidisciplinary approach to the care of vascular patients.

Surg Clin N Am 93 (2013) xvii–xix
http://dx.doi.org/10.1016/j.suc.2013.06.004
0039-6109/13/$ – see front matter Published by Elsevier Inc.

surgical.theclinics.com

Claudication of the lower extremities is present in up to 9% of patients over the age of 65. The review of the current state of diagnosis, prevention, and treatment is discussed by Dr Henke and colleagues from the University of Michigan. This article helps us understand how vascular disease is a continuous and systemic problem that can further progress into an advanced form of arterial occlusive disease. Dr Blecha and coworkers (from the University of Chicago) outline the diagnosis as well as the current open and endovascular options of treatment for patients with critical limb ischemia. Identification and treatment of risk factors, including hyperlipidemia, diabetes, and smoking, are of paramount importance.

Carotid artery disease is one of the most preventable causes of stroke. Dr Rodriguez and colleagues from Northwestern University discuss extensively the current modalities of diagnosis and treatment of carotid artery occlusive disease.

Atherosclerotic arterial occlusive diseases, such as Burger disease, Takayasu autoimmune arteritis, giant cell arteritis, and polyarteritis nodosa, are outlined in the fifth article. Dr Chaer and colleagues from the University of Pittsburgh discuss in detail the pathogenesis, clinical presentation, and treatment for each clinical entity.

Aneurysmal diseases of the thoracic, abdominal aorta, and peripheral arterial aneurysms are discussed by Dr Hoel (from Northwestern University), Dr Yamanouchi and colleagues (from the University of Wisconsin), and Dr Hall (from the University of Chicago), respectively. The treatment modality for aneurysmal disease in all anatomic territories has significantly shifted toward minimally invasive endovascular therapy. The next territory to be conquered seems to be the aortic arch. There are experimental grafts that are being tested in Europe.

Dr Bobadilla from the University of Kentucky reviews the clinical presentation, diagnosis, and treatment of acute and chronic mesenteric ischemia. This early diagnosis of acute mesenteric ischemia defines survival, however, it remains a great challenge. Open, endovascular, and hybrid options of treatment are discussed.

On vascular trauma, a detailed description of vascular territory is presented by Dr Mell and coworkers (from Stanford University). Early diagnosis and treatment are of paramount importance and newer endovascular treatment modalities are also well outlined. Technology has contributed along with refined surgical techniques to reducing morbidity and mortality from vascular injuries.

The article authored by Dr Brown and colleagues (from the Medical College of Wisconsin) discusses in detail all aspects of varicose vein disease and other forms of superficial venous disease of the lower extremities. This disease affects millions of Americans and is a frequent cause of significant morbidity. The diagnosis is simple and the current noninvasive treatment modalities, including laser, radiofrequency ablation, and sclerotherapy, are discussed in depth.

Venous thromboembolic (VTE) disease is a source of significant morbidity and mortality as well as cost. This remains one of the closely monitored outcome measures. VTE prevention, diagnosis, and treatment are well covered in the article by Dr Hoch and coworkers from the University of Wisconsin School of Medicine and Public Health.

Dialysis access is one of the most common vascular procedures performed by general surgeons. Dr Rose and colleagues from Howard University discuss in detail the importance of the multidisciplinary approach to the care of these hemodialysis-dependent patients. Dialysis access surveillance for the detection of early access failure and other complications has been the standard of care. The Dialysis Outcomes Quality Initiative has contributed to higher expectations of care that all providers have to adhere to.

I hope the readers will find this issue of comprehensive reviews useful to their clinical practice. Last, but not least, I would like to thank all the authors for providing us with outstanding articles.

Girma Tefera, MD
Division of Vascular Surgery, Department of Surgery
University of Wisconsin School of Medicine and Public Health
600 Highland Avenue, CSC Suite G5/325
Madison, WI 53792, USA

E-mail address:
tefera@surgery.wisc.edu

Noninvasive Imaging Workup of Patients with Vascular Disease

Christopher J. François, MD

KEYWORDS

• Cardiovascular disease • Patient workup • Diagnostic imaging • Angiography

KEY POINTS

- In hemodynamcially stable patients with acute onset of symptoms requiring an urgent diagnosis, computed tomographic angiography (CTA) is recommended.
- In hemodynamically unstable patients who may have acute aortic dissection or rupturing aneurysm, ultrasonography (US) and echocardiography can readily be performed at the bedside.
- Follow-up of patients with known aortic aneurysm or dissection can be done with CTA or magnetic resonance angiography (MRA).
- In patients with chronic symptoms that could be related to mesenteric ischemia or renal artery stenosis, initial screening can be performed with US.
- Definitive diagnosis of and preoperative planning for chronic mesenteric ischemia and renal artery stenosis is done with CTA or MRA.

INTRODUCTION

The diagnostic workup of patients with cardiovascular disease is frequently challenging and requires a multimodality approach to appropriately determine management; this is particularly true for diseases of the thoracoabdominal circulation. Depending on the presenting symptoms and their acuity, the noninvasive diagnostic imaging strategies can include radiography, ultrasonography (US), computed tomography (CT), and magnetic resonance (MR) imaging. Although a complete review of the different techniques and their use for all potential vascular pathologies is beyond its scope, this article provides an introduction to the use of these imaging modalities for commonly encountered diseases of the aorta, mesenteric arteries, and renal arteries, focusing on how the acuity of presentation and likelihood of disease affects the workup of patients with known or suspected vascular disease.

Department of Radiology, University of Wisconsin School of Medicine and Public Health, 600 Highland Avenue, Madison, WI 53562, USA
E-mail address: cfrancois@uwhealth.org

Surg Clin N Am 93 (2013) 741–760
http://dx.doi.org/10.1016/j.suc.2013.04.004
0039-6109/13/$ – see front matter © 2013 Elsevier Inc. All rights reserved.

surgical.theclinics.com

Aorta

Aortic aneurysms and acute aortic syndrome (AAS) are 2 of the most common diseases of the aorta repaired by surgical or endovascular techniques. The workup of patients with suspected aortic aneurysms and AAS largely depends on the acuity of symptoms and the index of suspicion that these present. In general, the greater the acuity of presentation and the higher the pretest probability of detecting disease, the more important it is to proceed with studies that are readily available, expedient, and with a high negative predictive value.

Aortic Aneurysms

Aortic aneurysms are defined as local or diffuse dilation of the aorta to 50% or more of the normal aortic diameter. Aortic aneurysms are frequently detected incidentally on radiographic imaging performed for other purposes. The appearance of aortic aneurysms on a radiograph depends on their location and configuration. For example, thoracic aortic aneurysms (TAA) will cause displacement of the mediastinal contours laterally to the right or left, depending on whether the ascending (**Fig. 1**) or descending (**Fig. 2**) aorta is dilated, respectively. Abdominal aortic aneurysms are typically not seen on abdominal radiographs unless they are very large and displace normal abdominal structures peripherally (**Fig. 3**). Although aortic dilation can be suspected based on abnormal contours on chest and abdominal radiographs, plain radiography is neither sensitive nor specific enough to confidently confirm or exclude the diagnosis of TAA or AAA.

For more definitive screening of aortic size in patients with suspected aortic aneurysm,[1,2] US for AAA and echocardiography for TAA are more appropriate than radiographs. In fact, US (**Fig. 4**) has been recommended as a screening tool for the detection of AAA in male patients younger than 65 years.[3] When performed, US should for evaluation of the aorta and as a dedicated aortic study, using standardized techniques to minimize interobserver and intraobserver variability in measurement.[4] Every attempt should be made to image the entire thoracic or abdominal aorta, with

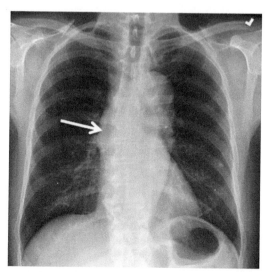

Fig. 1. Frontal chest radiograph of ascending thoracic aortic aneurysm. Right mediastinal border is laterally displaced (*arrow*).

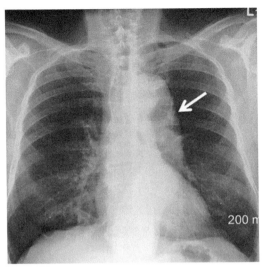

Fig. 2. Frontal chest radiograph of descending thoracic aortic aneurysm. Left mediastinal border is laterally displaced (*arrow*).

measurements of maximum wall-to-wall dimension. Of note, US typically underestimates the size of the aorta relative to computed tomographic angiography (CTA) by approximately 4 mm.[5] In addition, US is limited in evaluating aortas in patients who are obese or in evaluating the complete extent of complex TAA and AAA. Even though

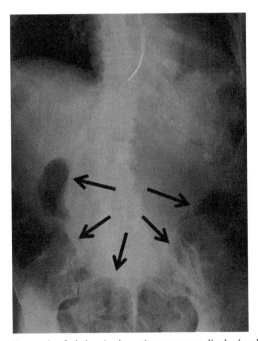

Fig. 3. Abdominal radiograph of abdominal aortic aneurysm displacing bowel loops peripherally in mid abdomen (*arrows*).

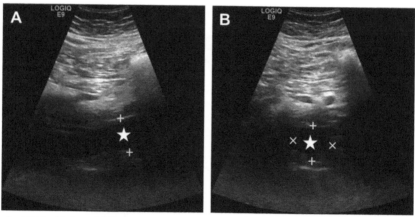

Fig. 4. (*A*) Sagittal and (*B*) transverse ultrasonographic images of 3.6 × 3.2-cm abdominal aortic aneurysm (*star*).

US and echocardiography can be used to follow patients with simple aneurysms, for more complex aortic aneurysms or before repair, CTA or MR angiography (MRA) (**Fig. 5**) is necessary to evaluate the entire extent of the aneurysm and its relationship to branch vessels.

Although US is portable and can be performed at the bedside in patients who are hemodynamically unstable, it is neither sensitive nor specific enough to completely exclude rupture or impending rupture. In patients with suspected impending rupture (**Fig. 6**) or rupture (**Fig. 7**) of an aortic aneurysm who are hemodynamically stable, CTA is the imaging modality of choice to completely evaluate the aorta.[1] In patients with AAA it is important to evaluate the thoracic aorta as well because of the increased incidence of TAA in patients with AAA,[6] especially women and elderly patients.[7]

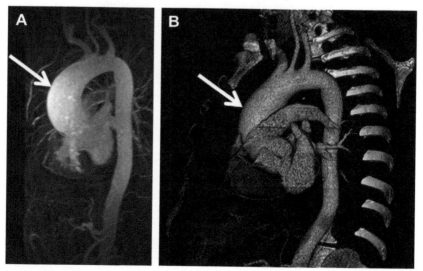

Fig. 5. (*A*) Magnetic resonance angiography (MRA) and (*B*) computed tomographic angiography (CTA) images of ascending thoracic aortic aneurysm (*arrow*).

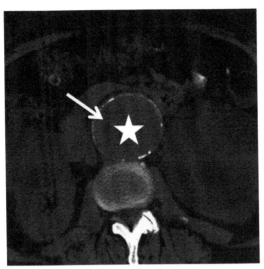

Fig. 6. Abdominal aortic aneurysm (*star*) with impending rupture. Noncontrast computed tomography (CT) of the abdomen reveals hyperdense crescent sign (*arrow*) associated with impending rupture.

CTA is currently the clinical standard of reference for the diagnosis and pretreatment planning of TAA and AAA.[8] For patients with ascending TAA, the examination should be performed using cardiac gating to minimize artifact related to cardiac motion (**Fig. 8**). In patients with large aneurysms, a large amount of thrombus may be present within the aneurysm sac; in such cases it is critical that measurements be made from the source data or by using multiplanar reformation rather than volume-rendering

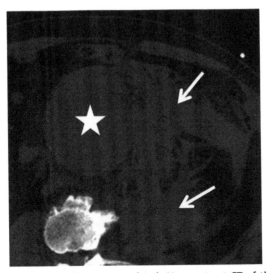

Fig. 7. Ruptured abdominal aortic aneurysm (*star*). Noncontrast CT of the abdomen shows hemorrhage around the aorta and in the retroperitoneum (*arrows*).

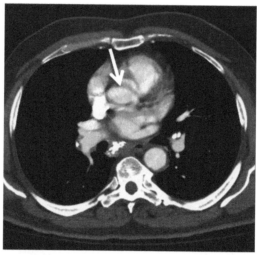

Fig. 8. To evaluate the ascending aorta, image acquisition should be gated to the electrocardiogram to avoid cardiac motion artifact (*arrow*), which can simulate aortic dissection.

or maximum-intensity projection images because these modalities will show only the lumen, leading to underestimation of the true size of the aorta (**Fig. 9**).

Noncontrast-enhanced (NCE) CT is typically sufficient for following known aortic aneurysms in patients who have suboptimal US imaging. NCE CT is also adequate for detection of impending rupture or rupture.[9] However, for preoperative planning,

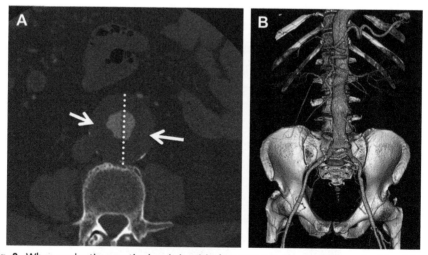

Fig. 9. When evaluating aortic size, it is critical to measure the aorta from double oblique multiplanar reformatted images (*A*) rather than volume-rendered (*B*) or maximum-intensity projection images. Although volume-rendered and maximum-intensity projection images nicely depict the anatomy, they can potentially underestimate the size of the aorta if there is a significant amount of thrombus within the aneurysm or false lumen (*arrows*). Measurements of aorta size should be from outer wall to outer wall (*dotted line*).

contrast-enhanced (CE) CTA is necessary to assess vessel patency and the presence of atherosclerotic plaque and thrombus.

CE and NCE MRA are alternatives for the diagnosis and follow-up of TAA and AAA.[10] With improved scanner hardware and software, imaging times have been greatly reduced[11] such that a complete MRA of the thoracoabdominal aorta can be completed within a single breath-hold (**Fig. 10**). Benefits of MRA relative to CTA are the lack of ionizing radiation, particularly in younger and female patients, and the fact that nephrotoxic contrast agents are not necessary. Although CE MRA is generally safer than CE CTA for patients with renal dysfunction, in patients with severe renal failure (estimated glomerular filtration rate <30 mL/kg/min) caution should be exercised because of the association between exposure to gadolinium-based contrast agents and nephrogenic systemic fibrosis.[12] In these patients for whom both CT and MR contrast agents may be harmful, NCE MRA techniques are a viable alternative.

Acute Aorta Syndrome

AAS, which includes aortic dissection, intramural hematoma, and penetrating atherosclerotic ulcer, are life-threatening conditions that require rapid and accurate diagnosis. Patients frequently present with a sudden onset of chest pain that radiates to the back. Alternatively, patients may present with findings primarily related to

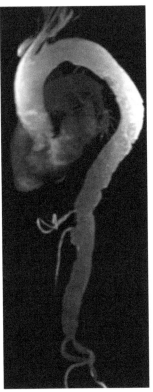

Fig. 10. Contrast-enhanced MRA of the entire aorta performed on a 3.0-T scanner using a 32-channel coil and parallel imaging to accelerate acquisition to approximately 18 seconds.

malperfusion of one of the branches off the aorta. A complete discussion of the role of noninvasive imaging for the evaluation and management of patients with AAS is beyond the scope of this article, which instead briefly highlights the roles of radiography, US, CTA, and MRA in the diagnosis and follow-up of patients with suspected or known AAS.

Chest radiography is recommended in all patients presenting with chest pain because it is rapid, inexpensive, and provides valuable information regarding the presence or absence of a variety of cardiovascular and noncardiovascular causes of acute chest pain.[13] Findings of aortic dissection on chest radiography include mediastinal widening, obscuration of the aortopulmonary window, thickening of the paratracheal stripe, and displacement of intimal calcifications (**Fig. 11**).[14,15] However, these findings are nonspecific, and up to 20% of patients with aortic dissection will have no findings of aortic dissection on chest radiography. Therefore, a negative chest radiograph should not preclude further workup to establish the diagnosis.[16,17]

In patients who are hemodynamically unstable, echocardiography is particularly useful in assessing for the presence of ascending aortic dissection.[18] Transthoracic echocardiography (TTE) is more sensitive and specific than chest radiography for the detection of dissections of the ascending thoracic aorta. TTE can also identify complications of aortic dissection such as aortic valve regurgitation, myocardial infarction, and cardiac tamponade. However, TTE is suboptimal for the evaluation of the descending thoracic aorta, and a negative TTE should not preclude further investigation in patients who may have AAS.[19] Transesophageal echocardiography (TEE) (**Fig. 12**), on the other hand, is much more accurate than TTE for the diagnosis of dissections of the ascending and descending thoracic aortic. The sensitivity of TEE in diagnosing aortic dissection approaches 100%.[20]

CE CTA is the diagnostic imaging modality of choice for the evaluation of patients with acute chest pain that could be related to AAS. This choice holds especially true now that most emergency departments have access to CT scanning 24 hours a day, and frequently have dedicated CT scanners within the department. To

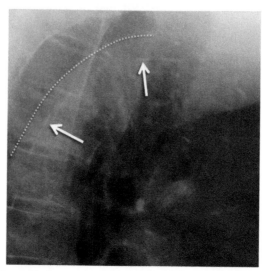

Fig. 11. Chest radiograph in aortic dissection showing displaced intimal calcifications (*arrows*). The outer wall of the aorta is indicated by the dotted line.

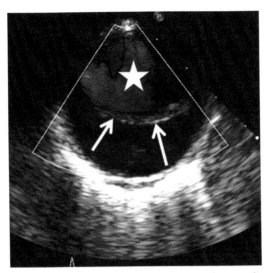

Fig. 12. Transesophageal echocardiography of a patient with ascending aortic dissection. The intimal flap (*arrows*) separates the true lumen (*star*) from the false lumen. The true lumen has much more flow than the false lumen, as indicated by the presence of color within the true lumen and absence of color in the false lumen.

differentiate between aortic dissection and intramural hematoma (**Fig. 13**), an NCE CT scan should be performed initially, before the administration of intravenous contrast. In a large meta-analysis, CE CTA had a sensitivity of 100% and specificity of 98% for the detection of aortic dissection.[20] In addition to detecting the presence of aortic dissection (**Fig. 14**), CE CTA is useful for evaluating the extent of the dissection, localizing tears in the intima, and assessing side-branch involvement and relative end-organ perfusion.

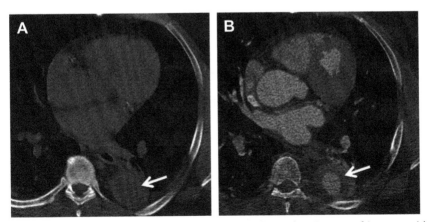

Fig. 13. (*A*) Noncontrast-enhanced and (*B*) contrast-enhanced CT images of intramural hematoma. The presence of circumferential high attenuation within the wall of the descending aorta (*arrows*) is much more conspicuous on the noncontrast-enhanced image (*A*) than on the contrast-enhanced image (*B*).

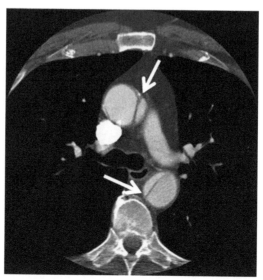

Fig. 14. Contrast-enhanced CTA of aortic dissection involving the ascending and descending thoracic aorta. The intimal flap (*arrows*) appears as a low-density linear structure within the lumen of the aorta.

In patients in whom CE CTA is contraindicated, MRA is nearly as accurate as CTA for the diagnosis of AAS. The sensitivity and specificity of MRA for the diagnosis of aortic dissection is nearly 100%.[20] As with aortic aneurysms, the speed of CE MRA in detecting aortic dissection has been dramatically improved as a result of new scanner hardware and sequence design. It is now possible to scan the entire thoracic aorta within approximately 15 to 20 seconds (**Fig. 15**).

MESENTERIC ISCHEMIA

Although mesenteric ischemia is relatively rare, it is associated with a high rate of morbidity and mortality, particularly in patients with acute mesenteric ischemia. Because the presenting symptoms are usually vague, the workup and diagnosis of mesenteric ischemia is frequently delayed, leading to an increased incidence of complications. In patients presenting with acute abdominal pain the differential diagnosis is extensive, and includes a larger number of nonvascular causes of abdominal pain than for vascular abnormalities. This situation differs to that in patients with chronic mesenteric ischemia, who usually present with postprandial abdominal pain, weight loss, and food intolerance.

Acute Mesenteric Ischemia

In patients with acute abdominal pain, the initial workup typically starts with abdominal radiographs. In patients with acute mesenteric ischemia, the initial abdominal radiographs are usually negative or nonspecific. Not until the ischemia has progressed to bowel infarction do the radiographs demonstrate signs of bowel ischemia.[21,22] Typical features of acute mesenteric ischemia that can be seen on radiographs include dilated loops of bowel, pneumatosis intestinalis (**Fig. 16**), hepatic portal venous gas, and pneumoperitoneum.

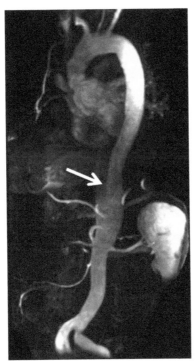

Fig. 15. MRA of the thoracoabdominal aorta acquired in a patient with chronic aortic dissection (*arrow*). Using parallel imaging, the length of acquisition was 18 seconds using 20 mL of gadolinium-based contrast agent.

CTA is the preferred imaging modality for the rapid and noninvasive diagnosis of acute mesenteric ischemia.[23–25] Not only can CTA be used to assess the vasculature for stenosis, embolism, or occlusion (**Fig. 17**), but it is more sensitive for demonstration of the secondary signs of bowel ischemia, including bowel-wall thickening, stranding of the fat around the intestines, and pneumatosis.[26] CTA can also differentiate between arterial and venous causes of acute mesenteric ischemia. The sensitivity and specificity of CTA for the diagnosis of acute mesenteric ischemia are 96% and 94%, respectively.

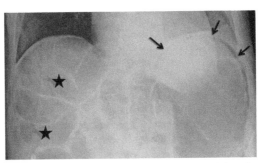

Fig. 16. Acute mesenteric ischemia with dilated loops of bowel (*stars*) and pneumatosis intestinalis (*arrows*).

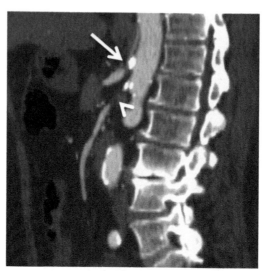

Fig. 17. Sagittal reformatted image from CTA in patient with acute thrombosis of the superior mesenteric (*arrowhead*) and celiac (*arrow*) arteries.

MRA is sensitive and specific for the detection of vascular stenosis and occlusions, including the origins of the celiac, superior mesenteric, and inferior mesenteric arteries. However, its role in the workup of patients with acute abdominal pain is limited because of the longer scan times and lesser sensitivity for detection of the secondary signs of bowel ischemia.

Although US can detect proximal stenosis or occlusion of the celiac and superior mesenteric arteries well,[27] it has a limited role in the evaluation of the mesenteric circulation in patients presenting with acute mesenteric ischemia, owing to the limitations in evaluating the distal mesenteric vessels and the bowel wall. However, US is frequently performed in patients with acute abdominal pain to evaluate for nonvascular etiology such as acute cholecystitis, choledocholithiasis, appendicitis, or pancreatitis.

Chronic Mesenteric Ischemia

Patients with chronic mesenteric ischemia usually present with postprandial abdominal pain with or without weight loss and food intolerance. Atherosclerotic disease is the most common cause of chronic mesenteric ischemia. Other, less common, causes include fibromuscular dysplasia, median arcuate ligament syndrome, and vasculitis. In these patients, abdominal radiographs have very little to no impact on management. As such, a normal abdominal radiograph does not exclude chronic mesenteric ischemia.

B-mode and Doppler US is a more useful method for screening patients with suspected chronic mesenteric ischemia, even though visualization of the mesenteric vessels is quite challenging technically because of overlying bowel gas. Peak systolic velocities greater than 275 cm/s in the superior mesenteric artery and 200 cm/s in the celiac artery are suggestive of severe stenosis, and indicate a need for additional anatomic imaging evaluation.[28,29] US is also beneficial in identifying additional potential causes of chronic abdominal pain, including nephrolithiasis, choledocholithiasis, and chronic pancreatitis.

For the definitive diagnosis of celiac and superior mesenteric artery stenosis, CTA or MRA[30] is recommended. The sensitivity and specificity of CTA and MRA for the diagnosis of chronic mesenteric ischemia is greater than 90%. Findings on both CTA and MRA include focal stenoses or occlusions at the origins of the mesenteric vessels caused by atherosclerotic disease (**Fig. 18**). CTA and MRA may depict findings that indicate nonatherosclerotic causes as well (**Fig. 19**). A benefit of MRA relative to CTA is that flow quantification can be performed in the mesenteric circulation before and after a meal challenge to detect the changes in blood flow to the gastrointestinal tract.[31,32] In patients with chronic mesenteric ischemia, postprandial blood flow increases significantly less than in healthy controls.

RENAL ARTERIES

Hypertension is a common problem that affects an increasing number of the adult population. The overwhelming majority of patients with hypertension are considered to have essential hypertension that is not due to other secondary causes. Of the secondary causes of hypertension, renal artery stenosis (RAS) is the most frequently encountered. The workup of patients with suspected renovascular hypertension should focus on those with a high index of suspicion based on the presence of an abdominal bruit, malignant or rapidly increasing hypertension, onset after the age of 50 years, refractory hypertension, or worsening renal function while on angiotensin-converting enzyme inhibitors.[33] Acute renal artery stenosis or occlusion secondary to embolism or dissection is less common than chronic RAS secondary to atherosclerotic disease.

The initial evaluation of patients with suspected RAS is frequently with Doppler US (**Fig. 20**) because it is inexpensive and does not require contrast or ionizing radiation. Findings of RAS on Doppler US include elevated peak systolic velocities in the main renal arteries,[34] diminished systolic to diastolic velocity ratio ("parva and tarda"

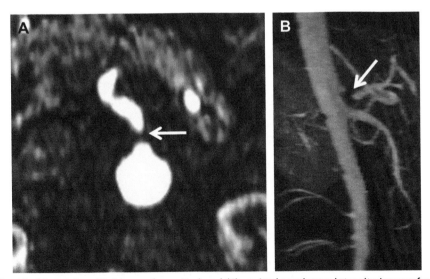

Fig. 18. (*A*) Axial multiplanar reformatted and (*B*) sagittal maximum-intensity images from contrast-enhanced MRA in patient with chronic mesenteric ischemia secondary to occlusion of the celiac artery (*arrow*).

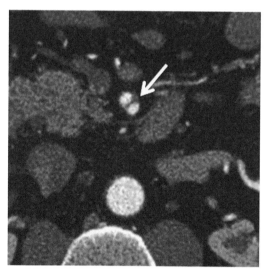

Fig. 19. Chronic mesenteric ischemia secondary to systemic arterial mediolysis. CTA reveals a dissection in the superior mesenteric artery (*arrow*).

waveform, **Fig. 21**), a prolonged early systolic acceleration time, and loss of the early systolic peak.

Evaluation of the renal arteries with MRA is safe and accurate, with an average sensitivity and specificity of 97% and 85%.[35] MRA of the renal arteries can be performed with[36] or without[37–40] contrast enhancement. In addition to morphologic evaluation of the arterial anatomy (**Figs. 22** and **23**), flow-sensitive MR sequences

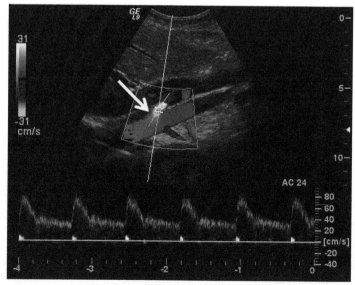

Fig. 20. Normal renal Doppler ultrasound to normal flow velocities in the proximal renal artery (*arrow*).

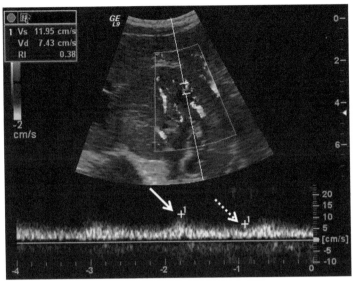

Fig. 21. "Parva and tarda" waveform with decreased peak systolic (*solid arrow*) to diastolic (*dashed arrow*) flow in the arcuate renal arteries.

can be used to detect elevations in flow velocities or areas of flow turbulence distal to stenoses.[37,41–43] Newer 3-dimensional, cine flow-sensitive MR methods may enable accurate quantification pressure gradients across renal artery stenoses noninvasively.[44]

CTA is also highly accurate for the detection of RAS, with sensitivities and specificities greater than 90%.[35] Disadvantages of CTA relative to US and MRA include the

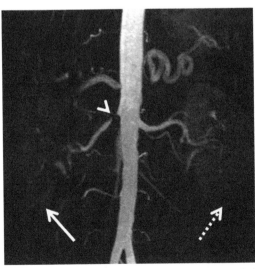

Fig. 22. Contrast-enhanced MRA of severe right renal artery stenosis (*arrowhead*) causing decreased perfusion of the right kidney (*solid arrow*) relative to the left kidney (*dashed arrow*).

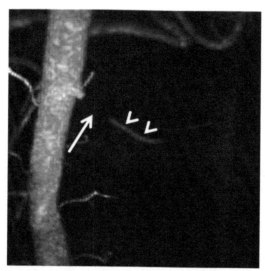

Fig. 23. Contrast-enhanced MRA of acute left renal artery stenosis (*arrow*) caused by embolism. Arrowheads indicate the more distal renal artery.

need for nephrotoxic contrast agents and ionizing radiation. However, CTA is more rapid than MRA and US and usually provides a better depiction of the branch renal arteries than MRA, which can be important in evaluating patients suspected of having fibromuscular dysplasia (**Fig. 24**). In addition, CTA is more accurate than MRA for evaluating the patency of renal artery stents (**Fig. 25**).

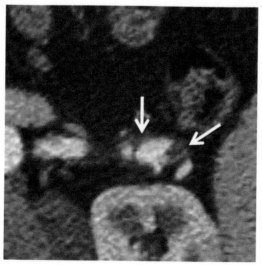

Fig. 24. CTA of fibromuscular dysplasia (FMD) involving the left renal artery. There are multiple stenoses (*arrows*), characteristic of FMD.

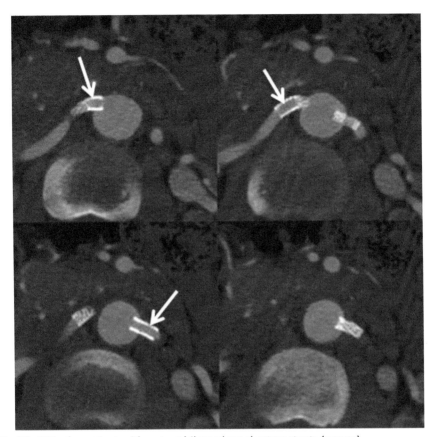

Fig. 25. CTA of a patient with patent bilateral renal artery stents (*arrows*).

SUMMARY

The workup of patients with vascular diseases greatly depends on the acuity of the symptoms. In patients who are acutely ill, a diagnosis is required rapidly and with a high level of accuracy. Chest and abdominal radiographs can be obtained fairly quickly and inexpensively. However, these tend to be less sensitive and specific than other cross-sectional imaging studies in establishing the cause of the acute presentation. In patients who are hemodynamically stable, CTA is the diagnostic imaging modality of choice for the workup of those with suspected aortic aneurysm rupture, AAS, acute mesenteric ischemia, or acute renal infarction. In patients who are hemodynamically unstable, echocardiography and ultrasonography are noninvasive alternatives that can be performed at the bedside.

In patients with a more chronic presentation or who are being evaluated for screening purposes, US is an appropriate first step in the workup of suspected aortic aneurysms, chronic mesenteric ischemia, and RAS. In patients with suboptimal US evaluations, CTA and MRA are accurate noninvasive strategies for accurate delineation of the vascular anatomy and morphology. In addition, CTA and MRA can be used for preoperative planning in lieu of invasive catheter angiography.

REFERENCES

1. Desjardins B, Dill KE, Flamm SD, et al. ACR Appropriateness Criteria® pulsatile abdominal mass, suspected abdominal aortic aneurysm. Int J Cardiovasc Imaging 2013;29(1):177–83.
2. Lederle FA, Johnson GR, Wilson SE, et al. The aneurysm detection and management study screening program: validation cohort and final results. Aneurysm Detection and Management Veterans Affairs Cooperative Study Investigators. Arch Intern Med 2000;160(10):1425–30.
3. Fleming C, Whitlock EP, Beil TL, et al. Screening for abdominal aortic aneurysm: a best-evidence systematic review for the U.S. Preventive Services Task Force. Ann Intern Med 2005;142(3):203–11.
4. Singh K, Bonaa KH, Solberg S, et al. Intra- and interobserver variability in ultrasound measurements of abdominal aortic diameter. The Tromso Study. Eur J Vasc Endovasc Surg 1998;15(6):497–504.
5. Manning BJ, Kristmundsson T, Sonesson B, et al. Abdominal aortic aneurysm diameter: a comparison of ultrasound measurements with those from standard and three-dimensional computed tomography reconstruction. J Vasc Surg 2009;50(2):263–8.
6. Larsson E, Vishnevskaya L, Kalin B, et al. High frequency of thoracic aneurysms in patients with abdominal aortic aneurysms. Ann Surg 2011;253(1):180–4.
7. Hultgren R, Larsson E, Wahlgren CM, et al. Female and elderly abdominal aortic aneurysm patients more commonly have concurrent thoracic aortic aneurysm. Ann Vasc Surg 2012;26(7):918–23.
8. Diehm N, Herrmann P, Dinkel HP. Multidetector CT angiography versus digital subtraction angiography for aortoiliac length measurements prior to endovascular AAA repair. J Endovasc Ther 2004;11(5):527–34.
9. Rakita D, Newatia A, Hines JJ, et al. Spectrum of CT findings in rupture and impending rupture of abdominal aortic aneurysms. Radiographics 2007;27(2):497–507.
10. Atar E, Belenky A, Hadad M, et al. MR angiography for abdominal and thoracic aortic aneurysms: assessment before endovascular repair in patients with impaired renal function. AJR Am J Roentgenol 2006;186(2):386–93.
11. Wilson GJ, Hoogeveen RM, Willinek WA, et al. Parallel imaging in MR angiography. Top Magn Reson Imaging 2004;15(3):169–85.
12. Sadowski EA, Bennett LK, Chan MR, et al. Nephrogenic systemic fibrosis: risk factors and incidence estimation. Radiology 2007;243(1):148–57.
13. Gomes AS, Bettmann MA, Boxt LM, et al. Acute chest pain—suspected aortic dissection. American College of Radiology. ACR Appropriateness Criteria. Radiology 2000;215(Suppl):1–5.
14. Eyler WR, Clark MD. Dissecting aneurysms of the aorta: roentgen manifestations including a comparison with other types of aneurysms. Radiology 1965;85(6):1047–57.
15. Fultz PJ, Melville D, Ekanej A, et al. Nontraumatic rupture of the thoracic aorta: chest radiographic features of an often unrecognized condition. AJR Am J Roentgenol 1998;171(2):351–7.
16. Jagannath AS, Sos TA, Lockhart SH, et al. Aortic dissection: a statistical analysis of the usefulness of plain chest radiographic findings. AJR Am J Roentgenol 1986;147(6):1123–6.
17. von Kodolitsch Y, Nienaber CA, Dieckmann C, et al. Chest radiography for the diagnosis of acute aortic syndrome. Am J Med 2004;116(2):73–7.

18. Shah BN, Ahmadvazir S, Pabla JS, et al. The role of urgent transthoracic echocardiography in the evaluation of patients presenting with acute chest pain. Eur J Emerg Med 2012;19(5):277–83.
19. Meredith EL, Masani ND. Echocardiography in the emergency assessment of acute aortic syndromes. Eur J Echocardiogr 2009;10(1):i31–9.
20. Shiga T, Wajima Z, Apfel CC, et al. Diagnostic accuracy of transesophageal echocardiography, helical computed tomography, and magnetic resonance imaging for suspected thoracic aortic dissection: systematic review and meta-analysis. Arch Intern Med 2006;166(13):1350–6.
21. Wolf EL, Sprayregen S, Bakal CW. Radiology in intestinal ischemia. Plain film, contrast, and other imaging studies. Surg Clin North Am 1992;72(1):107–24.
22. Wadman M, Syk I, Elmstahl B, et al. Abdominal plain film findings in acute ischemic bowel disease differ with age. Acta Radiol 2006;47(3):238–43.
23. Shih MC, Hagspiel KD. CTA and MRA in mesenteric ischemia: part 1, role in diagnosis and differential diagnosis. AJR Am J Roentgenol 2007;188(2):452–61.
24. Kirkpatrick ID, Kroeker MA, Greenberg HM. Biphasic CT with mesenteric CT angiography in the evaluation of acute mesenteric ischemia: initial experience. Radiology 2003;229(1):91–8.
25. Turkbey B, Akpinar E, Cil B, et al. Utility of multidetector CT in an emergency setting in acute mesenteric ischemia. Diagn Interv Radiol 2009;15(4):256–61.
26. Alpern MB, Glazer GM, Francis IR. Ischemic or infarcted bowel: CT findings. Radiology 1988;166(1 Pt 1):149–52.
27. Danse EM, Van Beers BE, Goffette P, et al. Acute intestinal ischemia due to occlusion of the superior mesenteric artery: detection with Doppler sonography. J Ultrasound Med 1996;15(4):323–6.
28. Bowersox JC, Zwolak RM, Walsh DB, et al. Duplex ultrasonography in the diagnosis of celiac and mesenteric artery occlusive disease. J Vasc Surg 1991;14(6):780–6 [discussion: 786–8].
29. Moneta GL, Yeager RA, Dalman R, et al. Duplex ultrasound criteria for diagnosis of splanchnic artery stenosis or occlusion. J Vasc Surg 1991;14(4):511–8 [discussion: 518–20].
30. Meaney JF, Prince MR, Nostrant TT, et al. Gadolinium-enhanced MR angiography of visceral arteries in patients with suspected chronic mesenteric ischemia. J Magn Reson Imaging 1997;7(1):171–6.
31. Burkart DJ, Johnson CD, Reading CC, et al. MR measurements of mesenteric venous flow: prospective evaluation in healthy volunteers and patients with suspected chronic mesenteric ischemia. Radiology 1995;194(3):801–6.
32. Li KC, Hopkins KL, Dalman RL, et al. Simultaneous measurement of flow in the superior mesenteric vein and artery with cine phase-contrast MR imaging: value in diagnosis of chronic mesenteric ischemia. Work in progress. Radiology 1995;194(2):327–30.
33. Amis ES Jr, Bigongiari LR, Bluth EI, et al. Radiologic investigation of patients with renovascular hypertension. American College of Radiology. ACR Appropriateness Criteria. Radiology 2000;215(Suppl):663–70.
34. Postma CT, van Aalen J, de Boo T, et al. Doppler ultrasound scanning in the detection of renal artery stenosis in hypertensive patients. Br J Radiol 1992;65(778):857–60.
35. Vasbinder GB, Nelemans PJ, Kessels AG, et al. Diagnostic tests for renal artery stenosis in patients suspected of having renovascular hypertension: a meta-analysis. Ann Intern Med 2001;135(6):401–11.

36. Fain SB, King BF, Breen JF, et al. High-spatial-resolution contrast-enhanced MR angiography of the renal arteries: a prospective comparison with digital subtraction angiography. Radiology 2001;218(2):481–90.
37. Francois CJ, Lum DP, Johnson KM, et al. Renal arteries: isotropic, high-spatial-resolution, unenhanced MR angiography with three-dimensional radial phase contrast. Radiology 2011;258(1):254–60.
38. Herborn CU, Watkins DM, Runge VM, et al. Renal arteries: comparison of steady-state free precession MR angiography and contrast-enhanced MR angiography. Radiology 2006;239(1):263–8.
39. Maki JH, Wilson GJ, Eubank WB, et al. Navigator-gated MR angiography of the renal arteries: a potential screening tool for renal artery stenosis. AJR Am J Roentgenol 2007;188(6):W540–6.
40. Wyttenbach R, Braghetti A, Wyss M, et al. Renal artery assessment with nonenhanced steady-state free precession versus contrast-enhanced MR angiography. Radiology 2007;245(1):186–95.
41. Westenberg JJ, van der Geest RJ, Wasser MN, et al. Stenosis quantification from post-stenotic signal loss in phase-contrast MRA datasets of flow phantoms and renal arteries. Int J Card Imaging 1999;15(6):483–93.
42. Schoenberg SO, Just A, Bock M, et al. Noninvasive analysis of renal artery blood flow dynamics with MR cine phase-contrast flow measurements. Am J Physiol 1997;272(5 Pt 2):H2477–84.
43. Schoenberg SO, Knopp MV, Bock M, et al. Renal artery stenosis: grading of hemodynamic changes with cine phase-contrast MR blood flow measurements. Radiology 1997;203(1):45–53.
44. Bley TA, Johnson KM, Francois CJ, et al. Noninvasive assessment of transstenotic pressure gradients in porcine renal artery stenoses by using vastly undersampled phase-contrast MR angiography. Radiology 2011;261(1):266–73.

Contemporary and Optimal Medical Management of Peripheral Arterial Disease

Matthew C. Tattersall, DO, Heather M. Johnson, MD,
Peter J. Mason, MD, MPH*

KEYWORDS

- Peripheral arterial disease • Claudication • Cardiovascular disease risk
- Supervised exercise therapy • Optimal medical therapy

KEY POINTS

- Atherosclerotic lower extremity peripheral arterial disease (PAD) is a highly prevalent condition associated with a significant increase in risk of all-cause mortality and cardiovascular morbidity and mortality.
- PAD is underdiagnosed and undertreated.
- Treatment is focused on 2 primary objectives: (1) lowering cardiovascular risk and cardiovascular disease (CVD) event rates and (2) improvement in symptoms and quality of life.
- Contemporary multidisciplinary and intersociety guidelines exist to optimal medical therapy.
- Substantial evidence supports the implementation of tobacco cessation counseling and pharmacotherapy to help achieve tobacco abstinence, antiplatelet therapy, HMG-CoA reductase inhibitors (statins) therapy and antihypertensive therapy in patients with PAD for the purpose of lowering cardiovascular event rates and improving survival.
- For patients with claudication, supervised exercise therapy and cilostazol improve measures of walking performance and quality of life.

BACKGROUND

PAD refers to the stenosis, occlusion, or aneurysmal change of upper extremity and/or lower extremity arteries.[1,2] Although the term, PAD, can be used to categorize a variety of disease entities and presentations, the acute and chronic conditions associated with atherosclerosis are the most common. The focus of this review is on the epidemiology, risk factors, and medical management of nonacute atherosclerotic lower extremity PAD.

Division of Cardiovascular Medicine, University of Wisconsin School of Medicine and Public Health, Clinic Science Center, MC 3248, 600 Highland Avenue, Madison, WI 53792, USA
* Corresponding author.
E-mail address: pjmason@medicine.wisc.edu

Surg Clin N Am 93 (2013) 761–778
http://dx.doi.org/10.1016/j.suc.2013.04.009
0039-6109/13/$ – see front matter © 2013 Elsevier Inc. All rights reserved.

surgical.theclinics.com

EPIDEMIOLOGY

PAD affects more than 8 million adults in the United States alone.[3] PAD is a disease of aging, with an increase in disease prevalence from 10% in individuals aged 65 to more than 30% in octogenarians.[4,5] Concomitant PAD is highly prevalent in individuals with new or established cerebrovascular or coronary artery disease, with prevalence rates greater than 30%.[6,7] Many studies have demonstrated equal prevalence among genders but there is a well-described ethnic disparity, with PAD afflicting non-Hispanic African Americans and Mexican Americans at a higher rate than non-Hispanic whites.[4] Even after controlling for traditional risk factors, PAD prevalence is 2-fold higher in non-Hispanic African Americans compared with non-Hispanic whites.[4,8]

PAD is associated with significant morbidity and mortality, with more than 14,000 US deaths attributable to PAD in 2011.[3] Studies have indicated that regardless of symptom status, the presence of PAD or a low ankle-brachial index (ABI) (<0.9) is associated with a more than 2-fold increase in total mortality, cardiovascular mortality, and coronary events.[9–11]

PAD is an under-recognized condition. The classical clinical presentation of PAD is lower extremity claudication. Historically, claudication has been defined using the Rose questionnaire[12]:

- Pain involving 1 or both calves
- Provoked by exertion
- Not present at rest
- Prompts patient to stop exertion
- Must abate within 10 minutes of rest
- No abatement in leg pain during continued exertion

Less than 10% of patients afflicted with PAD, however, present with typical claudication symptoms.[5] A majority of patients with PAD are either asymptomatic or present with atypical leg pain and a minority of patients present with acute or limb threatening conditions:

- Asymptomatic approximately 40%
- Atypical leg pain approximately 50%
- Typical claudication less than approximately 10%
- Critical limb ischemia approximately 1%–3%
- Acute limb ischemia less than 1%

Recent analyses have indicated that the diagnosis of PAD is missed in 85% to 90% of patients when relying only on clinical history or a screening questionnaire.[13]

PATHOPHYSIOLOGY

Claudication symptoms occur due to a mismatch in oxygen demand and delivery in the skeletal muscles. Arterial insufficiency and PAD most often occur due to insidious progression in the severity of atherosclerosis, but other processes can also cause reduced arterial blood flow (**Box 1**). The presence and severity of symptoms are also affected by other physiologic factors (muscle mechanics and energy metabolism, endothelial function, collateral blood flow, oxygen delivery, and carrying capacity) and patient factors (age, weight, and conditioning). Atherosclerotic PAD is a marker of a progressive systemic process; therefore, even asymptomatic disease and borderline reduction in ABI values (0.9–1.0) are associated with a significantly increased risk in all-cause mortality and cardiovascular morbidity and mortality.[5,11,14,15]

Box 1
Causes of peripheral arterial disease
Atherosclerosis
Arterial thromboembolism
Cardioembolism
Degenerative diseases
• Marfan syndrome
• Ehlers-Danlos syndrome
Dysplastic disease
• Fibromuscular dysplasia
Vasculitis
• Large: giant cell arteritis
• Medium: polyarteritis nodosa
• Small: rheumatoid arthritis, systemic lupus erythematosus
Buerger disease
Inherited thrombophilias
Entrapment syndromes

SCREENING AND DIAGNOSIS

Given the frequency of asymptomatic and atypical presentations of PAD, with the low sensitivity of disease detection by history alone, accurate diagnosis hinges on effective screening of patients at risk for PAD. Patients considered at high risk for PAD and who should be considered for screening include[1,16]

- People under age 50 with diabetes and 1 additional atherosclerotic risk factor
- People aged 50 and older with diabetes and/or smoking history
- Anyone greater than 65 years of age
- Those with known vascular disease in other arterial systems (coronary, carotid, and renal)
- Those with reduced or abnormal pulses on physical examination
- Those with symptoms concerning for PAD

The ABI is a simple, inexpensive, and noninvasive test that provides clinicians with information regarding PAD diagnosis and severity. The ABI is considered by some the fifth vital sign and is performed by measuring the ratio between the highest ankle (dorsalis pedis and posterior tibial arteries) systolic blood pressure and the highest arm (brachial) systolic blood pressure. Typically, systolic blood pressures are 8% to 15% higher in the lower extremities, which results in an ABI greater than 1.0.[17] ABI values between 1.0 and 1.4 are normal, and greater than or equal to 1.4 indicate noncompressible vessels. Mild, moderate, and severe arterial insufficiency is present when ABI values are between 0.7 and 0.9, 0.4 and 0.7, and less than 0.4, respectively. Recent guidelines and publications have recommended the inclusion of the borderline reduced category (0.9–1.0) to reflect the importance of both subclinical disease and the limitations of the resting ABI.[16,18]

The ABI has excellent test characteristics, with a reported sensitivity and specificity, compared with angiography, of greater than 90%.[19,20] When the resting ABI is normal or borderline reduced, a postexercise ABI can be used to aid diagnosis, help distinguish between claudication and pseudoclaudication, and provide an assessment of functional status.[1] Beyond the ABI, other modalities are helpful in the diagnosis of PAD and include pulse volume recording, continuous wave Doppler ultrasound, duplex ultrasound, magnetic resonance angiography, CT angiography, and contrast angiography.

RISK FACTORS

The risk factors for atherosclerotic PAD are similar to the risk factors that promote atherosclerotic changes in other arterial vascular beds, with differences in the magnitude of risk conferred by each risk factor on PAD development.

Smoking

Smoking is the most powerful risk factor for the development of PAD. Observational studies demonstrate that smoking is a more potent risk factor for the development of PAD than for the development of coronary artery disease.[21] The mechanism of effect is not entirely understood because tobacco's impact on the development of PAD is only partially explained by its pathophysiologic modification of traditional cardiovascular risk factors.[22] Smoking has deleterious effects on endothelial function, alters vascular tone, and promotes inflammation and erythrocytosis, which alter the rheologic properties of blood.[23] Smoking confers a 2-fold to 6-fold increased risk of developing PAD and there is a dose-dependent effect with smoking and risk of incident PAD.[21] Smokers with PAD also experience worse disease-specific outcomes, with higher rates of critical limb ischemia and amputation, higher procedural complications, and increased bypass graft failure.[24,25] Smoking cessation improves overall survival and this effect becomes apparent 1 year after cessation.[26] Secondhand smoke exposure is also important and a dose-dependent relationship between exposure to secondhand smoke and risk of PAD has been demonstrated.[27]

Diabetes Mellitus

Diabetes mellitus (DM) is a potent risk factor for the development of PAD. Studies have demonstrated that DM confers at least a 2-fold increased risk of PAD.[1,4] There also seems to be a continuous increase in PAD risk based on glycemic control. One meta-analysis found that for every 1% increase in hemoglobin (Hgb) A1c, there was a 30% increase in risk of incident PAD.[28] Patients with DM are at particularly high risk for presenting with late PAD manifestations, including neuropathy, impaired microcirculation, altered skin integrity, and impaired immune response, which all contribute to the development of ischemic complications. Patients with diabetes and PAD have higher mortality rates at younger ages and are 5 times more likely to undergo amputation compared with nondiabetics.[29] As opposed to smokers, who have a higher association of PAD development in the arterial vessels above the knee, patients with DM have a higher association of PAD development below the knee.[29,30] In addition to the metabolic effects of DM with other CVD risk factors (eg, hypertension and dyslipidemia), DM promotes development of atherosclerosis through at least 2 mechanisms: (1) hyperglycemia, hyperinsulinemia, and free fatty acid production–impaired nitric oxide signaling and endothelial dysfunction and (2) hyperglycemia oxidative stress and platelet aggregation, which alters the rheologic properties of blood.[30]

Hypertension

Elevated blood pressure is a significant risk factor for the development of PAD. In the Framingham Heart Study, there was an increase in the development of intermittent claudication by 2-fold in men and 4-fold in women with hypertension.[31] The coexistence of hypertension and PAD is common, with more than 50% of those with PAD having concomitant hypertension.[32] Both conditions are associated with an increased risk of cardiovascular events and death. In the Systolic Hypertension in the Elderly (SHEP) Trial, men and women with systolic hypertension and ankle arm indices less than or equal to 0.9 had significantly increased risk of both total and CVD mortality (odds ratio [OR] 2.8–3.3).[33]

Hyperlipidemia

An increased risk of PAD has been associated with dyslipidemia in several studies.[5,34,35] Analogous to coronary atherosclerosis, there have been many studies highlighting the relationship between PAD and low high-density lipoprotein, elevated total cholesterol, and elevated low-density lipoprotein cholesterol (LDL-C).[1] There is a continuous relationship between lipid abnormalities and risk of PAD, with a 10% increase in incident PAD for each 10-mg/dL increase in total cholesterol.[5]

Effect of Multiple Risk Factors

A recent report of the Health Professionals Follow-Up Study, which prospectively evaluated more than 40,000 individuals over a period of 2 decades, indicated that the combination of smoking, hypertension, hyperlipidemia, and DM accounted for the vast majority of incident PAD. Each condition was an independent risk factor for PAD development and the magnitude of risk was both graded (duration of exposure) and additive, with increasing risk noted with combinations of each risk factor. Together, these 4 conditions explained a significant majority of incident PAD, with a 75% population attributable risk, defined as the proportion of disease that would not occur if these risk factors were eliminated.[36]

Nontraditional Risk Factors

Although the aforementioned risk factors confer the majority of risk, other nontraditional risk factors are associated with PAD.[1] Most notably, elevated homocysteine levels have been shown associated with a 2-fold increased risk in vascular disease development.[37] Prospective studies have indicated that there is a graded response to homocysteine levels and risk of all-cause mortality and CVD mortality.[38] There remains, however, no evidence that lowering homocysteine levels leads to a decline in cardiovascular events.[39]

Inflammation is associated with and is known to hasten the progression of PAD. In the Edinburgh Artery Study, C-reactive protein, interleukin (IL)-6, and intercellular adhesion molecule were all associated with and accelerated the progression of PAD.[40] Of these inflammatory markers, IL-6 had the strongest association and was an independent predictor of PAD progression. The investigators postulated that this may be the dual inflammation and procoagulant effects that IL-6 possesses. In a nested case control study of the Physicians' Health Study, C-reactive protein was found a strong predictor of PAD development, with additive predictive ability above traditional risk factors.[41]

MEDICAL TREATMENT

Complete recommendations for the optimal medical management of patients with PAD are in the recently published and updated American College of Cardiology Foundation/American Heart Association (ACCF/AHA) task force guidelines on the management of patients with PAD, which were developed in collaboration with the Society for

Cardiovascular Angiography and Interventions, Society of Interventional Radiology, Society for Vascular Medicine, and Society for Vascular Surgery.[1,16] According to these guidelines, all patients with PAD should undergo comprehensive lifestyle modifications to reduce the overall risk of adverse cardiovascular events.[1,16] Behavioral modifications to achieve a target body mass index less than 25 kg/m^2, adoption of a cardiovascular healthy diet with reductions in dietary total and saturated fat, and daily aerobic exercise are fundamental to a heart and vascular healthy lifestyle. Many patients require, however, a more tailored counseling approach to risk factor modification and may also require initiation of pharmacotherapy.

Tobacco Cessation

Smoking cessation provides the cornerstone in efforts to decrease risk of all-cause and cardiovascular mortality. Smoking cessation reduces the rate of PAD progression and the incidence of vascular complications (amputation and limb ischemia) and may help reduce claudication severity. Tobacco cessation, however, is not easily accomplished and counseling by a health care professional as well as pharmacologic assistance is often required and is of proved benefit.

Counseling on the importance of tobacco cessation is both mandatory and effective. Even brief counseling has proved influential; unfortunately, less than 50% of patients are offered assistance with tobacco cessation in primary care.[13] Vascular specialists are uniquely positioned to have an impact on tobacco use and have a responsibility in this regard. Intensive counseling and structured programs are most effective, with 1-year quit rates approaching 20%.[42] In a recent study of patients with PAD, 6-month quit rates were significantly higher among those who received intensive counseling compared with brief point-of-care counseling (21.3% vs 6.8%, $P = .023$). Intensive counseling consisted of 6 counseling sessions over 5 months in which education, cognitive-behavioral counseling, identification of quit dates, and social support were all delineated.[43]

Multimodality interventions that include pharmacotherapy are the most effective, with cessation rates approaching 44%,[44] and there are 3 medications with proved benefit in achieving tobacco cessation:

1. Nicotine replacement therapy
2. Bupropion
3. Varenicline (Chantix)

Nicotine replacement has an important role in assisting patients with tobacco cessation. A Cochrane review of 150 tobacco cessation trials found that use of nicotine replacement was associated with a significant 50% to 70% increase in the rate of maintaining abstinence from tobacco compared with placebo at 6 months.[45,46] The method of nicotine replacement (chewing gum, transdermal patches, nasal spray, inhalers, and tablets) did not alter efficacy.[45,46]

Another key pharmacologic agent to aid tobacco cessation is the antidepressant, bupropion. Bupropion is a unique aminoketone antidepressant agent that has a weak inhibitory effect on norepinephrine and dopamine reuptake. The exact mechanism of action in smoking cessation, however, remains somewhat unclear.[47]

In a double-blind, placebo-controlled trial comparing bupropion therapy with or without nicotine replacement, bupropion produced a statistically significant increase in the rate of abstinence at 12 months (30.3% in the bupropion group vs 15.6% in the placebo, $P<.001$). Although the combination of bupropion and nicotine replacement yielded the highest abstinence rates (35.5%), the difference between quit rates with bupropion alone or in combination with nicotine replacement was not statistically significant.[48]

Varenicline (Chantix) is an $\alpha4\beta2$–nicotinic acetylcholine receptor partial agonist and, compared with available alternatives, has demonstrated superior rates of smoking cessation. By stimulating dopamine release in the brain and inhibiting nicotine binding to the nicotine receptor, varenicline helps reduce withdrawal symptoms and nicotine cravings and decreases the reinforcement and reward associated with tobacco use. Compared with placebo, varenicline has demonstrated superior short-term and long-term quit rates.[49] In 1 randomized, placebo-controlled trial comparing varenicline with bupropion, varenicline produced the highest rates of abstinence at 1 year after treatment.[44]

Smoking cessation is perhaps the most important modifiable risk factor in the battle against PAD development and progression and the recently updated ACCF/AHA PAD treatment guidelines provide the following class I recommendations[16]:

- Any current or former smoker should be asked about tobacco status at every visit.
- Patients who smoke should be assisted with a counseling and a cessation plan that includes referral to smoking cessation and/or pharmacologic aid.
- Unless clinically contraindicated, patients who smoke should be offered 1 or more of the following pharmacotherapeutic agents: nicotine replacement, bupropion, and varenicline.

Diabetes Mellitus Management

Although DM confers a significant risk of PAD development, trials evaluating glycemic control have not demonstrated a protective effect with tight glycemic control. The Diabetes Control and Complications Trial found a significant reduction in the microvascular complications of DM with tight glycemic control, whereas the reduction in macrovascular complications did not reach statistical significance.[50] Other studies have examined the effect of tight glycemic control on the development of CVD, with many of these trials including PAD in the composite endpoints (**Table 1**).[51–56] Although there seems to be consistency in the evidence that tight glycemic control reduces microvascular complications, the evidence continues to be lacking with regards to macrovascular events. Current ACCF/AHA PAD treatment guidelines (**Table 2**) provide the following recommendation:

- HgBA1c <7% for prevention of microvascular sequelae and potential benefits with respect to macrovascular complications of DM (class IIa, level C).[1,16]

In addition to glycemic control, the American Diabetes Association recommends:

- An annual evaluation for the presence of PAD in all patients with diabetes.
- For patients with diabetes older than 50 years, a screening ABI examination is recommended and this study should be repeated every 5 years if the initial result is normal or borderline reduced.
- Finally, all patients with diabetes and PAD should be evaluated regularly for the presence of peripheral neuropathy and should receive preventive foot care to help minimize the risk of developing ischemic complications and limb loss.[30]

Blood Pressure Control

As defined by the Seventh Report of the Joint National Committee on Prevention, Detection, Evaluation, and Treatment of High Blood Pressure, hypertension is a systolic blood pressure greater than or equal to 140 mm Hg and diastolic blood pressure

Table 1
Glycemic control and macrovascular endpoints

Study	Population	Primary Macrovascular Endpoints	Intervention	Outcomes
PROactive[51]	Type 2 DM	ACS, nonfatal MI, endovascular/surgical revascularization on leg arteries, or amputation	Pioglitazone vs placebo	Nonsignificant 10% reduction in macrovascular events
VADT[52]	Type 2 DM	MI, stroke, CVD death, CHF, PVD surgery, inoperable CAD, or amputation	1.5% Reduction in HgbA1c	No significant benefit in intensive glycemic control on composite outcome
UKPDS survivor cohort[53]	Type 2 DM	Death from MI, stroke, or PVD	FPG <108 mg/dL	~10-y Follow-up of original trial: intensive glycemic control reduced MI but not PAD
UKPDS[54]	Type 2 DM	Death from MI, stroke, or PVD	FPG <108 mg/dL	Nonsignificant reduction in PAD RR 0.65 (95% CI, 0.36–1.18).
ACCORD[55]	Type 2 DM	Nonfatal MI, nonfatal stroke, or CVD death	HgbA1c <6.0%	Increased mortality in intensive glycemic control group
ADVANCE[56]	Type 2 DM	Composite of macrovascular and microvascular events	HgbA1c <6.5%	No significant effect on macrovascular events; reduction in combined macrovascular and microvascular events

Abbreviations: ACCORD, action to control cardiovascular risk in diabetes; ACS, acute coronary syndrome; ADVANCE, action in diabetes and vascular disease. Preterax and Diamicron Modified Release Controlled Evaluation; CAD, coronary artery disease; CHF, congestive heart failure; FPG, fasting plasma glucose; MI, myocardial infarction; PROactive, PROspective pioglitAzone clinincal trial in macroVascular events; PVD, peripheral vascular disease; RR, relative risk; UKPDS, united kingdom prospective diabetes study; VADT, veterans affairs diabetes trial.

greater than or equal to 90 mm Hg.[57] Blood pressure modification in patients with PAD has 2 goals:

- First, to reduce sequelae of PAD, such as amputation
- Second, to reduce cardiovascular events, such as myocardial infarction, stroke, and cardiovascular death

In adult patients with type 2 DM in the United Kingdom Prospective Diabetes Study Group 36 study, the risk of both microvascular and macrovascular complications of DM were reduced with tight blood pressure control.[58] In this study, all-cause mortality and DM complications were reduced by 12% for each 10–mm Hg reduction in systolic blood pressure. Furthermore, the risk of lower extremity amputation or death from PAD was reduced by 16% for each 10–mm Hg decrease in systolic blood

Table 2
Guideline-recommended medical interventions for reducing cardiovascular risk and improving symptoms in patients with PAD

Clinical Category	Guideline-Recommended Interventions
Reduce cardiovascular risk and event rates	
Smoking cessation[16]	Screen for and counsel smokers every clinical visit Pharmacologic (varenicline, bupropion, nicotine replacement) therapy should be offered unless contraindicated Behavioral modification therapy offered
Antiplatelet therapy[16]	Aspirin or clopidogrel in symptomatic PAD for reduction of cardiovascular events (clopidogrel is an alternative to aspirin)
Antihypertensive therapy[57]	Treat blood pressure to <140/90 mm Hg and <130/80 mm Hg in diabetics and patients with chronic kidney disease
Lipid-lowering therapy[67]	Treat LDL-C to goal <100 mg/dL or <70 mg/dL in patients at high vascular risk (eg, multisystem atherosclerotic disease)
Diabetes treatment[30,a]	Optimize glycemic control: goal HgbA1c <7% Annual evaluation for the presence of PAD and peripheral neuropathy, screening ABI for patients with diabetes >50 y of age, and regular preventive foot care
Improve PAD symptoms and quality of life	
Exercise therapy[1]	Supervised exercise therapy for at least 30–45 min 3 times weekly for at least 12 wk
Cilostazol[1]	To improve claudication symptoms and increase walking distance in patients without concomitant heart failure

[a] Diabetes control has not been demonstrated to reduce cardiovascular event rates but has been shown to decrease important complications of microvascular disease (eg, retinopathy, neuropathy, and nephropathy).

pressure. These results were seen despite adjustment for potential confounders, such as age at diagnosis of DM, ethnic group, smoking status, presence of albuminuria, HgBA1c, high-density lipoprotein and LDL-C, and triglycerides.[58]

Blood pressure control in patients with PAD is further supported by the results of the Heart Outcomes Prevention Evaluation study, where the use of ramipril compared to placebo resulted in a 20% relative risk reduction in the composite end point of myocardial infarction, stroke, or vascular death.[1,59] The current ACCF/AHA PAD treatment guidelines recommend

- Antihypertensive medication to achieve a goal of <140/90 mm Hg in nondiabetics and <130/80 mm Hg in patients with diabetes and/or chronic kidney disease (class I, level of evidence A)[1,16]
- Current PAD specific treatment guidelines recommend the use of angiotensin converting enzyme inhibitors (class IIa, level of evidence B)[1,16]

Although of historic concern, there are few data to support the relationship between β-blocker therapy and worsened symptoms of claudication.[60] β-Blocker therapy is indicated in patients with coronary atherosclerosis and has been demonstrated to reduce the risk of myocardial infarction and death.[61]

Lipid Lowering

The use of HMG-CoA reductase inhibitors (statins) is associated with significant benefits in primary and secondary prevention of CVD. Although the magnitude of this effect is well documented for coronary artery disease, less is known for PAD. The Heart Protection Study enrolled high-risk subjects, randomizing them to simvastatin 40 mg daily versus placebo. At study completion, simvastatin resulted in a significant reduction in mean LDL-C (88.9 mg/dL vs 127.6 mg/dL with placebo), all-cause mortality, and cardiovascular events.[62] A subgroup analysis of PAD patients within the Heart Protection Study demonstrated a 22% relative risk reduction in the rate of first major vascular event, and this observation was noted regardless of the initial baseline LDL-C.[62,63]

Although the overall risk reduction conferred by HMG-CoA reductase inhibitors is large, this medication class remains grossly underused among patients with PAD.[64,65] The treatment gap is not only present in patients with mild PAD. Data from the Bypass versus Angioplasty in severe Ischaemia of the Leg trial demonstrated that only 33% of patients with severe PAD were on statin therapy.[66]

The Adult Treatment Panel III guidelines consider PAD a CVD risk equivalent and recommend the following LDL-C treatment goals in patients with PAD:

- Low-density lipoprotein value <100 mg/dL (class I, level of evidence B)
- Low-density lipoprotein value <70 mg/dL if at increased risk of ischemic events (class IIA, level of evidence B) or with evidence of multisystem vascular disease.[1,67]

Antiplatelet Therapies

Aspirin therapy

Aspirin therapy in patients with PAD has long been a mainstay of best medical therapy. Early studies, such as the meta-analysis performed by Antithrombotic Trialists' Collaboration, demonstrated a significant benefit of daily aspirin use in high-risk vascular patients, with an overall reduction in cardiovascular events (stroke, myocardial infarction, and vascular-related death). In an analysis of a subgroup of patients with PAD (N = 9214), there was a significant 23% proportional reduction in major vascular events.[68]

More contemporary trials have called into question the benefit of aspirin use in primary CVD prevention, specifically among patients with asymptomatic PAD. The Aspirin for Asymptomatic Atherosclerosis trial was a randomized, double-blinded, placebo-controlled trial that evaluated the role of aspirin in prevention of cardiovascular events in asymptomatic patients with low ABI who were free of baseline CVD. No statistically significant reduction in major cardiovascular events was demonstrated with the use of 100 mg of aspirin daily versus placebo.[69] Two recent trials evaluating the role of aspirin in patients with diabetes and asymptomatic PAD have failed to demonstrate a significant benefit in cardiovascular event reduction.[70,71] Finally, a recent meta-analysis looking at aspirin use in the prevention of cardiovascular events in patients with PAD demonstrated a nonsignificant reduction in cardiovascular events.[72]

In contrast to the findings discussed previously, the Critical Leg Ischaemia Prevention Study enrolled symptomatic and asymptomatic patients with PAD and randomized them to aspirin or placebo. This study found a reduction in the incidence of vascular events in the aspirin group by 26%; however, this study was terminated early because it did not meet the prespecified enrollment.[73]

Thienopyridines

Clopidogrel, ticlopidine, and prasugrel are thienopyridine class agents that reduce platelet aggregation through inhibition of the platelet surface P2Y12 receptor.[74] Clopidogrel is the most commonly used thienopyridine antiplatelet agent and is the focus of this discussion. Clopidogrel has recently become available in generic formulation and has the most abundant efficacy and safety data.

In one of the early clopidogrel trials, Clopidogrel versus Aspirin in Patients at Risk of Ischaemic Events (CAPRIE), clopidogrel was compared with 325 mg of aspirin therapy in more than 19,000 high-vascular-risk patients. Clopidogrel was associated with a significant reduction in the combined endpoint (ischemic stroke, myocardial infarction, or and vascular death) compared with aspirin (5.32% vs 5.83%, $P = .04$).[75] Within the subgroup of patients with PAD (N = 6452), there was a 24% relative risk reduction in cardiovascular events.[75] Given the positive results of the CAPRIE study, there was clinical equipoise to evaluate the impact of dual antiplatelet therapy with both aspirin and clopidogrel in high-cardiovascular-risk patients. In the Clopidogrel and Aspirin versus Aspirin Alone for the Prevention of Atherothrombotic Events trial performed by the CHARISMA investigators, dual antiplatelet therapy with both clopidogrel and low-dose aspirin versus low-dose aspirin alone was evaluated in 15,603 high-cardiovascular-risk patients.[76] Overall, the dual antiplatelet strategy did not reduce the primary endpoint, which was a composite endpoint of myocardial infarction, stroke, or cardiovascular death.[76]

The current ACCF/AHA PAD treatment guidelines provide the following recommendations for antiplatelet therapy:

- Aspirin or clopidogrel therapy for patients with symptomatic PAD (class I, level of evidence A). Clopidogrel is recommended as an alternative to aspirin (class IB).
- Aspirin or clopidogrel therapy for patients with asymptomatic PAD (class IIA, level of evidence C).
- Dual antiplatelet therapy (eg, aspirin and clopidogrel) for patients with symptomatic PAD at high cardiovascular risk and low bleeding risk (class IIB).[16]

Warfarin has no role in the prevention of cardiovascular events in patients with PAD; low-dose aspirin (eg, 81 mg daily) is preferred to maintain cardiovascular benefit and minimize toxicity, and all aspirin formulations are considered equally effective.

Cilostazol

Cilostazol is a phosphodiesterase III inhibitor that increases cyclic adenosine monophosphate levels. The increase in cyclic adenosine monophosphate levels is associated with arterial vasodilatation, decreased platelet aggregation, reduced vascular smooth muscle proliferation, increased nitric oxide signaling, increase high-density lipoprotein levels, and decreases in triglyceride levels.[77,78] Cilostazol has been demonstrated in multiple randomized trials to improve walking distance in patients with intermittent claudication and it may also reduce rates of restenosis and revascularization. A meta-analysis of 7 randomized controlled trials that included more than 1500 patients with moderate to severe PAD demonstrated significant improvement in walking distance with use of cilostazol.[79] In another analysis of 9 randomized controlled trials, the use of cilostazol (100 mg twice daily) was associated with a 50% improvement in maximal walking distance from baseline.[80] The use of cilostazol has a proved long-term safety profile but is contraindicated in patients with reduced left ventricular systolic function and has limitations with respect to its side-effect profile and patient compliance.[81,82]

Current ACCF/AHA PAD treatment guidelines recommend

- Cilostazol (class IA) to improve claudication symptoms and increase walking distance in patients with lower extremity PAD and intermittent claudication[1,16]

Exercise Therapy

Patients with symptomatic and asymptomatic PAD have reduced functional capacity and quality of life and faster rates of mobility loss compared with patients without

PAD.[83–85] Supervised exercise therapy has been shown to improve measures of walking performance, claudication severity, and quality of life.[86,87] Postulated mechanisms for the benefits of exercise therapy include promotion of angiogenesis, improved skeletal muscle metabolism, increased muscle strength, improved endothelial function, and altered gait.

The magnitude of benefit conferred by supervised exercise for patients with intermittent claudication was summarized in a meta-analysis of 21 studies that demonstrated a 179% increase in initial claudication distance and 122% increase in maximal claudication distance.[88] The Claudication: Exercise versus Endoluminal Revascularization study demonstrated that compared with endovascular therapy, supervised exercise therapy significantly improves peak walking time and similarly improves quality of life measurements for patients with symptomatic aortoiliac disease.[89] The benefits of supervised exercise therapy are not, however, limited to patients with symptomatic PAD. In a study evaluating exercise therapy compared with resistance training and placebo on walking distance in patients with reduced ABI values, a treadmill exercise training program significantly improved 6-minute walk times, treadmill walking performance, brachial flow-mediated dilation (measure of endothelial dysfunction), and physical functioning scores in patients with symptomatic and asymptomatic PAD.[87] Additionally, regular exercise has been shown to reduce the risk of CVD through decreases in blood pressure, blood glucose, lipids, and inflammatory markers.

Current ACCF/AHA PAD treatment guidelines recommend

- Supervised exercise therapy for all patients with claudication (class IA)[1,16]
- Components of an effective exercise program that include supervised exercise (walking to the point of near maximal pain) for at least 30 to 45 minutes, 3 to 4 times a week, for a minimum of 12 weeks[1,16]

Unfortunately, unsupervised exercise therapy has not proved equal to supervised programs and the lack of insurance reimbursement for the latter has greatly limited its availability and use.

SUMMARY

PAD is an underdiagnosed and undertreated condition that is associated with a considerable increase in morbidity and mortality. Patients with PAD, regardless of symptom status, are at high risk of future cardiovascular events and mortality and require aggressive medical intervention and education. This is not always achieved in the primary care setting. Unfortunately, by the time PAD is diagnosed, the deleterious effects and risks associated with the condition have become well established. Therefore, vascular specialists fill a critical and influential role for the patient and primary care provider, because they often become involved in a patient's care at a period of sensitivity and potential responsiveness to guideline-recommended therapy.

Therapeutic interventions should almost universally be implemented and serve the primary goals of

- Lowering cardiovascular risk and cardiovascular event rates
- Improving symptoms and quality of life

The first objective is pursued through aggressive risk factor modification, including tobacco cessation, blood pressure control, lipid lowering, control of DM, and initiation of antiplatelet therapy. For patients with stable, symptomatic PAD, the recommended approach toward the second objective is initiation of supervised exercise therapy and cilostazol and pursuit of revascularization when medical therapy has failed.

REFERENCES

1. Hirsch AT, Haskal ZJ, Hertzer NR, et al. ACC/AHA 2005 Practice Guidelines for the management of patients with peripheral arterial disease (lower extremity, renal, mesenteric, and abdominal aortic): a collaborative report from the American Association for Vascular Surgery/Society for Vascular Surgery, Society for Cardiovascular Angiography and Interventions, Society for Vascular Medicine and Biology, Society of Interventional Radiology, and the ACC/AHA Task Force on Practice Guidelines (Writing Committee to Develop Guidelines for the Management of Patients With Peripheral Arterial Disease): endorsed by the American Association of Cardiovascular and Pulmonary Rehabilitation; National Heart, Lung, and Blood Institute; Society for Vascular Nursing; TransAtlantic Inter-Society Consensus; and Vascular Disease Foundation. Circulation 2006; 113(11):e463–654.
2. Hiatt WR, Goldstone J, Smith SC Jr, et al. Atherosclerotic Peripheral Vascular Disease Symposium II: nomenclature for vascular diseases. Circulation 2008; 118(25):2826–9.
3. Roger VL, Go AS, Lloyd-Jones DM, et al. Heart disease and stroke statistics—2012 update: a report from the American Heart Association. Circulation 2012; 125(1):e2–220.
4. Ostchega Y, Paulose-Ram R, Dillon CF, et al. Prevalence of peripheral arterial disease and risk factors in persons aged 60 and older: data from the National Health and Nutrition Examination Survey 1999-2004. J Am Geriatr Soc 2007; 55(4):583–9.
5. Newman AB, Siscovick DS, Manolio TA, et al. Ankle-arm index as a marker of atherosclerosis in the Cardiovascular Health Study. Cardiovascular Heart Study (CHS) Collaborative Research Group. Circulation 1993;88(3):837–45.
6. Agnelli G, Cimminiello C, Meneghetti G, et al. Low ankle-brachial index predicts an adverse 1-year outcome after acute coronary and cerebrovascular events. J Thromb Haemost 2006;4(12):2599–606.
7. Busch MA, Lutz K, Rohl JE, et al. Low ankle-brachial index predicts cardiovascular risk after acute ischemic stroke or transient ischemic attack. Stroke 2009; 40(12):3700–5.
8. Allison MA, Criqui MH, McClelland RL, et al. The effect of novel cardiovascular risk factors on the ethnic-specific odds for peripheral arterial disease in the Multi-Ethnic Study of Atherosclerosis (MESA). J Am Coll Cardiol 2006;48(6): 1190–7.
9. Fowkes FG, Murray GD, Butcher I, et al. Ankle brachial index combined with Framingham Risk Score to predict cardiovascular events and mortality: a meta-analysis. JAMA 2008;300(2):197–208.
10. Heald CL, Fowkes FG, Murray GD, et al. Risk of mortality and cardiovascular disease associated with the ankle-brachial index: systematic review. Atherosclerosis 2006;189(1):61–9.
11. Resnick HE, Lindsay RS, McDermott MM, et al. Relationship of high and low ankle brachial index to all-cause and cardiovascular disease mortality: the Strong Heart Study. Circulation 2004;109(6):733–9.
12. Rose GA. The diagnosis of ischaemic heart pain and intermittent claudication in field surveys. Bull World Health Organ 1962;27:645–58.

13. Hirsch AT, Criqui MH, Treat-Jacobson D, et al. Peripheral arterial disease detection, awareness, and treatment in primary care. JAMA 2001;286(11):1317–24.

14. Diehm C, Allenberg JR, Pittrow D, et al. Mortality and vascular morbidity in older adults with asymptomatic versus symptomatic peripheral artery disease. Circulation 2009;120(21):2053–61.

15. McDermott MM, Guralnik JM, Ferrucci L, et al. Asymptomatic peripheral arterial disease is associated with more adverse lower extremity characteristics than intermittent claudication. Circulation 2008;117(19):2484–91.

16. Rooke TW, Hirsch AT, Misra S, et al. 2011 ACCF/AHA Focused Update of the Guideline for the Management of Patients With Peripheral Artery Disease (updating the 2005 guideline): a report of the American College of Cardiology Foundation/American Heart Association Task Force on Practice Guidelines. J Am Coll Cardiol 2011;58(19):2020–45.

17. McDermott MM. The magnitude of the problem of peripheral arterial disease: epidemiology and clinical significance. Cleve Clin J Med 2006;73(Suppl 4): S2–7.

18. Aboyans V, Criqui MH, Abraham P, et al. Measurement and Interpretation of the Ankle-Brachial Index: a Scientific Statement From the American Heart Association. Circulation 2012;126(24):2890–909.

19. Fowkes FG. The measurement of atherosclerotic peripheral arterial disease in epidemiological surveys. Int J Epidemiol 1988;17(2):248–54.

20. Feigelson HS, Criqui MH, Fronek A, et al. Screening for peripheral arterial disease: the sensitivity, specificity, and predictive value of noninvasive tests in a defined population. Am J Epidemiol 1994;140(6):526–34.

21. Fowkes FG, Housley E, Riemersma RA, et al. Smoking, lipids, glucose intolerance, and blood pressure as risk factors for peripheral atherosclerosis compared with ischemic heart disease in the Edinburgh Artery Study. Am J Epidemiol 1992;135(4):331–40.

22. Price JF, Mowbray PI, Lee AJ, et al. Relationship between smoking and cardiovascular risk factors in the development of peripheral arterial disease and coronary artery disease: Edinburgh Artery Study. Eur Heart J 1999;20(5):344–53.

23. Krupski WC. The peripheral vascular consequences of smoking. Ann Vasc Surg 1991;5(3):291–304.

24. Shammas NW. Epidemiology, classification, and modifiable risk factors of peripheral arterial disease. Vasc Health Risk Manag 2007;3(2):229–34.

25. Bartholomew JR, Olin JW. Pathophysiology of peripheral arterial disease and risk factors for its development. Cleve Clin J Med 2006;73(Suppl 4):S8–14.

26. Jonason T, Bergstrom R. Cessation of smoking in patients with intermittent claudication. Effects on the risk of peripheral vascular complications, myocardial infarction and mortality. Acta Med Scand 1987;221(3):253–60.

27. He Y, Lam TH, Jiang B, et al. Passive smoking and risk of peripheral arterial disease and ischemic stroke in Chinese women who never smoked. Circulation 2008;118(15):1535–40.

28. Selvin E, Marinopoulos S, Berkenblit G, et al. Meta-analysis: glycosylated hemoglobin and cardiovascular disease in diabetes mellitus. Ann Intern Med 2004; 141(6):421–31.

29. Jude EB, Oyibo SO, Chalmers N, et al. Peripheral arterial disease in diabetic and nondiabetic patients: a comparison of severity and outcome. Diabetes Care 2001;24(8):1433–7.

30. American Diabetes Association. Peripheral arterial disease in people with diabetes. Diabetes Care 2003;26(12):3333–41.

31. Kannel WB, McGee DL. Update on some epidemiologic features of intermittent claudication: the Framingham Study. J Am Geriatr Soc 1985;33(1):13–8.
32. Olin JW. Hypertension and peripheral arterial disease. Vasc Med 2005;10(3): 241–6.
33. Newman AB, Tyrrell KS, Kuller LH. Mortality over four years in SHEP participants with a low ankle-arm index. J Am Geriatr Soc 1997;45(12):1472–8.
34. Bradby GV, Valente AJ, Walton KW. Serum high-density lipoproteins in peripheral vascular disease. Lancet 1978;2(8103):1271–4.
35. Cardia G, Grisorio D, Impedovo G, et al. Plasma lipids as a risk factor in peripheral vascular disease. Angiology 1990;41(1):19–22.
36. Joosten MM, Pai JK, Bertoia ML, et al. Associations between conventional cardiovascular risk factors and risk of peripheral artery disease in men. JAMA 2012;308(16):1660–7.
37. Boushey CJ, Beresford SA, Omenn GS, et al. A quantitative assessment of plasma homocysteine as a risk factor for vascular disease. Probable benefits of increasing folic acid intakes. JAMA 1995;274(13):1049–57.
38. Taylor LM Jr, Moneta GL, Sexton GJ, et al. Prospective blinded study of the relationship between plasma homocysteine and progression of symptomatic peripheral arterial disease. J Vasc Surg 1999;29(1):8–19 [discussion: 19–21].
39. Lonn E, Yusuf S, Arnold MJ, et al. Homocysteine lowering with folic acid and B vitamins in vascular disease. N Engl J Med 2006;354(15):1567–77.
40. Tzoulaki I, Murray GD, Lee AJ, et al. C-reactive protein, interleukin-6, and soluble adhesion molecules as predictors of progressive peripheral atherosclerosis in the general population: Edinburgh Artery Study. Circulation 2005;112(7):976–83.
41. Ridker PM, Stampfer MJ, Rifai N. Novel risk factors for systemic atherosclerosis: a comparison of C-reactive protein, fibrinogen, homocysteine, lipoprotein(a), and standard cholesterol screening as predictors of peripheral arterial disease. JAMA 2001;285(19):2481–5.
42. Clinical Practice Guideline Treating Tobacco Use and Dependence 2008 Update Panel, Liaisons, and Staff. A clinical practice guideline for treating tobacco use and dependence: 2008 update. A U.S. Public Health Service report. Am J Prev Med 2008;35(2):158–76.
43. Hennrikus D, Joseph AM, Lando HA, et al. Effectiveness of a smoking cessation program for peripheral artery disease patients: a randomized controlled trial. J Am Coll Cardiol 2010;56(25):2105–12.
44. Jorenby DE, Hays JT, Rigotti NA, et al. Efficacy of varenicline, an alpha4beta2 nicotinic acetylcholine receptor partial agonist, vs placebo or sustained-release bupropion for smoking cessation: a randomized controlled trial. JAMA 2006;296(1):56–63.
45. Stead LF, Perera R, Bullen C, et al. Nicotine replacement therapy for smoking cessation. Cochrane Database Syst Rev 2012;(11):CD000146.
46. Silagy C, Lancaster T, Stead L, et al. Nicotine replacement therapy for smoking cessation. Cochrane Database Syst Rev 2004;(3):CD000146.
47. Ferris R, White HL, Cooper BR. Some neurochemical properties of a new antidepressant, bupropion hydrochloride (Wellbutrin(R)). Drug Dev Res 1981;1: 21–35.
48. Jorenby DE, Leischow SJ, Nides MA, et al. A controlled trial of sustained-release bupropion, a nicotine patch, or both for smoking cessation. N Engl J Med 1999; 340(9):685–91.
49. Nides M, Oncken C, Gonzales D, et al. Smoking cessation with varenicline, a selective alpha4beta2 nicotinic receptor partial agonist: results from a 7-week,

randomized, placebo- and bupropion-controlled trial with 1-year follow-up. Arch Intern Med 2006;166(15):1561–8.

50. The effect of intensive treatment of diabetes on the development and progression of long-term complications in insulin-dependent diabetes mellitus. The Diabetes Control and Complications Trial Research Group. N Engl J Med 1993; 329(14):977–86.

51. Dormandy JA, Charbonnel B, Eckland DJ, et al. Secondary prevention of macrovascular events in patients with type 2 diabetes in the PROactive Study (PROspective pioglitAzone Clinical Trial In macroVascular Events): a randomised controlled trial. Lancet 2005;366(9493):1279–89.

52. Duckworth W, Abraira C, Moritz T, et al. Glucose control and vascular complications in veterans with type 2 diabetes. N Engl J Med 2009;360(2):129–39.

53. Holman RR, Paul SK, Bethel MA, et al. 10-year follow-up of intensive glucose control in type 2 diabetes. N Engl J Med 2008;359(15):1577–89.

54. Intensive blood-glucose control with sulphonylureas or insulin compared with conventional treatment and risk of complications in patients with type 2 diabetes (UKPDS 33). UK Prospective Diabetes Study (UKPDS) Group. Lancet 1998; 352(9131):837–53.

55. Gerstein HC, Miller ME, Byington RP, et al. Effects of intensive glucose lowering in type 2 diabetes. N Engl J Med 2008;358(24):2545–59.

56. Patel A, MacMahon S, Chalmers J, et al. Intensive blood glucose control and vascular outcomes in patients with type 2 diabetes. N Engl J Med 2008; 358(24):2560–72.

57. Chobanian AV, Bakris GL, Black HR, et al. Seventh report of the Joint National Committee on Prevention, Detection, Evaluation, and Treatment of High Blood Pressure. Hypertension 2003;42(6):1206–52.

58. Adler AI, Stratton IM, Neil HA, et al. Association of systolic blood pressure with macrovascular and microvascular complications of type 2 diabetes (UKPDS 36): prospective observational study. BMJ 2000;321(7258):412–9.

59. Yusuf S, Sleight P, Pogue J, et al. Effects of an angiotensin-converting-enzyme inhibitor, ramipril, on cardiovascular events in high-risk patients. The Heart Outcomes Prevention Evaluation Study Investigators. N Engl J Med 2000;342(3): 145–53.

60. Radack K, Deck C. Beta-adrenergic blocker therapy does not worsen intermittent claudication in subjects with peripheral arterial disease. A meta-analysis of randomized controlled trials. Arch Intern Med 1991;151(9):1769–76.

61. Hennekens CH, Albert CM, Godfried SL, et al. Adjunctive drug therapy of acute myocardial infarction—evidence from clinical trials. N Engl J Med 1996;335(22): 1660–7.

62. Heart Protection Study Collaborative Group. MRC/BHF Heart Protection Study of cholesterol lowering with simvastatin in 20,536 high-risk individuals: a randomised placebo-controlled trial. Lancet 2002;360(9326):7–22.

63. Heart Protection Study Collaborative Group. Randomized trial of the effects of cholesterol-lowering with simvastatin on peripheral vascular and other major vascular outcomes in 20,536 people with peripheral arterial disease and other high-risk conditions. J Vasc Surg 2007;45(4):645–54 [discussion: 653–4].

64. Rehring TF, Sandhoff BG, Stolcpart RS, et al. Atherosclerotic risk factor control in patients with peripheral arterial disease. J Vasc Surg 2005;41(5):816–22.

65. Owens CD, Conte MS. Medical management of peripheral arterial disease: bridging the "gap"? Circulation 2012;126(11):1319–21.

66. Adam DJ, Beard JD, Cleveland T, et al. Bypass versus angioplasty in severe ischaemia of the leg (BASIL): multicentre, randomised controlled trial. Lancet 2005;366(9501):1925–34.
67. Expert Panel on Detection, Evaluation, Treatment of High Blood Cholesterol in Adults. Executive Summary of The Third Report of The National Cholesterol Education Program (NCEP) Expert Panel on Detection, Evaluation, And Treatment of High Blood Cholesterol In Adults (Adult Treatment Panel III). JAMA 2001;285(19):2486–97.
68. Antithrombotic Trialists' Collaboration. Collaborative meta-analysis of randomised trials of antiplatelet therapy for prevention of death, myocardial infarction, and stroke in high risk patients. BMJ 2002;324(7329):71–86.
69. Fowkes FG, Price JF, Stewart MC, et al. Aspirin for prevention of cardiovascular events in a general population screened for a low ankle brachial index: a randomized controlled trial. JAMA 2010;303(9):841–8.
70. Belch J, MacCuish A, Campbell I, et al. The prevention of progression of arterial disease and diabetes (POPADAD) trial: factorial randomised placebo controlled trial of aspirin and antioxidants in patients with diabetes and asymptomatic peripheral arterial disease. BMJ 2008;337:a1840.
71. Ogawa H, Nakayama M, Morimoto T, et al. Low-dose aspirin for primary prevention of atherosclerotic events in patients with type 2 diabetes: a randomized controlled trial. JAMA 2008;300(18):2134–41.
72. Berger JS, Krantz MJ, Kittelson JM, et al. Aspirin for the prevention of cardiovascular events in patients with peripheral artery disease: a meta-analysis of randomized trials. JAMA 2009;301(18):1909–19.
73. Catalano M, Born G, Peto R. Prevention of serious vascular events by aspirin amongst patients with peripheral arterial disease: randomized, double-blind trial. J Intern Med 2007;261(3):276–84.
74. Mills DC, Puri R, Hu CJ, et al. Clopidogrel inhibits the binding of ADP analogues to the receptor mediating inhibition of platelet adenylate cyclase. Arterioscler Thromb 1992;12(4):430–6.
75. CAPRIE Steering Committee. A randomised, blinded, trial of clopidogrel versus aspirin in patients at risk of ischaemic events (CAPRIE). CAPRIE Steering Committee. Lancet 1996;348(9038):1329–39.
76. Bhatt DL, Fox KA, Hacke W, et al. Clopidogrel and aspirin versus aspirin alone for the prevention of atherothrombotic events. N Engl J Med 2006;354(16):1706–17.
77. Elam MB, Heckman J, Crouse JR, et al. Effect of the novel antiplatelet agent cilostazol on plasma lipoproteins in patients with intermittent claudication. Arterioscler Thromb Vasc Biol 1998;18(12):1942–7.
78. Ota H, Eto M, Kano MR, et al. Cilostazol inhibits oxidative stress-induced premature senescence via upregulation of Sirt1 in human endothelial cells. Arterioscler Thromb Vasc Biol 2008;28(9):1634–9.
79. Robless P, Mikhailidis DP, Stansby GP. Cilostazol for peripheral arterial disease. Cochrane Database Syst Rev 2008;(1):CD003748.
80. Pande RL, Hiatt WR, Zhang P, et al. A pooled analysis of the durability and predictors of treatment response of cilostazol in patients with intermittent claudication. Vasc Med 2010;15(3):181–8.
81. Packer M, Carver JR, Rodeheffer RJ, et al. Effect of oral milrinone on mortality in severe chronic heart failure. The PROMISE Study Research Group. N Engl J Med 1991;325(21):1468–75.

82. Hiatt WR, Money SR, Brass EP. Long-term safety of cilostazol in patients with peripheral artery disease: the CASTLE study (Cilostazol: a Study in Long-term Effects). J Vasc Surg 2008;47(2):330–6.
83. McDermott MM, Greenland P, Liu K, et al. The ankle brachial index is associated with leg function and physical activity: the Walking and Leg Circulation Study. Ann Intern Med 2002;136(12):873–83.
84. McDermott MM, Liu K, Greenland P, et al. Functional decline in peripheral arterial disease: associations with the ankle brachial index and leg symptoms. JAMA 2004;292(4):453–61.
85. McDermott MM, Guralnik JM, Tian L, et al. Baseline functional performance predicts the rate of mobility loss in persons with peripheral arterial disease. J Am Coll Cardiol 2007;50(10):974–82.
86. Bendermacher BL, Willigendael EM, Nicolai SP, et al. Supervised exercise therapy for intermittent claudication in a community-based setting is as effective as clinic-based. J Vasc Surg 2007;45(6):1192–6.
87. McDermott MM, Ades P, Guralnik JM, et al. Treadmill exercise and resistance training in patients with peripheral arterial disease with and without intermittent claudication: a randomized controlled trial. JAMA 2009;301(2):165–74.
88. Gardner AW, Poehlman ET. Exercise rehabilitation programs for the treatment of claudication pain. A meta-analysis. JAMA 1995;274(12):975–80.
89. Murphy TP, Cutlip DE, Regensteiner JG, et al. Supervised exercise versus primary stenting for claudication resulting from aortoiliac peripheral artery disease: six-month outcomes from the claudication: exercise versus endoluminal revascularization (CLEVER) study. Circulation 2012;125(1):130–9.

Diagnosis, Prevention, and Treatment of Claudication

Jordan P. Knepper, MD, Peter K. Henke, MD*

KEYWORDS

- Claudication • Atherosclerosis • Peripheral arterial disease

KEY POINTS

- Claudication is a marker for systemic atherosclerosis, which mandates proper medical therapy and risk factor reduction.
- Increasing use of invasive therapies for patients with claudication has possible risks including thrombosis and progression to critical limb ischemia, and as such, providers must advise patients appropriately.
- For patients with true lifestyle limitations, consideration of the lesion length and location needs to be considered when offering endovascular or surgical revascularization.
- In those patients undergoing revascularization for claudication, long-term follow-up of the repair is essential.

BACKGROUND

Lower extremity chronic ischemia due to atherosclerosis represents the continuum of peripheral arterial disease (PAD), encompassing intermittent claudication (ranging from mild to lifestyle-limiting), rest pain, and tissue loss. Traditionally, the indication for invasive intervention has been critical limb ischemia (CLI), including those with rest pain and/or tissue loss, as a means to prevent amputation.

The Trans-Atlantic Inter-Society Consensus (TASC II) guideline regarding PAD was published in 2007, and defines claudication as muscle discomfort in the lower extremities, which is relieved by rest within 10 minutes.[1]

The frequency of claudication ranges with age, from 0.6% in a group of 45- to 54-year-olds, to 2.5% in 55- to 64-year-olds and 8.8% in 65- to 74-year-olds.[2] Importantly, there are other reasons for claudication, as studies have noted that only 16% to 20% people with symptoms have noninvasive evidence of PAD-related claudication. PAD is defined as an at rest ankle brachial index (ABI) of less than 0.9.[3]

Section of Vascular Surgery, University of Michigan, CVC - 5463, 1500 East Medical Center Drive, SPC-5867, Ann Arbor, MI 48109, USA
* Corresponding author.
E-mail address: henke@umich.edu

Surg Clin N Am 93 (2013) 779–788
http://dx.doi.org/10.1016/j.suc.2013.04.005
0039-6109/13/$ – see front matter © 2013 Elsevier Inc. All rights reserved.

surgical.theclinics.com

Given the systemic nature of atherosclerosis understanding the natural history of PAD related to claudication is important for determining clinical decisions. Although angiographic progression may be seen in more than 60% of patients,[2] only 2% of patients presenting with claudication will eventually progress to amputation in the 5 years following diagnosis.[3] This indicates a relatively benign nature of claudication, and highlights the importance of diagnosis for medical but rarely surgical intervention. In contrast, those with CLI have an amputation rate approaching 12% at just 3 months,[4] and endoluminal or open surgical procedures are commonly indicated.

Symptoms may be related to degree and length of stenosis, or in the case of plaque rupture and thrombosis, they may relate to segmental arterial occlusion. The specific pathophysiology of PAD progression is associated with genetics, modifiable (eg, smoking) and nonmodifiable (eg, gender) risk factors, and age. As with so many diseases, risk factor reduction to stabilize mild disease (ie, claudication) is paramount.

DIAGNOSIS OF CLAUDICATION

An accurate history is essential as the initial phase of evaluation, as multiple etiologies exist for limb pain and fatigue (**Table 1**). Claudication presents as pain with ambulation/exertion in the calf, thigh, and/or buttock, depending on the location and extent of the arterial lesions.[2] The symptoms are reproducible with a given level of activity or distance, and they do not depend on position. The clinical presentation is not often classic, and claudication may coexist with other etiologies of limb pain. However, pain radiating down the back of the whole leg, or pain localized to major joints, is usually not vascular in origin. Multiple causes for limb pain often coexist in those with PAD given age and sometimes debility.[5]

Once a history suggestive of claudication has been elicited, noninvasive vascular studies should be obtained. The primary means of establishing the diagnosis of claudication uses ABIs.[6] This test can be done in any office with a hand-held Doppler, and is the occlusive systolic pressure of the posterior tibial and dorsalis pedis artery divided by the highest systolic arm pressure. An ABI of less than 0.9 at rest indicates a vascular origin to the patient's limb symptoms.[7] Although ABIs are sensitive for most patients with a diagnosis of PAD, patients with end-stage renal disease or longstanding diabetes may have medial calcification and noncompressible vessels, typically causing the ABI to be greater than 1.5. In these patients with invalid ABIs, toe brachial indices (TBIs) may be useful, as digital vessels are often preserved. If these values are abnormal, one can consider PAD as a source of claudication in these patients.

Table 1 Differential diagnosis of lower limb pain		
Class	**Pathophysiology**	**Distinguishing Features**
Musculoskeletal	Osteoarthritis	Focal to joints, may be positional
	Myopathies	May have autoimmune markers and occur at rest
Neuropathic	Sensory neuropathy	Often position, burning in quality and not related to activity
	Lumbar radiculopathy	May be positional and related to a history of back pain
Venous	Venous claudication	Swelling, often described as bursting
Other	Includes chronic compartment syndrome	More often in athletes often young

In patients with mild claudication, resting ABI maybe normal. However, if these patients are exercised, and repeat measurements are taken, decreased indices may be found and may help further elicit proximal mild PAD. A typical scenario is well compensated for aortoiliac disease. In general, proximal arterial occlusions are more disabling for patients than distal occlusions, despite often similar ABI values.

Although physical examination may be able to discern at which level normal pulsations stop, the level can be better determined in an objective manner using segmental pressures and waveforms to localize the level of disease, whether it be at iliac, femoral-popliteal or distal artery levels, or multiple segments.[2]

Once the diagnosis of PAD is established, further imaging is warranted if the patient has an indication for a revascularization procedure. Duplex ultrasound provides imaging in B-mode, which can also provide direct imaging of stenosis or occlusions, and often supplements segmental pressures.[2] However, operative decisions are not commonly made solely on duplex imaging.

The use of computerized tomography angiography (CT-A) has become common for the diagnostic imaging of PAD. However, CT-A is limited for resolution of below the knee arteries in patients with highly calcified distal vessels.[8] Magnetic resonance imaging has been evaluated for PAD, and has good sensitivity and specificity.[9] However, gadolinium can harm renal function, and there is often wide variance among centers' expertise in reformatting images.[10]

Contrast angiography remains the gold standard in patients with PAD, as it provides a means of direct vascular imaging without interference seen in other techniques, as well as a platform for possible intervention. Iodinated contrast agents have the potential for nephrotoxicity, but alternative contrast agents have also been used successfully intra-arterially, namely CO_2.[2]

MEDICAL MANAGEMENT

Patients with a diagnosis of claudication have a significant atherosclerotic burden. In these patients, medical management is appropriate, regardless of underlying condition or future plans for intervention (**Table 2**). In fact, it is the authors' opinion that the most important reason for diagnosing claudication related to PAD is to ensure that these patients are on the appropriate cardioprotective medications.

The basic clinical approach includes smoking cessation, an ambulation program, antiplatelet therapy, and cholesterol reduction, as will be discussed in detail. Hypertension is ubiquitous and will not be specifically discussed in relation to PAD claudication, but suffice it say that uncontrolled hypertension does increase the risk of progression.[11] Similarly, diabetics should have intensive blood glucose control to decrease macrovascular cardiovascular complications.

Table 2
Medications for PAD patients

Medication	Mechanism of Action	Reason for Use
Aspirin	Platelet inhibition	Reduction of atherothrombotic events
Clopidogrel	Platelet Inhibition	Slightly better than aspirin at risk reduction
Statins	Cholesterol reduction/ anti-inflammatory	Improved outcome, stabilize disease progression
Naftidrofuryl	Vasoactive (serotonin inhibitor)	Improved walking distance
Cilostazol	Vasoactive (phosphodiesterase type 3 inhibitor)	Improved walking distance

For the establishment of baseline status, many authors argue that the patient should undergo basic laboratory tests, including blood count, basic metabolic fasting panels, hemoglobin A-1C, and renal function analysis.[12] Lipid and liver function panels are also important in some cases, especially when considering statin therapy.[2]

Antiplatelet therapy is a mainstay for patients with PAD. Aspirin, 50 to 100 mg/d, is recommended for patients for primary and secondary prevention of atherothrombosis.[13,14] Other antiplatelet agents have been studied. For example, the CAPRIE study suggested a small benefit of clopidogrel over aspirin, with an 8.7% relative risk reduction of strokes, myocardial infarction (MI), or other causes of vascular death.[15] However, clopidigrel is costlier than aspirin. No evidence exists yet for new-generation antiplatelet agents for patients with claudication.

Smoking cessation is among the most important interventions for patients with PAD, and it can be accomplished via several means. The impact of smoking on PAD is the strongest single factor, increasing the odds of developing symptomatic PAD by 3.4, as determined from a prospective longitudinal trial.[16] The use of varenicline has the strongest evidence, with a large prospective trial showing 4-week abstinence rates of 44% as compared with 17% for placebo.[17] Nicotine patches and buproprion are also useful medications that may allow the patient to successfully wean his or her addiction to nicotine. The reader is referred to update detailed guidelines for more comprehensive review.[18]

Many studies have evaluated the relationship between structured walking programs and outcomes in PAD. This generally involves walking 30 to 40 minutes, stopping as necessary, 4 to 5 times per week. A recent review evaluated 25 randomized control trials with the primary outcomes of maximum walking distance and pain-free walking distance assessed. This meta-analysis concluded that a supervised walking program was effective in improving mean walking distance and pain-free walking distance in patients with intermittent claudication. The pooled results evaluating individual aspects of the walking regimen did not identify any of the individual exercise components as being independently associated with the improvement. These findings suggest the presence of a walking program alone was sufficient to improve symptoms,[19] and confirm the importance of a structured walking program as the foundation of medical therapy for claudication related to PAD.

Another essential medication that patients with PAD claudication should be prescribed is an HMG-CoA reductase agent, or statin. These agents have level 1 evidence to support their use in PAD patients, and they are primarily cardioprotective. In a large randomized controlled trial (RCT) trial, a 16% relative risk reduction was observed regardless of low-density lipoprotein (LDL) levels, and a 20% decrease in need for peripheral arterial reconstructions was observed with 40 mg/d of simvastatin.[20] Moreover, there is some evidence that these agents may improve walking distance also.[21]

Although claudication can be improved with the structured therapies mentioned, some patients remain symptomatic. In these patients refractory to a structured walking program, additional medical therapies may be of benefit. A recently described therapy for the medical management of PAD is naftidrofuryl. Naftidrofuryl is a vasoactive compound that blocks serotonin. It has been used intravenously and was previously studied for CLI. More recently it has been administered by an oral route as a treatment for claudication. A recent Cochrane review examined the utility of this compound and evaluated outcomes, inlcuding all-cause mortality, reduction of pain, progression of disease, and change in ABIs.[22] Another systematic review evaluated the effect of medical therapies on the treatment of intermittent claudication and ranked naftidrofuryl as the best among medication-based therapies, with the greatest increase in mean walking distance and pain-free walking distance.[23] A contributing clinical trial showed a 92% improvement in pain-free walking distance in the treatment group versus a 17% increase in the placebo group.[24] However, this therapy is not yet widely available.

Cilostazol is commonly used for claudication and is effective. Cilostazol is a phosphodiesterase type 3 inhibitor, and its effectiveness is likely based on its action as a vasodilator, as well as having mild antiplatelet effects.[25] An RCT of cilostazol showed doubling of absolute walking distance,[26] but it did not show a significant increase in either exercise or resting ABIs. In the systematic review presented previously, the authors found cilostazol to be the second-most effective pharmacologic means of management of intermittent claudication symptoms.[23] These findings support the TASC II recommendations for the use of cilostazol 100 mg twice daily as first-line treatment for improvement of symptoms in patients with claudication. However, patients with severe cardiac diastolic dysfunction and congestive heart failure should not receive this therapy.[3]

Medical management can successfully treat the symptoms of most patients with claudication and remains safe due to the low progression to limb threat. This remains the preferred treatment strategy in most claudication patients.

ENDOVASCULAR MANAGEMENT

In patients with lifestyle-limiting claudication refractory to medical therapy, endovascular therapy is often the first-line therapy, given the presumed lower morbidity as compared with open surgery. A meta-analysis of the efficacy of endovascular therapy compared with noninvasive therapies, such as medical therapy and supervised exercise, in patients with intermittent claudication has been performed.[27] The data were combined and calculated using ABIs and walking distance in a pooled sample of nearly 900 patients. Although there was much heterogeneity in the population studied, quantitative data suggest that endovascular therapy improved outcomes as measured by ABIs in walking distance alone; however, amputation rates and other outcomes related to long-term complications of intervention were not measured. A Cochrane review comparing exercise and medical management versus percutaneous transluminal angioplasty produced 11 articles that were found suitable for analysis: those who received endovascular intervention, those received supervised exercise therapy, and those who received both therapies. The review concluded that patients with claudication who underwent a supervised exercise program had equivalent functional outcomes to those patients who received percutaneous interventions; however, those who received both had slightly higher quality-of-life scores.[19]

Comparisons of endovascular techniques have been done. Several studies have evaluated balloon angioplasty alone in lower extremity segments compared with angioplasty with stenting. A review found 24 studies about this topic available for meta-analysis and included 934 patients, 452 of whom underwent balloon angioplasty and 482 of whom underwent angioplasty plus stenting. The study evaluated the 1 year outcomes in these patients and concluded that at 1 year there was no significant increase in ABIs with the addition of stenting. Patency rates were not statistically different, leading to the conclusion that there was no difference between the 2 therapies at 1 year.[28] Another study examined the difference between self-expanding stents after an RCT showed that there was less restenosis with use of self-expanding stents compared with balloon angioplasty alone. Most of these patients underwent intervention for claudication, and there was a primary patency rate of 52%. The investigators noted that stents failed more often in patients with TASC D lesions and when poor run-off existed.[29]

A Cochrane analysis was further undertaken to examine the role of stenting versus angioplasty alone in claudication. This pooled analysis of clinical trials found that in the femoropopliteal segment disease there was no statistical difference between the groups in patency rates or secondary outcomes at 1 year.[30]

Covered stent grafts in femoropopliteal occlusive disease are sometimes used in lieu of open surgical bypass. An RCT of covered stent grafting of femoropopliteal segment for occlusive disease as compared with open prosthetic bypass showed similar patency and complications with 2-year follow-up.[31] These authors did find that patients with poor outflow and TASC D lesions were more likely to have treatment failure. Although initial technical success was documented in this study, caution should be taken. A recent series of patients treated with covered stent grafts showed many of these patients were treated for claudication, and graft thrombosis occurred at a significant rate and converted these claudicants, with relatively benign disease, to limb threatening ischemia. These thromboses resulted in multiple reinterventions.[32]

The treatment of PAD by endoluminal techniques has markedly increased over the last decade. From this section, one can see that stenting versus angioplasty alone is likely a matter of preference of the operator; however, care must be taken in intervening in patients with claudication, as the risk of thrombosis and conversion to higher-grade limb ischemia remains a real possibility. Lastly, many new technologies have come and gone (eg, cryoplasty and laser atherectomy), as there has been little evidence that they are more effective than standard angioplasty and stenting, and they are oftentimes much more costly.

SURGICAL MANAGEMENT

Some large clinical trials have shown that endovascular interventions have a similar outcome to open surgery.[33] Although this outcome might be similar, some studies also indicate more procedures for claudication are being performed, and the outcomes have remained consistent.[34] Most surgical procedures for inflow, or aortoiliac disease, involve prosthetic grafts with good durability and outcomes as compared with endolumial procedures.[35] In those suitable for aortofemoral bypassing, end-to-side as compared with end-to-end anastomoses have similar long-term outcomes and are the authors' preference.

The principles of infrainguinal bypass will be briefly reviewed. First, the threshold should be high when offering a surgical bypass for claudication, as that is a nonlimb-threatening problem. A failed bypass can convert a claudicant to a patient with CLI. Second, the autologous vein is the first, second, and third choice for conduit. Prosthetic grafts are inferior over time,[36] and if they occlude, this risk of limb threat is higher as compared with vein graft failure.[37] Saphenous vein of greater than 3 mm is ideal and directly impacts long-term patency.[38] Third, most bypasses for claudicants are femoral to popliteal, although occasionally a femoral-to-tibial bypass is required for isolated popliteal occlusions. Fourth, after the bypass has been completed, it is the authors' practice to perform intraoperative duplex to assess the vein graft and the anastomotic sites. This is also recommended lifelong to follow the graft for later stenoses. Fifth, the configuration of the graft, reversed, in situ, or translocated nonreversed, is the surgeon's choice; all are acceptable and yield similar results in most series. Lastly, it is important that the patient be on antiplatelet therapy and statin therapy, as both increase graft patency in the long term.[39,40]

International therapies are changing for PAD. Administrative data were used to compare endovascular intervention to open surgical bypass in over 500,000 patients from 1999 to 2007 who received percutaneous intervention, lower extremity bypass,

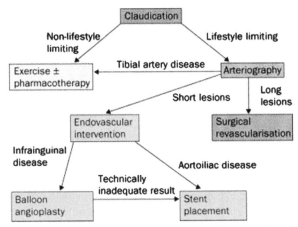

Fig. 1. Treatment algorithm for claudication. (*From* Ouriel K. Peripheral arterial disease. Lancet 2001;358:1257–64.)

or aortobifemoral bypass.[41] The sample included a large number of patients with claudication. Notably, percutaneous intervention had increased threefold over the study period. From a cost standpoint, it was determined that angioplasty had a significantly higher cost than bypass grafting for claudication. Additionally, in-hospital mortality was similar for the percutaneous and bypass groups. However, the in-hospital amputation rate was significantly higher for the endovascular group, compared with either the bypass group or the aortic bypass group.

As international management is preformed increasingly for claudication, it is important to also understand patient-centered outcomes. A clinical trial assessing quality of life found slightly improved quality of life in bypass patients, but those with occluded graft and resultant amputation found this effect diminished.[42]

NOVEL TREATMENTS

Trials that involve angiogenesis (gene therapies and cell therapies) for use in PAD have primarily focused on CLI patients. A meta-analysis of these RCTs showed the pooled response rate for placebo was not significantly different for claudicants. However, they did find significant differences in those with CLI.[43] Finally, ixmyelocel-T phase 2 clinical trial reports show clinical promise for this treatment in CLI, but phase 3 trials and further data regarding claudication have yet to be published.[44]

SUMMARY

Although the mainstay of treatment for claudication remains medical, there appears to be some justification for intervention in selected patients. (**Fig. 1**)[2] presents a logical algorithm.

Claudication is a marker for systemic atherosclerosis, which mandates proper medical therapy and risk factor reduction. Increasing use of invasive therapies for patients with claudication has possible risks including thrombosis and progression to CLI, and as such, providers must advise patients appropriately. For patients with true lifestyle limitations, the lesion length and location needs to be considered when offering endovascular or surgical revascularization for patients. In those patients undergoing revascularization for claudication, long-term follow-up of the repair is essential.

REFERENCES

1. Norgren L, Hiatt WR, Dormandy JA, et al. Inter-society consensus for the management of peripheral arterial disease (tasc ii). Eur J Vasc Endovasc Surg 2007;33(Suppl 1):S1–75.
2. Ouriel K. Peripheral arterial disease. Lancet 2001;358:1257–64.
3. Norgren L, Hiatt WR, Dormandy JA, et al. Inter-society consensus for the management of peripheral arterial disease (tasc ii). J Vasc Surg 2007;45(Suppl S): S5–67.
4. Long-term mortality and its predictors in patients with critical leg ischaemia. The I.C.A.I. Group (Gruppo Di Studio Dell'ischemia Cronica Critica Degli Arti Inferiori). The Study Group of Criticial Chronic Ischemia of the Lower Exremities. Eur J Vasc Endovasc Surg 1997;14:91–5.
5. McDermott MM, Fried L, Simonsick E, et al. Asymptomatic peripheral arterial disease is independently associated with impaired lower extremity functioning: the women's health and aging study. Circulation 2000;101:1007–12.
6. Rutherford RB, Baker JD, Ernst C, et al. Recommended standards for reports dealing with lower extremity ischemia: revised version. J Vasc Surg 1997;26:517–38.
7. Ouriel K, Zarins CK. Doppler ankle pressure: an evaluation of three methods of expression. Arch Surg 1982;117:1297–300.
8. Napoli A, Anzidei M, Zaccagna F, et al. Peripheral arterial occlusive disease: diagnostic performance and effect on therapeutic management of 64-section ct angiography. Radiology 2011;261:976–86.
9. Huber A, Heuck A, Baur A, et al. Dynamic contrast-enhanced mr angiography from the distal aorta to the ankle joint with a step-by-step technique. AJR Am J Roentgenol 2000;175:1291–8.
10. Au K, Singh MK, Bodukam V, et al. Atherosclerosis in systemic sclerosis: a systematic review and meta-analysis. Arthritis Rheum 2011;63:2078–90.
11. Ness J, Aronow WS, Ahn C. Prevalence of coronary artery disease, ischemic stroke, and symptomatic peripheral arterial disease and of associated risk factors in older men and women with and without diabetes mellitus. Prev Cardiol 2000;3:160–2.
12. Pararajasingam R, Nasim A, Sutton C, et al. The role of screening blood tests in patients with arterial disease attending vascular outpatients. Eur J Vasc Endovasc Surg 1998;16:513–6.
13. Patrono C, Andreotti F, Arnesen H, et al. Antiplatelet agents for the treatment and prevention of atherothrombosis. Eur Heart J 2011;32:2922–32.
14. Collaborative overview of randomised trials of antiplatelet therapy–I: prevention of death, myocardial infarction, and stroke by prolonged antiplatelet therapy in various categories of patients. Antiplatelet trialists' collaboration. BMJ 1994; 308:81–106.
15. A randomised, blinded, trial of clopidogrel versus aspirin in patients at risk of ischaemic events (CAPRIE). CAPRIE Steering Committee. Lancet 1996;348: 1329–39.
16. Aboyans V, Criqui MH, Denenberg JO, et al. Risk factors for progression of peripheral arterial disease in large and small vessels. Circulation 2006;113:2623–9.
17. Gonzales D, Rennard SI, Nides M, et al. Varenicline, an alpha4beta2 nicotinic acetylcholine receptor partial agonist, vs sustained-release bupropion and placebo for smoking cessation: a randomized controlled trial. JAMA 2006;296:47–55.
18. Rooke TW, Hirsch AT, Misra S, et al. 2011 ACCF/AHA focused update of the guideline for the management of patients with peripheral artery disease (updating the 2005 guideline): a report of the American College of Cardiology

Foundation/American Heart Association task force on practice guidelines. J Am Coll Cardiol 2011;58:2020–45.

19. Frans FA, Bipat S, Reekers JA, et al. Systematic review of exercise training or percutaneous transluminal angioplasty for intermittent claudication. Br J Surg 2012;99:16–28.
20. MRC/BHF heart protection study of cholesterol lowering with simvastatin in 20,536 high-risk individuals: a randomised placebo-controlled trial. Lancet 2002;360:7–22.
21. Aung PP, Maxwell HG, Jepson RG, et al. Lipid-lowering for peripheral arterial disease of the lower limb. Cochrane Database Syst Rev 2007;(4):CD000123.
22. Smith FB, Bradbury A, Fowkes G. Intravenous naftidrofuryl for critical limb ischaemia. Cochrane Database Syst Rev 2012;(7):CD002070.
23. Stevens JW, Simpson E, Harnan S, et al. Systematic review of the efficacy of cilostazol, naftidrofuryl oxalate and pentoxifylline for the treatment of intermittent claudication. Br J Surg 2012;99:1630–8.
24. Kieffer E, Bahnini A, Mouren X, et al. A new study demonstrates the efficacy of naftidrofuryl in the treatment of intermittent claudication. Findings of the naftidrofuryl clinical ischemia study (ncis). Int Angiol 2001;20:58–65.
25. Vodnala D, Rajagopalan S, Brook RD. Medical management of the patient with intermittent claudication. Cardiol Clin 2011;29:363–79.
26. Money SR, Herd JA, Isaacsohn JL, et al. Effect of cilostazol on walking distances in patients with intermittent claudication caused by peripheral vascular disease. J Vasc Surg 1998;27:267–74 [discussion: 274–5].
27. Ahimastos AA, Pappas EP, Buttner PG, et al. A meta-analysis of the outcome of endovascular and noninvasive therapies in the treatment of intermittent claudication. J Vasc Surg 2011;54:1511–21.
28. Mwipatayi BP, Hockings A, Hofmann M, et al. Balloon angioplasty compared with stenting for treatment of femoropopliteal occlusive disease: a meta-analysis. J Vasc Surg 2008;47:461–9.
29. Ihnat DM, Duong ST, Taylor ZC, et al. Contemporary outcomes after superficial femoral artery angioplasty and stenting: the influence of tasc classification and runoff score. J Vasc Surg 2008;47:967–74.
30. Bachoo P, Thorpe PA, Maxwell H, et al. Endovascular stents for intermittent claudication. Cochrane Database Syst Rev 2010;(1):CD003228.
31. Kedora J, Hohmann S, Garrett W, et al. Randomized comparison of percutaneous viabahn stent grafts vs prosthetic femoral-popliteal bypass in the treatment of superficial femoral arterial occlusive disease. J Vasc Surg 2007;45:10–6 [discussion: 16].
32. Johnston PC, Vartanian SM, Runge SJ, et al. Risk factors for clinical failure after stent graft treatment for femoropopliteal occlusive disease. J Vasc Surg 2012;56:998–1006, 1007.e1001 [discussion: 1006–7].
33. Adam DJ, Beard JD, Cleveland T, et al. Bypass versus angioplasty in severe ischaemia of the leg (basil): multicentre, randomised controlled trial. Lancet 2005;366:1925–34.
34. Simons JP, Schanzer A, Nolan BW, et al. Outcomes and practice patterns in patients undergoing lower extremity bypass. J Vasc Surg 2012;55:1629–36.
35. Burke CR, Henke PK, Hernandez R, et al. A contemporary comparison of aortofemoral bypass and aortoiliac stenting in the treatment of aortoiliac occlusive disease. Ann Vasc Surg 2010;24:4–13.
36. Pereira CE, Albers M, Romiti M, et al. Meta-analysis of femoropopliteal bypass grafts for lower extremity arterial insufficiency. J Vasc Surg 2006;44:510–7.

37. Jackson MR, Belott TP, Dickason T, et al. The consequences of a failed femoro-popliteal bypass grafting: comparison of saphenous vein and PTFE grafts. J Vasc Surg 2000;32:498–504, 504–5.

38. Nguyen LL, Hevelone N, Rogers SO, et al. Disparity in outcomes of surgical revascularization for limb salvage: race and gender are synergistic determinants of vein graft failure and limb loss. Circulation 2009;119:123–30.

39. Henke PK, Blackburn S, Proctor MC, et al. Patients undergoing infrainguinal bypass to treat atherosclerotic vascular disease are underprescribed cardioprotective medications: effect on graft patency, limb salvage, and mortality. J Vasc Surg 2004;39:357–65.

40. Tangelder MJ, Lawson JA, Algra A, et al. Systematic review of randomized controlled trials of aspirin and oral anticoagulants in the prevention of graft occlusion and ischemic events after infrainguinal bypass surgery. J Vasc Surg 1999;30:701–9.

41. Sachs T, Pomposelli F, Hamdan A, et al. Trends in the national outcomes and costs for claudication and limb threatening ischemia: angioplasty vs bypass graft. J Vasc Surg 2011;54:1021–1031.e1021.

42. Tangelder MJ, McDonnel J, Van Busschbach JJ, et al. Quality of life after infrainguinal bypass grafting surgery. Dutch Bypass Oral Anticoagulants or Aspirin (BOA) study group. J Vasc Surg 1999;29:913–9.

43. De Haro J, Acin F, Lopez-Quintana A, et al. Meta-analysis of randomized, controlled clinical trials in angiogenesis: gene and cell therapy in peripheral arterial disease. Heart Vessels 2009;24:321–8.

44. Powell RJ, Marston WA, Berceli SA, et al. Cellular therapy with ixmyelocel-t to treat critical limb ischemia: the randomized, double-blind, placebo-controlled restore-cli trial. Mol Ther 2012;20:1280–6.

Critical Limb Ischemia

Matthew J. Blecha, MD

KEYWORDS

- Acute limb ischemia • Critical limb ischemia • Lower extremity revascularization
- Arterial occlusive disease • Lower extremity angioplasty • PAD

KEY POINTS

- Acute limb ischemia should be suspected in patients with new-onset limb pain and a cool, pulseless extremity on physical examination.
- Acute limb ischemia is a surgical emergency, necessitating emergent heparinization and revascularization to prevent limb loss.
- Critical limb ischemia is defined clinically by ischemic rest pain or tissue loss in conjunction with either ankle-brachial index less than 0.4 or toe pressure less than 30 mm Hg.
- Management of critical limb ischemia includes optimization of medical therapy, arterial imaging, and revascularization, with the goal of achieving in-line flow to the affected limb when tissue loss is present.
- As a guiding principle, short-segment arterial stenosis or occlusions are treated with angioplasty and long-segment arterial occlusions are treated with surgical bypass in patients with critical limb ischemia.

INTRODUCTION

Critical limb ischemia refers to the clinical state of advanced arterial occlusive disease, placing an extremity at risk for gangrene and limb loss. This article reviews the etiologies, diagnosis, and treatment of critical limb ischemia. Critical limb ischemia has 2 broad clinical subcategories that are vital to differentiate:

1. Acute limb ischemia
2. Chronic arterial occlusive disease

Acute limb ischemia refers to the acute arterial thrombosis of an extremity, resulting in an abrupt cessation of flow to the extremity. Acute limb ischemia is a surgical emergency mandating urgent extremity revascularization to avoid the need for amputation. The potential sources of acute limb ischemia are arterial embolus, in situ arterial

Disclosures: No financial or conflict disclosures.
Section of Vascular Surgery and Endovascular Therapy, The University of Chicago Medical Center, 5841 South Maryland Avenue, MC 5028, Suite J555, Chicago, IL 60637, USA
E-mail address: matthew.blecha@yahoo.com

thrombosis in the setting of advanced chronic arterial occlusive disease, and major arterial trauma.

Chronic arterial occlusive disease with critical limb ischemia is the condition of progressive atherosclerosis, creating a state of extremity hypoperfusion with insufficient tissue oxygenation. Chronic arterial occlusive disease warrants prompt treatment but is not an emergent state, allowing for thorough imaging, patient risk stratification, and planning of revascularization. Pathologies other than atherosclerosis can result in chronic arterial occlusive disease and are briefly reviewed.

ACUTE LIMB ISCHEMIA
Treatment Steps for Acute Limb Ischemia

1. Confirm diagnosis with physical examination and arterial imaging
2. Initiate anticoagulation therapy
3. Perform revascularization
4. Monitor post procedure for compartment syndrome and rhabdomyolysis
5. Evaluate the patient for potential embolic sources and continue therapeutic anticoagulation

Diagnosis of Acute Limb Ischemia

The clinical hallmark of acute limb ischemia is the acute onset of extremity pain in conjunction with absent pulses in the affected extremity. The severity of pain symptoms can vary dramatically depending on the etiology of the acute arterial occlusion. Patients who experience acute limb ischemia secondary to an arterial embolism versus patients who experience in situ arterial thrombosis in the setting of chronic arterial occlusive disease can have dramatically different clinical presentations.

Occlusive arterial embolism to an otherwise normal arterial bed will nearly universally result in the abrupt onset of severe pain in the affected extremity. These patients lack collateral vessels around the flush occlusion, making the affected limb completely devoid of any arterial flow. The physical examination findings in this state are the presence of bounding "water hammer" pulses proximal to the occlusion and absent pulses distal to the occlusion. The distal extremity will be cool to touch, and after 3 to 4 hours may have neurologic abnormalities (sensory loss followed by motor loss). The limb is pale with poor capillary refill. The contralateral limb in this situation will typically have normal pulses, unless the patient has underlying peripheral artery occlusive disease (PAD). Revascularization within 6 hours is critical to avoid limb loss.

In situ arterial thrombosis secondary to worsening chronic occlusive disease may present in a more indolent fashion. These patients experience acute primary vessel thrombosis due to either plaque rupture and secondary to arterial thrombosis, or due to a critically low-velocity flow state resulting in intra-arterial thrombosis. Although the primary symptom is limb pain, the acuity may be more vague than in patients with embolism. Physical examination findings will still be a cool, pulseless foot, often with dependent rubor instead of pallor. The contralateral pulse and Doppler examination are typically abnormal, as atherosclerosis affects both limbs. The severity of pain symptoms is inversely proportional to the quality of collateral arterial flow around the occlusion.

Emergent arterial imaging is indicated for any patient presenting with acute-onset limb pain and absent pulses. Imaging options include duplex ultrasound, computed tomography angiography (CTA), magnetic resonance angiography (MRA), and invasive diagnostic angiogram.

Duplex ultrasound is rapid, can be performed at the bedside, and has near 100% sensitivity for diagnosing complete arterial occlusion. Ankle-brachial index (ABI) will be near zero for patients with acute limb ischemia. Evaluating aorto-iliac inflow and tibial arterial outflow vessels may be suboptimal with duplex alone.

CTA has the benefit of rapid availability and high-quality imaging, which allows for precise planning of revascularization. CTA provides imaging of the entire arterial tree from the aortic inflow to the digital level. CTA typically requires 150 mL of iodinated contrast and therefore has to be used with caution in patients with baseline renal insufficiency (glomerular filtration rate <40). For patients with renal insufficiency, aggressive hydration before and after examination with sodium bicarbonate is recommended for CTA or invasive angiography.[1]

MRA has a limited role in acute limb ischemia, as the examination can be lengthy (45–60 minutes), is less often available outside regular work hours, and generally has poorer arterial imaging than 64 (or greater) slice CTA.

Invasive angiography has the advantage of allowing for simultaneous percutaneous revascularization with both mechanical thrombectomy and thrombolytic therapy.

After revascularization for embolism, patients should undergo echocardiography and aortic imaging after the limb is revascularized to investigate the proximal source of embolus.

Treatment of Acute Limb Ischemia

Before engaging in any revascularization for acute limb ischemia, the treating surgeon should perform a global patient evaluation with confirmation of ambulatory status, relative quality of life, and surgical risk. A 30-day amputation rate of 15%[2,3] is discussed with the patient and family.

Once quality arterial imaging has been obtained, urgent revascularization is undertaken with the goal of achieving uninterrupted in-line flow from the aorta to the affected extremity. The goal of lower extremity revascularization is to have at least one tibial artery patent with angiographic confirmation of outflow to the foot. In the upper extremity, outflow to the hand via the radial or ulnar artery (ideally both) with filling of the palmar arch is the treatment goal.

If no contraindication to anticoagulation exists, the patient should be given an intravenous (IV) heparin bolus of 100 U/kg followed by IV heparin infusion of 15 U/kg with a goal partial thromboplastin time (PTT) of 60 to 80. If a continuous thrombolytic therapy drip is initiated, then heparin dose should be reduced to prevent bleeding complications. This dosing, as well as contraindications to anticoagulation and thrombolytic therapy are discussed later in this article.

There are 2 primary treatment options for acute limb ischemia:

1. Percutaneous thrombolytic therapy with adjunctive mechanical thrombectomy
2. Surgical thrombectomy with as-needed adjunctive bypass or endarterectomy

Option 1 for Acute Limb Ischemia: Endovascular Percutaneous Thrombectomy and Thrombolysis

Arterial access should be achieved proximal to the arterial occlusion. Most commonly, contralateral retrograde common femoral arterial access is achieved followed by angiogram of the aorto-iliac system. The primary predictor of success for percutaneous revascularization of acute limb ischemia is successful guidewire crossing through the thrombus burden. If the thrombus burden extends proximally to the aortic bifurcation, then brachial artery access may be necessary to achieve guidewire and catheter passage into the thrombus.

This is followed by catheter and sheath selection of the affected limb's iliac arterial system. Through this sheath, dedicated lower extremity angiography can then be performed. A hydrophilic glidewire with supporting 4-Fr supporting catheter can then be used to cross into the arterial thrombus. The guidewire should be passed as distally as possible, then the angiojet catheter (Medrad/Possis, Minneapolis, MN, USA) can be passed over the guidewire, activated through the thrombus burden, and the thrombus treated with both tissue plasminogen activator (TPA) bolus of 5 mg and mechanical pulse spray/suctioning with the catheter (**Fig. 1**).[4] **Fig. 2** illustrates an acute iliac artery embolus treated with percutaneous mechanical thrombectomy.

For mechanical thrombectomy of the iliac, common femoral, superficial femoral, and popliteal arteries, 0.035-inch glidewires and 6-Fr thrombectomy catheters can be used. When treating tibial thrombus, smaller caliber 0.018-inch guidewires with 3-Fr angiojet thrombectomy catheter are used. The mechanical thrombectomy catheters will typically create a flow channel of adequate diameter to reperfuse the limb. Residual thrombus can then be treated as needed with continuous TPA drip of 0.05 to 0.1 U/kg per hour. Thrombolytic drip is performed through "side-hole" infusion catheters invested into the region of thrombus (**Fig. 3**). Moderate-dose IV heparin drip is also administered while patients are receiving TPA infusion. Fibrinogen level, PTT, international normalized ratio, and hemoglobin should be checked every 6 hours while the TPA drip is ongoing. TPA should be held for fibrinogen level below 100 mg/dL and heparinized saline infused through the catheter until the next angiogram should this occur. PTT goal while the TPA drip is ongoing is 30 to 50 seconds. Higher levels are associated with increased bleeding risk.

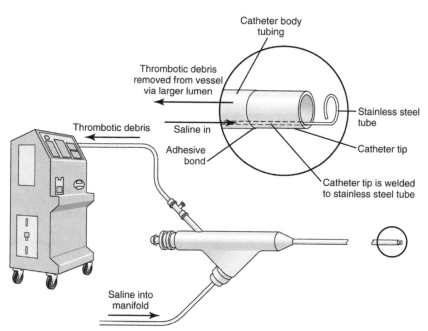

Fig. 1. Angiojet catheter for percutaneous mechanical thrombectomy. (*From* Kasirajan K. Acute ischemia: treatment. In: Cronenwett JL, Johnston KW, editors. Rutherford's Vascular Surgery. 7th Edition. Philadelphia: Elsevier; 2010; with permission.)

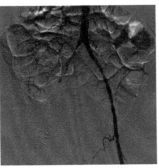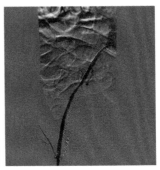

Fig. 2. Acute arterial embolus to the right distal common iliac artery seen on the image on the left. After a 5-mg TPA bolus and percutaneous mechanical thrombectomy with angiojet device, successful resolution of the occlusion is seen on the right. The underlying external iliac stenosis would be subsequently treated with angioplasty.

Once follow-up angiography confirms successful lysis of the thrombus burden, any underlying arterial occlusive disease can be identified and treated percutaneously with angioplasty, or if necessary surgically with bypass or endarterectomy.

Unlike anticoagulants and antiplatelet medications (heparins, warfarin, thrombin inhibitors, factor Xa inhibitors, aspirin, clopidogrel), which serve to prevent thrombus formation, TPA directly induces lysis of a fibrin-based clot, creating significant bleeding risks for anyone with recent endothelial injury. Contraindications to thrombolytic therapy include the following[5–7]:

- Cerebrovascular accident (CVA) within 3 months
- Intracranial tumor or other gross pathology
- Intrathoracic, abdominal, pelvic, or thoracic surgery within 3 weeks

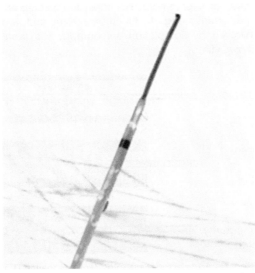

Fig. 3. Thrombolytic infusion "sidehole" catheter. (*Courtesy of* Angiodynamics, Inc, Latham, NY.)

- Major trauma within 3 weeks
- Severe (systolic blood pressure >180 mm Hg) hypertension that cannot be controlled with medication
- Cirrhosis with coagulation abnormality

Patients with acute limb ischemia who are not candidates for thrombolytic therapy should undergo emergent surgical revascularization.

Option 2 for Acute Limb Ischemia: Open Surgical Thrombectomy With As-Needed Adjunctive Revascularization or Thrombolytic Therapy

Treatment of acute arterial embolus

For patients experiencing acute embolus to an otherwise normal arterial tree, surgical embolectomy provides rapid revascularization and is an outstanding treatment option. The recommended exposure sites for acute embolus are based on anatomic location and extent of thrombus burden. Recommended dissection sites are the following:

- Lower extremity embolus with patent iliac, common femoral, and profunda femoral arteries: Below-knee popliteal artery cutdown with retrograde and antegrade Fogarty balloon thrombectomy. This dissection site allows for selective Fogarty balloon catheter thrombectomy of both the anterior tibial artery and the tibio-peroneal trunk.
- Lower extremity embolus with occluded common femoral artery: Common femoral artery cutdown with Fogarty balloon thrombectomy of the iliac, profunda femoral, and distal arteries. Secondary cutdown at the below-knee popliteal artery to expose the origin of the tibial vessels may also be necessary after the inflow thrombectomy if remote thrombectomy does not result in at least one tibial artery being widely patent to the foot.
- Upper extremity embolus: Brachial artery cutdown at the antecubital level just above the bifurcation with control of the proximal radial and ulnar arteries.

Muscular fascia should never be closed after surgical thrombectomy because of the risk for compartment syndrome. Appropriate Fogarty balloon sizes are No. 5 for iliac and subclavian arteries; No. 4 for femoral, popliteal, and brachial arteries; and No. 3 for tibial, radial, and ulnar arteries (**Fig. 4**). All embolectomy and thrombectomy procedures should be followed by completion angiography with confirmation of in-line flow to the affected distal limb.

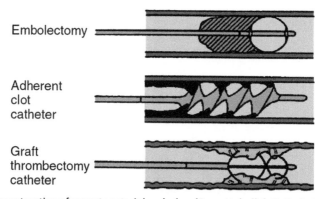

Embolectomy

Adherent
clot
catheter

Graft
thrombectomy
catheter

Fig. 4. Treatment options for acute arterial embolus. (*From* Hoballah JJ. Technique: open surgical. In: Cronenwett JL, Johnston KW, editors. Rutherford's Vascular Surgery. 7th Edition. Philadelphia: Elsevier; 2010; with permission.)

If thrombectomy is unsuccessful at the tibial artery level, intraoperative direct intra-arterial distal thrombolytic therapy can be performed. A sheath or catheter can be placed in an antegrade fashion down the proximal arterial system and 5 mg of TPA injected directly into the thrombosed tibial vessel. Ten minutes later, secondary angiogram is performed to evaluate the efficacy of the TPA.

Surgical treatment of acute limb ischemia in setting of chronic arterial occlusive disease

Surgical treatment of acute limb ischemia secondary to arterial thrombosis in the setting of coexisting chronic arterial occlusive disease is a far more challenging scenario than acute embolus. It can be difficult to discern, based on angiography or CTA, which vessels have been occluded for several months and which arteries are acutely occluded. These patients, as mentioned previously, may present with more subtle onset of pain. Essentially they are patients with chronic arterial occlusive disease (discussed later in this article) who have developed arterial thrombosis and reached a critical threshold of tissue ischemia.

Surgical treatment for these patients is "whatever it takes" to achieve in-line flow to affected extremity. The treatment armamentarium includes thrombectomy, bypass, endarterectomy, thrombolytic therapy, angioplasty, and stenting. Treatment is individualized to patient anatomy. Dissection should be performed at the level of the most distal inflow artery that has uninterrupted proximal in-line flow. From here, attempts at distal thrombectomy can be made with the understanding that distal outflow vessel exposure, further thrombectomy, and bypass may be necessary based on post-thrombectomy angiographic findings. Similarly, based on post-thrombectomy imaging, subsequent sheath insertion with angioplasty can be performed if anatomically feasible. Ensuring patency of the profunda femoral artery should always be attempted to potentially prevent limb loss in the event of revascularization failure.

Percutaneous Versus Open Surgical Revascularization in Acute Limb Ischemia

Limb salvage and mortality rates were equivalent in the 2 largest randomized trials (Surgery vs Thrombolysis for Ischemic Lower Extremity [STILE] and Thrombolysis or Peripheral Arterial Surgery [TOPAS] II trials) comparing surgical thrombectomy to percutaneous thrombolysis.[2,3] The endovascular limb in these trials, however, relied on thrombolysis alone without initial percutaneous mechanical thrombectomy. Mechanical thrombectomy achieves rapid revascularization and typically removes more than 90% of the acute thrombus burden within minutes while avoiding the morbidity of open vascular surgery.[8] The author's strong preference is to treat all patients with acute limb ischemia (without contraindication to TPA) with percutaneous mechanical thrombectomy and as-needed continued percutaneous thrombolytic drip.

Monitoring and Treatment for Post Revascularization Compartment Syndrome and Rhabdomyolysis

Compartment syndrome

Patients undergoing revascularization for acute limb ischemia are at high risk for calf compartment syndrome. Reperfusion edema and the confined space of the anterior, lateral, and deep/superficial posterior compartments can result in venous compression, worsening edema, and ultimately neurologic ischemia. Risk for compartment syndrome is highest for patients with a lack of collateral vessels (embolus or trauma in a normal arterial tree) and for patients with prolonged ischemia before revascularization.

The anterior and lateral compartments are the most common first symptomatic distribution, presenting with peroneal nerve distribution sensory deficit on the dorsum of the foot. The most reliable physical exam finding in compartment syndrome is pain with passive extension of the muscles of the involved compartment.

Any suspicion for compartment syndrome warrants either immediate 4-compartment fasciotomy (**Fig. 5**) or measuring of compartment pressures. Any post revascularization compartment pressure greater than 30 mm Hg warrants fasciotomy. To avoid permanent neurologic injury, error should always be made on the side of full 4-compartment fasciotomy when concerning symptoms or signs of compartment syndrome exist.

Rhabdomyolysis

Patients with prolonged (greater than 6 hours) acute limb ischemia are at risk for acute renal tubular necrosis due to recirculation of the necrotic muscle breakdown product myoglobin. Oliguria and discolored (pink or red) urine should raise suspicion for rhabdomyolysis. Diagnosis can be confirmed with urine myoglobin level. Urine microscopy will be negative for red blood cells but urine dip will be positive for blood. Treatment is IV hydration, diuresis with mannitol, and alkalinization of urine with IV bicarbonate.[9] Urine myoglobin levels may not be rapidly attainable in many hospitals. Similar to compartment syndrome, it is safest to empirically treat rhabdomyolysis if the diagnosis is in question.

CRITICAL LIMB ISCHEMIA SECONDARY TO CHRONIC ARTERIAL OCCLUSIVE DISEASE
Definition and Epidemiology

Chronic arterial occlusive disease can reach a critical threshold, placing patients at risk for major lower extremity amputation. Clinically, critical limb ischemia is defined by specified hemodynamic findings in conjunction with either of the following:

1. Ischemic rest pain
2. Lower extremity ulceration with hemodynamic findings incompatible with wound healing.[10]

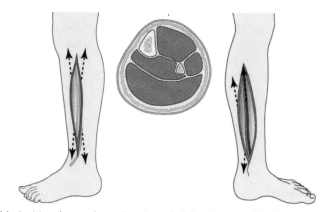

Fig. 5. Double-incision (anterolateral and medial) fasciotomy of the lower leg. A longitudinal incision lateral to the tibia and overlying the intermuscular septum is used to visualize the anterior and lateral compartments. Parallel fascial incisions are used to decompress these compartments. A medial incision immediately posterior to the tibia is used to access both posterior compartments. The soleus muscle must be detached from the tibia to decompress the deep posterior compartment. (*From* Janzing H, Broos P, Rommens P. Compartment syndrome as a complication of skin traction in children with femoral fractures. J Trauma 1996;41:156.)

Atherosclerosis is a multisystemic process placing patients with PAD at high risk for stroke, myocardial infarction, and renal failure. More than 90% of patients who are symptomatic from PAD have some degree of coronary artery disease (CAD), of which more than 60% is severe or advanced. Subsequently, patients with critical limb ischemia have a median 5-year survival of less than 5 years (**Fig. 6**).[11] The prevalence of PAD after age 70 is 14.5% in the United States.[12]

Etiology

More than 95% of chronic lower extremity arterial occlusive disease with limb threat is secondary to atherosclerotic stenosis or occlusions. Atherosclerotic risk factors with relative risk for symptomatic PAD are illustrated in (**Fig. 7**).[11] Other leading potential sources of chronic arterial occlusive disease are history of prior embolization, popliteal artery aneurysm with chronic thrombosis or emboli, popliteal artery entrapment syndrome, popliteal adventitial cystic disease, thromboangitis obliterans (Buerger disease), fibromuscular dysplasia, aortic coarctation, Takayasu arteritis, endofibrosis of the external iliac artery, persistent sciatic artery, and radiation injury.[13]

Levels of lower extremity arterial occlusive disease are anatomically categorized as follows:

- Inflow distribution: aortic, common iliac, external iliac arteries
- Femoral popliteal distribution: common femoral, superficial femoral, profunda femoral, and popliteal arteries
- Tibial distribution: anterior tibial, posterior tibial, peroneal, and pedal arteries

Most patients with critical limb ischemia have multisegment arterial occlusive disease. Tibial distribution disease confers the highest risk for major amputation. Tibial disease is most common in patients with diabetes and renal failure. Patients with diabetes and PAD have a ninefold higher amputation rate versus patients who are nondiabetic with PAD.[14]

Symptoms

Ischemic rest pain is pain in the foot at rest, particularly when the patient is laying flat or elevates the affected limb. The loss of gravity's supplemental effect on arterial flow to the foot creates a "tipping point" at which tissues in the foot become ischemic. Pain is

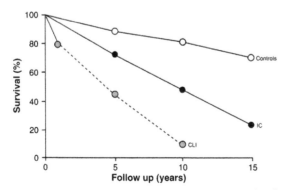

Fig. 6. Long-term survival for controls, patients with intermittent claudication, and critical limb ischemia. (*From* Norgren L, Hiatt WR, Dormandy JA, et al. TASC II Working Group. Inter-society consensus for the management of peripheral arterial disease (TASC II). J Vasc Surg 2007;45(Suppl S):S5–67; with permission.)

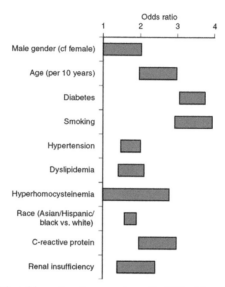

Fig. 7. Risk factors with odds ratios for symptomatic PAD. (*From* Norgren L, Hiatt WR, Dormandy JA, et al. TASC II Working Group. Inter-society consensus for the management of peripheral arterial disease (TASC II). J Vasc Surg 2007;45(Suppl S):S5–67; with permission.)

typically relieved with lowering of the affected extremity. Diabetic patients with coexisting neuropathy may not experience rest pain despite critically diminished arterial flow, because of chronic sensory loss.

Ulceration may be primarily ischemic or gangrenous. Other potential ulceration sources, such as neuropathy and venous stasis can be difficult to heal if inadequate perfusion exists.

Diagnosis

Multiple physical examination findings are associated with critical limb ischemia. Absent pedal pulses, dependent rubor of the foot, absent calf and pedal hair, cool sensation, and ulceration are all characteristic.

Noninvasive arterial Doppler examination with ankle and digital pressures have near 100% sensitivity in detecting chronic arterial occlusive disease. Arterial calcification, seen commonly in patients with diabetes or renal failure, may result in falsely elevated ankle pressure and ABI. However, Doppler waveforms and digital pressures are still reliable with vessel calcification and have excellent sensitivity for PAD. The hemodynamic criteria for critical limb ischemia are as follows:

1. ABI less than 0.4
2. Toe pressure less than 30 mm Hg

These findings are considered a threshold beneath which nonhealing of pedal ulceration can be expected. Simultaneous arterial duplex scanning can be performed in the vascular laboratory to evaluate the location and extent of infra-inguinal stenosis or occlusion. Toe pressures of less than 30 mm Hg are predictive of nonhealing of pedal ulceration in diabetic and nondiabetic patients alike (**Fig. 8**).[15]

Once the diagnosis of critical limb ischemia is made, patients with adequate risk for revascularization should undergo further arterial imaging. All revascularization must be

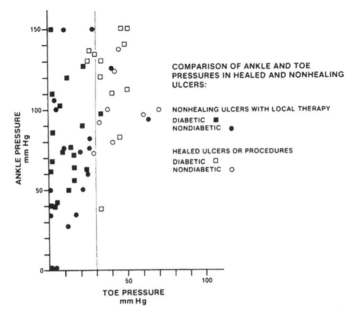

Fig. 8. Toe pressures of less than 30 mm Hg consistently predict nonhealing of pedal ulceration for diabetic and nondiabetic patients alike. (*Data from* Ramsey DE, Manke DA, Summer DS. Toe blood pressure: a valuable adjunct to ankle pressure measurement for assessing peripheral arterial disease. J Cardiovasc Surg 1983;24:43.)

based on quality arterial imaging from the abdominal aorta level to the foot of the affected extremity. Options include invasive diagnostic angiography with the potential for simultaneous endovascular intervention, CTA, MRA, and arterial duplex scanning. CTA and MRA provide adequate imaging on which inflow and femoral-popliteal artery revascularization can be planned. Tibial artery imaging with CTA and MRA is institutionally variable and can be difficult in CTA because of dense arterial calcification. The author's strong preference before performing any tibial-level revascularization is a preoperative subtraction angiogram achieved through a catheter inserted as distally as possible within the affected arterial tree (**Fig. 9**).

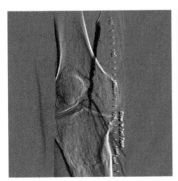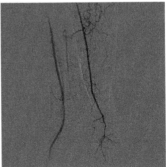

Fig. 9. Selective popliteal artery catheterization for patient with digital gangrene reveals complete occlusion of the below-knee popliteal and proximal tibial arteries (*right*) with reconstitution of the distal posterior tibial and anterior tibial arteries (*left*) as potential bypass targets. Distal SFA to posterior tibial artery bypass was ultimately performed.

Treatment Goals

Medical therapy

Initial evaluation should include global health assessment, with particular attention paid to any recent symptoms of CAD if open surgery is planned. Although essentially all patients with PAD have some element of CAD, asymptomatic patients have not been found to benefit from preoperative coronary revascularization.[16] Nevertheless, the prevalence of CAD in patients with PAD makes cardiac stress testing before major vascular surgery recommended.[17]

Risk factor modification is critical in preventing limb loss, myocardial infarction, stroke, and death in patients with symptomatic PAD. Medical management with survival benefit for patients with symptomatic PAD includes the following:

1. Antiplatelet therapy with either aspirin or clopidogrel[18,19]
2. Low-density lipoprotein cholesterol less than 100 mg/dL and HMG-COA reductase inhibitor (statin) medication use[20]
3. Tight blood sugar control for patients with diabetes, with HBA1C goal of lower than 7%[21]
4. Blood pressure control with particular benefit of angiotensin-converting enzyme inhibitor therapy[22]
5. Tobacco cessation[23–25]

Revascularization goal

Lower extremity revascularization to prevent amputation is recommended for ambulatory patients with critical limb ischemia. In the setting of tissue loss, the goal of revascularization is to achieve uninterrupted in-line flow to the area of ulceration. Anatomic findings, as well patient operative risk, are the primary determinants of what endovascular and surgical interventions are performed. General guiding principles of revascularization are as follows:

1. Endovascular therapy: stenosis at all arterial levels; short-segment occlusions in the iliac or superficial femoral artery (SFA) distribution
2. Surgical bypass: long-segment arterial occlusions
3. Surgical endarterectomy: occlusion or high-grade stenosis at the common femoral artery bifurcation level to preserve flow to both the SFA and profunda femoral artery

These are not hard rules for revascularization, and treatment must be individualized with consideration given to patient operative risk, life expectancy, adequacy of autogenous venous conduit for potential bypass, and individual operator expertise and comfort level with given procedures.

For patients with rest pain in the absence of ulceration, correction of in-flow disease alone is often adequate to remove the patient from the limb threat category without the need for more morbid distal bypass procedures. If inflow alone is corrected, patients should be carefully monitored postoperatively for persistent rest pain or ulceration development. If either of these occur, more distal revascularization should be performed to achieve in-line flow to the foot.

Endovascular therapy

The following is a simplified summary of endovascular revascularization steps:

1. Obtain arterial access and perform angiography
2. Pass a guidewire beyond areas of stenosis or occlusion
3. Confirm that the guidewire is in the true lumen of the distal arterial tree
4. Perform angioplasty, stent placement, or atherectomy over the guidewire

5. Confirm success of results with completion angiography

The angioplasty concept is depicted in **Fig. 10**.[26] The 2 primary indications for stent placement are residual stenosis after angioplasty or presence of dissection after angioplasty.

With respect to patency outcomes, stenosis fares better than occlusions and short-segment disease has improved patency to long-segment lesions.[27] Iliac percutaneous revascularization has primary and secondary patency rates of 67% and 80% at 5 years.[28]

An example of a short-segment SFA lesion well suited to angioplasty is seen in **Fig. 11**. Transluminal treatment patency rates for femoral-popliteal lesions are listed in **Table 1**.[29] Within the superficial femoral artery long segment TransAtlantic Inter-Society Consensus (TASC) class C and D occlusive disease has improved patency with primary stenting versus angioplasty alone (**Fig. 12**).[30]

Tibial-level angioplasty is also feasible, but has significantly poorer patency than iliac and SFA percutaneous interventions. Tibial angioplasty primary patency rates are less than 50% at 1 year.[31,32] **Fig. 13** illustrates a short-segment anterior tibial artery stenosis well suited to angioplasty in a patient with digital gangrene. Often patency is necessary only until pedal ulceration has healed, beyond which correction of above-knee disease may keep patients out of the limb threat category.

Access site complications represent the most frequent morbidity of endovascular procedures with bleeding, pseudoaneurysm, or arterial dissection and thrombosis inducing a complication that requires open surgical intervention after 1% to 2% of procedures.[33] Pseudoaneurysms larger than 2 cm can be treated percutaneously with thrombin injection under duplex ultrasound guidance: 1000 units of thrombin diluted in 3 mL of normal saline is injected to the pseudoaneurysm through a 21-gauge needle (**Fig. 14**).[34] Access site dissection resulting in arterial thrombosis is best treated with surgical thromboendarterectomy. Bleeding refractory to direct pressure and reversal of anticoagulation resulting in hemodynamic compromise, tense hematoma on the

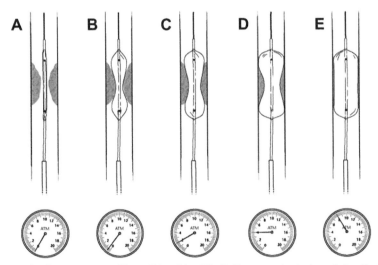

Fig. 10. Angioplasty concept. (*From* Schneider PA. Balloon angioplasty: minimally invasive autologous revascularization. In: Schneider PA, editor. Endovascular skills. New York: Marcel Dekker; 2003. p. 201–16; with permission.)

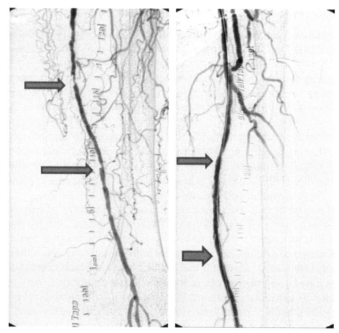

Fig. 11. Short-segment dual stenosis suitable for angioplasty in a patient with pedal ulceration. Pretreatment on the right and postangioplasty imaging on the left. *Arrows* pointing to occlusive disease segments.

skin, or transfusion requirement greater than 4 units of packed red blood cells should be treated with surgical arterial repair and hematoma drainage.

Open surgical therapy

Surgical bypass is performed for long-segment occlusive disease in acceptable risk patients with critical limb ischemia. All bypasses should be based on angiographic and hemodynamically confirmed normal inflow arteries. In the setting of tissue loss, the outflow target should provide in-line distal flow to the affected foot. The shortest-length bypass that provides in-line flow to the foot should be performed.

Aorto-iliac reconstructions are generally performed with prosthetic Dacron or polytetrafluoroethylene (PTFE) conduit. Open aorto-iliac reconstruction is preferred for

Table 1 Infrainguinal angioplasty outcomes of femoral-popliteal PTA patency			
Lesion and Treatment	**1-Y Patency, %**	**3-Y Patency, %**	**5-Y Patency, %**
Stenosis – PTA	77	61	55[a]
Stenosis – PTA + Stent	75	66	
Occlusion – PTA	65	48	42
Occlusion – PTA + Stent	73	64	

Abbreviation: PTA, percutaneous transluminal angioplasty.
[a] Versus 75% for above-knee vein bypass; versus 60% for above-knee polytetrafluoroethylene bypass.
From Norgren L, Hiatt WR, Dormandy JA, et al. TASC II Working Group. Inter-society consensus for the management of peripheral arterial disease (TASC II). J Vasc Surg 2007;45(Suppl S):S5–67; with permission.

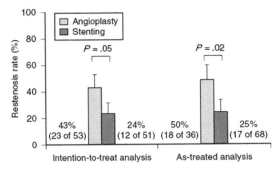

Fig. 12. Primary angioplasty versus primary combined angioplasty and stenting for TASC C and D occlusive lesions in the SFA/Popliteal artery distribution. (*Data from* Schillinger M, Sabeti S, Loewe C, et al. Balloon angioplasty versus implantation of nitinol stents in the superficial femoral artery. N Engl J Med 2006;354:1879–88.)

acceptable surgical risk patients with bilateral TASC C and D occlusive disease. An example of anatomy best treated with aorto-bifemoral artery bypass is depicted in **Fig. 15.** Primary patency for direct aorto-iliac reconstructions is excellent and approaches 90% in most series.[35–39]

Patients with high abdominal operative risk critical limb ischemia with advanced aorto-iliac occlusive disease that is not amenable to endovascular therapy can be treated with extra-anatomic bypass. Axillary bifemoral artery bypass (**Fig. 16**) can be performed with heavy sedation and local anesthesia and has 3-year patency rates

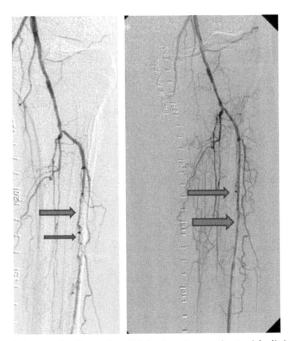

Fig. 13. Stenosis of the proximal anterior tibial artery in a patient with digital gangrene successfully treated with angioplasty. Pretreatment seen left and posttreatment on the right. *Arrows* pointing to occlusive disease segments.

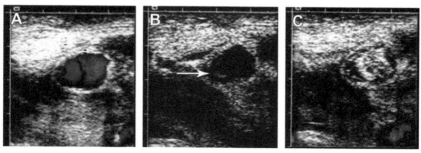

Fig. 14. Pseudoaneurysm thrombin injection. Duplex ultrasound of a femoral pseudoaneurysm. (A) Color-flow image demonstrating typical swirling flow in the pseudoaneurysm cavity. (B) This image, taken 18 seconds later with color flow turned off, shows the tip of a 22-gauge needle in the left lower portion of the pseudoaneurysm (*arrow*). After placement of the needle, color flow is turned back on and thrombin is injected. (C) Color-flow image 21 seconds later demonstrating that the pseudoaneurysm cavity is completely filled with echogenic thrombus. (*From* Kang SS, Labropoulos N, Mansour MA, et al. Percutaneous ultrasound guided thrombin injection: a new method for treating postcatheterization femoral pseudoaneurysms. J Vasc Surg 1998;27:1032–8; with permission.)

in the 70% to 80% range.[40–45] For unilateral iliac occlusion with patent contralateral iliac artery system, fem-fem bypass is an option (**Fig. 17**).

For infrainguinal long-segment arterial occlusions, surgical bypass with autogenous venous conduit provides the most durable revascularization. In addition to improved patency, autogenous vein does not have the graft infection potential of prosthetic conduit. A venous conduit of 3 mm or greater should be sought. Ipsilateral greater

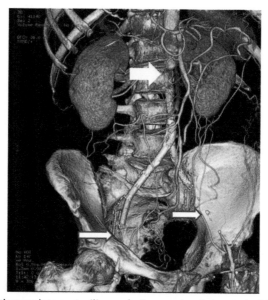

Fig. 15. Patient with complete aorto-iliac occlusion previously treated with covered stents at outside hospital, subsequently treated with aorto-bifemoral artery bypass with good success. *Arrows* pointing to occlusive disease segments.

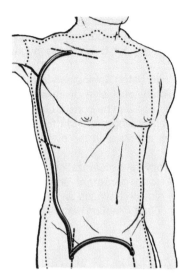

Fig. 16. Axillary bifemoral artery bypass. (*From* Schneider JR. Extra-anatomic bypass. In: Cronenwett JL, Johnston KW, editors. Rutherford's vascular surgery. 7th edition. Philadelphia: Elsevier; 2010; with permission.)

saphenous vein is the first preference. Other options include contralateral greater saphenous vein and upper extremity cephalic and basilic veins. In multiple randomized trials of infrainguinal bypass, autogenous venous conduit has demonstrated significantly better patency than PTFE and Dacron.[45–47] It is the author's practice to perform completion angiography in the operating room after all infrainguinal bypasses.

If no autogenous vein is available, then 6-mm-diameter PTFE or Dacron conduit is used for infrainguinal bypass. For bypasses to distal tibial arteries where wound breakdown is particularly common, cryopreserved cadaveric saphenous vein or composite sequential (proximal prosthetic and distal autogenous) conduit are useful to

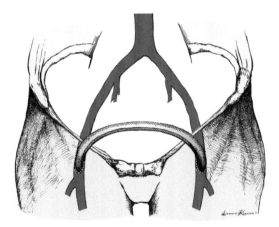

Fig. 17. Femoral-femoral artery bypass. (*From* Schneider JR. Extra-anatomic bypass. In: Cronenwett JL, Johnston KW, editors. Rutherford's vascular surgery. 7th edition. Philadelphia: Elsevier; 2010; with permission.)

reduce the incidence of exposed prosthetic bypass. Heparin-bonded PTFE conduit has illustrated modest improvement in prosthetic bypass patency relative to non–heparin-bonded historical patency for below-knee bypass in patients with critical limb ischemia.[48]

Thromboendarterectomy with patch angioplasty remains the gold standard treatment for common femoral artery occlusive disease. When concomitant bypass is needed, a long proximal graft hood can be constructed to serve effectively as a patch angioplasty. Preserving and optimizing profunda femoral artery outflow, particularly for patients with SFA disease, is critical in the event the SFA revascularization fails in the future.

Open surgical lower extremity revascularization does carry fairly high morbidity. Wound complications (20%) and persistent edema (20%) are common. Within 1 year, 10% of patients who received bypass experience graft thrombosis and 10% experience major amputation. Graft infection occurs following 1% to 2% of prosthetic conduit bypasses.[11]

Hybrid surgical therapy
Combinations of endovascular and open surgical therapies are frequently applicable to patients with critical limb ischemia with short-segment lesions in one anatomic distribution and more advanced lesions in another segment. The most frequent hybrid revascularization performed is iliac distribution angioplasty and stent placement in conjunction with infrainguinal bypass or common femoral endarterectomy. **Fig. 18** exhibits such anatomy and treatment. Similarly, outflow vessel angioplasty is an option when a short focal stenosis exists and the total bypass length can be significantly shortened by treating a distal lesion with endovascular therapy.

Surgical versus endovascular therapy in critical limb ischemia
The decreased morbidity associated with endovascular revascularization relative to open surgery has led many vascular specialists to adopt an endovascular first approach to treating critical limb ischemia. The primary advantage of surgical intervention over endovascular revascularization is durability of reconstruction, particularly for TASC C and D infrainguinal occlusions with vein graft 5-year patencies of more than 75%. Although 2-year primary patency for endovascular treatment of TASC D

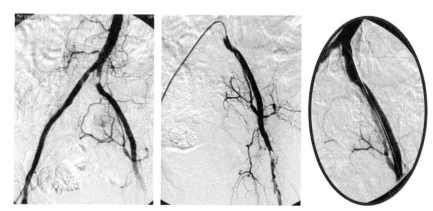

Fig. 18. Patient best treated with hybrid revascularization of common iliac angioplasty with above result followed by common femoral endarterectomy. The image on the left and center are pretreatment. Image on the right is post common iliac artery stent placement.

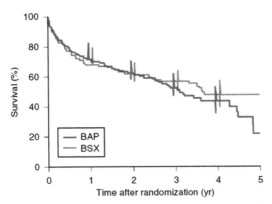

Fig. 19. Limb salvage rates in the bypass first versus angioplasty limbs of the BASIL trial. (*Data from* Adam DJ, Beard JD, Cleveland T, et al. Bypass vs angioplasty in severe ischaemia of the leg (BASIL): multicentre, randomised controlled trial. Lancet 2005;366:1925–34.)

SFA-popliteal lesions is just 28%, secondary patency with percutaneous reintervention is achieved in more than 80%, avoiding the need for major open surgery.[49]

The Bypass versus Angioplasty in Severe Ischaemia of the Leg (BASIL) trial represents the largest randomized trial comparing surgical bypass to endovascular therapy for lower extremity arterial occlusive disease. Limb salvage rates were found to be equivalent for endovascular versus open surgical bypass (**Fig. 19**).[50] Overall survival was similar between the 2 groups at 2 years, and there was a trend toward increased overall survival in the open surgical group after 2 years. Further, patients with failed angioplasty who crossed over into the surgical bypass cohort experienced a statistically significant higher amputation rate at all follow periods up to 6 years.[51]

Postrevascularization surveillance

Regardless of the type of revascularization performed, patients with critical limb ischemia should be followed with serial arterial duplex and ABI with digital pressures. Angioplasty and stenting sites are prone to re-stenosis. Lower extremity bypasses are vulnerable to neo-intimal hyperplasia-induced stenosis anywhere along the length of a vein bypass and near the anastomosis sites of prosthetic bypasses.[52–54] Stenoses are detected as areas of increased peak systolic velocity on Doppler analysis. A velocity ratio of greater than 3:1 between an area of stenosis and the proximal normal arterial segment indicates a 50% or greater stenosis. **Fig. 20** depicts a proximal

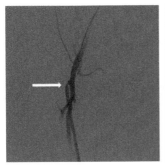 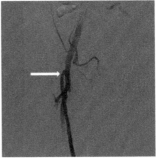

Fig. 20. Proximal femoral-popliteal artery bypass stenosis detected after drop in ABI treated with angioplasty. Preangioplasty seen on the left and post angioplasty images on the right. *Arrows* pointing to occlusive disease segments.

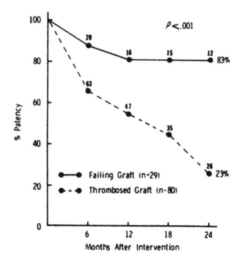

Fig. 21. A 24-month primary assisted patency versus secondary patency for lower extremity bypass, emphasizing the importance of treating underlying bypass graft stenosis before thrombosis occurs. (*From* Ascher E, Collier PE, Gupta SK, et al. Reoperation for PTFE bypass failure: the importance of distal outflow site and operative technique in determining outcome. J Vasc Surg 1987;5:298; with permission.)

femoral-popliteal bypass graft stenosis treated with angioplasty after a drop in ABI was detected. An absolute velocity of less than 40 cm per second in a bypass distal to a stenosis represents a threatened graft that should be imaged with CTA or angiography. Significant in-graft stenosis should be treated with transluminal angioplasty, surgical patch angioplasty, or revision jump graft. In addition, new atherosclerotic lesions in the native arteries proximal or distal to lower extremity bypasses should be treated to assist bypass patency.

There is profound benefit to correction of significant stenosis in a threatened bypass to maintain primary assisted patency. Once a bypass becomes thrombosed, secondary patency is reduced threefold relative to assisted primary patency for bypasses intervened on before thrombosis occurs (**Fig. 21**).[29] After revascularization, it is our practice to obtain arterial duplex scanning at 1, 3, 6, and 12 months after the procedure and every 6 months thereafter.

Nonreconstructable tibial occlusive disease and critical limb ischemia

Patients with nonreconstructable tibial distribution occlusive disease (no bypass targets) benefit from intermittent pneumatic compression treatment at the calf level.[55] This can be used as a last measure for attempt at limb salvage before major amputation in patients with critical limb ischemia. Further ongoing research in treating such patients is directed at angiogenesis via stem cell and growth factor implantation in the calf, as well as bone marrow stimulation with granulocyte colony stimulating factor (GCSF).[56]

REFERENCES

1. Merten GJ, Burgess WP, Gray LV, et al. Prevention of contrast-induced nephropathy with sodium bicarbonate: a randomized controlled trial. JAMA 2004;291:2328.
2. The STILE Trial: results of a prospective randomized trial evaluating surgery versus thrombolysis for ischemia of the lower extremity. Ann Surg 1994;220: 251–66.

3. Ouriel K, Veith FJ, Sasahara AA. A comparison of recombinant urokinase with vascular surgery as initial treatment for acute arterial occlusion of the legs for the Thrombolysis or Peripheral Arterial Surgery (TOPAS) investigators. N Engl J Med 1998;338:1105–11.
4. Sumi M, Ohki T. Rutherford's vascular surgery. Chapter 85, p. 2403. Image 158-1 A. Philadelphia: Elsevier; 2010.
5. Campbell WB, Rider BM, Szymanska TH. Current management of acute leg ischemia: results of audit by the Vascular Surgical Society of Great Britain and Ireland. Br J Surg 1998;85:1498–503.
6. Nypaver TJ, Whyte BR, Endean ED, et al. Nontraumatic lower-extremity acute arterial ischemia. Am J Surg 1998;176:147–52.
7. Pemberton M, Varty K, Nydahl S, et al. The surgical management of acute limb ischemia due to native vessel occlusion. Eur J Vasc Endovasc Surg 1999;17:72–6.
8. Kasirajan K, Gray B, Beavers FP, et al. Rheolytic thrombectomy in the management of acute and subacute limb threatening ischemia. J Vasc Interv Radiol 2001;12:413–21.
9. Eneas JF, Schoenfield BY, Humphreys MH. The effect of infusion of mannitol-sodium bicarbonate on the clinical course of myoglobinuria. Arch Intern Med 1979;139:801.
10. Rutherford RB, Baker JD, Ernst C, et al. Recommended standards for reports dealing with lower extremity ischemia: revised version. J Vasc Surg 1997; 26(3):517–38.
11. Norgren L, Hiatt WR, Dormandy JA, et al, TASC II Working Group. Inter-Society Consensus for the Management of Peripheral Arterial Disease (TASC II). J Vasc Surg 2007;45:S9A.
12. Selvin E, Erlinger TP. Prevalence of and risk factors for peripheral arterial disease in the United States: results from the National Health and Nutrition Examination Survey, 1999-2000. Circulation 2004;110:738–43.
13. Norgren L, Hiatt WR, Dormandy JA, et al, TASC II Working Group. Inter-society consensus for the management of peripheral arterial disease. J Vasc Surg 2007; 45(Suppl S):22.
14. Feinglass J, Brown JL, LoSasso A, et al. Rates of lower-extremity amputation and arterial reconstruction in the United States, 1979 to 1996. Am J Public Health 1999;89:1222.
15. Ramsey DE, Manke DA, Summer DS. Toe blood pressure: a valuable adjunct to ankle pressure measurement for assessing peripheral arterial disease. J Cardiovasc Surg 1983;24:43.
16. McFalls EO, Ward HB, Moritz TE, et al. Coronary-artery revascularization before elective major vascular surgery. N Engl J Med 2004;351:2795–804.
17. Fleisher LA, Beckman JA, Brown KA, et al. ACC/AHA 2007 guidelines on perioperative cardiovascular evaluation and care for noncardiac surgery: executive summary: a report of the American College of Cardiology/American Heart Association Task Force on Practice Guidelines (Writing Committee to Revise the 2002 Guidelines on Perioperative Cardiovascular Evaluation for Noncardiac Surgery) Developed in Collaboration With the American Society of Echocardiography, American Society of Nuclear Cardiology, Heart Rhythm Society, Society of Cardiovascular Anesthesiologists, Society for Cardiovascular Angiography and Interventions, Society for Vascular Medicine and Biology, and Society for Vascular Surgery. J Am Coll Cardiol 2007;50:1707–32.
18. ATC. Collaborative overview of randomised trials of antiplatelet therapy—I: prevention of death, myocardial infarction, and stroke by prolonged antiplatelet

therapy in various categories of patients. Antiplatelet Trialists' Collaboration. BMJ 1994;308:81–106.

19. CAPRIE Steering Committee. A randomised, blinded, trial of clopidogrel versus aspirin in patients at risk of ischaemic events (CAPRIE). Lancet 1996;348: 1329–39.

20. Heart Protection Study Collaborative Group. MRC/BHF Heart Protection Study of cholesterol lowering with simvastatin in 20,536 high-risk individuals: a randomised placebo-controlled trial. Lancet 2002;360:7–22.

21. The Diabetes Control and Complications Trial (DCCT) Research Group. Effect of intensive diabetes management on macrovascular events and risk factors in the Diabetes Control and Complications Trial. Am J Cardiol 1995;75:894–903.

22. Yusuf S, Sleight P, Pogue J, et al. Effects of an angiotensin-converting-enzyme inhibitor, ramipril, on cardiovascular events in high-risk patients. The Heart Outcomes Prevention Evaluation Study Investigators. N Engl J Med 2000;342:145–53.

23. Creager MA, Jones DW, Easton JD. Atherosclerotic Vascular Disease Conference: Writing Group V: medical decision making and therapy. Circulation 2004;109:2634–42.

24. Jonason T, Bergstrom R. Cessation of smoking in patients with intermittent claudication. Effects on the risk of peripheral vascular complications, myocardial infarction and mortality. Acta Med Scand 1987;221:253–60.

25. Faulkner KW, House AK, Castleden WM. The effect of cessation of smoking on the accumulative survival rates of patients with symptomatic peripheral vascular disease. Med J Aust 1983;1:217–9.

26. Sumi M, Ohki T. Rutherford's vascular surgery. Chapter 85, p. 1278. Image A and B. Philadelphia: Elsevier; 2010.

27. Taylor SM, Kalbaugh CA, Healy MG, et al. Do current outcomes justify more liberal use of revascularization for vasculogenic claudication? A single center experience of 1000 consecutively treated limbs. J Am Coll Surg 2008;6:1053–64.

28. Schurmann K, Mahnken A, Meyer J, et al. Long-term results 10 years after iliac arterial stent placement. Radiology 2002;224:731–8.

29. Ascher E, Collier PE, Gupta SK, et al. Reoperation for PTFE bypass failure: the importance of distal outflow site and operative technique in determining outcome. J Vasc Surg 1987;5:298.

30. Schillinger M, Sabeti S, Loewe C, et al. Balloon angioplasty versus implantation of nitinol stents in the superficial femoral artery. N Engl J Med 2006;354: 1879–88.

31. Ferraresi R, Centola M, Ferlini M, et al. Long-term outcomes after angioplasty of isolated, below-the-knee arteries in diabetic patients with critical limb ischaemia. Eur J Vasc Endovasc Surg 2009;37(3):336–42.

32. Conrad MF, Kang J, Cambria RP, et al. Infrapopliteal balloon angioplasty for the treatment of chronic occlusive disease. J Vasc Surg 2009;50(4):799–805.

33. Met R, Van Lienden KP, Koelemay MJ, et al. Subintimal angioplasty for peripheral arterial occlusive disease: a systematic review. Cardiovasc Intervent Radiol 2008;31(4):687–97.

34. Kang SS, Labropoulos N, Mansour MA, et al. Percutaneous ultrasound guided thrombin injection: a new method for treating postcatheterization femoral pseudoaneurysms. J Vasc Surg 1998;27:1032–8.

35. de Vries SO, Hunink MG. Results of aortic bifurcation grafts for aortoiliac occlusive disease: a meta-analysis. J Vasc Surg 1997;26:558.

36. McDaniel MD, Macdonal PD, Haver RA, et al. Published results of surgery for aortoiliac occlusive disease. Ann Vasc Surg 1997;11:425.

37. Onohara T, Komori K, Kume M, et al. Multivariate analysis of long-term results after an axillobifemoral and aortobifemoral bypass in patients with aortoiliac disease. J Cardiovasc Surg 2000;41:905.
38. Mingoli A, Sapienza P, Feldhaus RJ, et al. Comparison of femorofemoral and aortofemoral bypass for aortoiliac occlusive disease. J Cardiovasc Surg 2001; 42:381.
39. Dimick JB, Cowan JA, Henke PK, et al. Hospital volume-related difference in aorto-bifemoral bypass operative mortality in the United States. J Vasc Surg 2003;37:970.
40. Schneider JR. Comparison of axillofemoral and aortofemoral bypass for aortoiliac occlusive disease. J Vasc Surg 1996;23:270. Comment on Passman et al.
41. Harris EJ Jr, Taylor LM Jr, McConnell DB, et al. Clinical results of axillobifemoral bypass using externally supported polytetrafluoroethylene. J Vasc Surg 1990; 12:416–21.
42. El-Massry S, Saad E, Sauvage LR, et al. Axillofemoral bypass with externally supported, knitted Dacron grafts: a follow-up through twelve years. J Vasc Surg 1993;17:107–15.
43. Corbett CR, Taylor PR, Chilvers AS, et al. Axillofemoral bypass in poor risk patients with critical ischaemia. Ann R Coll Surg Engl 1984;66:170–2.
44. Dé P, Hepp W. Present role of extraanatomic bypass graft procedures for aortoiliac occlusive disease. Int Angiol 1991;10:224–8.
45. Klinkert P, Schepers A, Burger DH, et al. Vein versus polytetrafluoroethylene in above-knee femoropopliteal bypass grafting: five-year results of a randomized controlled trial. J Vasc Surg 2003;37:149–55.
46. Mills JL Sr. P values may lack power: the choice of conduit for above-knee femoropopliteal bypass graft. J Vasc Surg 2000;32:402–5.
47. Johnson WC, Lee KK. A comparative evaluation of polytetrafluoroethylene, umbilical vein, and saphenous vein bypass grafts for femoral-popliteal above-knee revascularization: a prospective randomized Department of Veterans Affairs cooperative study. J Vasc Surg 2000;32:268–77.
48. Dorigo W, Pulli R, Castelli P, et al, Propaten Italian Registry Group. A multicentric comparison between autologous saphenous vein and heparin-bonded expanded polytetrafluoroethylene (ePTFE) graft in the treatment of critical limb ischemia in diabetics. J Vasc Surg 2011;54(5):1332–8.
49. Baril DT, Chaer RA, Rhee RY, et al. Endovascular interventions for TASC II D femoropopliteal lesions. J Vasc Surg 2010;51(6):1406–12.
50. Adam DJ, Beard JD, Cleveland T, et al. Bypass versus angioplasty in severe ischaemia of the leg (BASIL): multicentre, randomised controlled trial. Lancet 2005;366:1925–34.
51. Bradbury A, Adam D, Bell J, et al. Bypass versus Angioplasty in Severe Ischaemia of the Leg (BASIL) trial: analysis of amputation free and overall survival by treatment received. J Vasc Surg 2010;51:18S–31S.
52. Mills JL, Fujitani RM, Taylor SM. The characteristics and anatomic distribution of lesions that cause reversed vein graft failure: a five-year prospective study. J Vasc Surg 1993;17:195–204, 276.
53. Mills JL. Mechanisms of vein graft failure: the location, distribution, and characteristics of lesions that predispose to graft failure. Semin Vasc Surg 1993;6: 78–91, 277.
54. Donaldson MC, Mannick JA, Whittemore AD. Causes of primary graft failure after in situ saphenous vein bypass grafting. J Vasc Surg 1992;15:113–8.

55. Kavros SJ, Delis KT, Turner NS, et al. Improving limb salvage in critical ischemia with intermittent pneumatic compression: a controlled study with 18-month follow-up. J Vasc Surg 2008;47:543–9.

56. Tateishi-Yuyama E, Matsubara H, Murohara T, et al. Therapeutic angiogenesis using cell transplantation (TACT) study investigators. Therapeutic angiogenesis for patients with limb ischemia by autologous transplantation of bone marrow cells; a pilot study and a randomized controlled trial. Lancet 2002;360:427–35.

Carotid Artery Occlusive Disease

Courtney Daly, MD, Heron E. Rodriguez, MD*

KEYWORDS

- Carotid • Stroke • Carotid endarterectomy • Carotid artery stent

KEY POINTS

- Clinically significant carotid stenosis can be effectively diagnosed by carotid duplex ultrasound. Limitations include heavily calcified plaques, contralateral carotid occlusion, and operator inexperience.
- Management of carotid occlusive disease requires optimal medical management in addition to surgical revascularization or endovascular revascularization in properly selected patients.
- The role of carotid endarterectomy (CEA) in the management of asymptomatic patients with carotid stenosis should be individualized. Neurologically asymptomatic patients with greater than 60% stenosis should be considered for CEA provided that the patient has a 3- to 5-year life expectancy, and perioperative stroke and death rates are less than 3%.
- For patients with symptomatic carotid stenosis greater than 50%, CEA or carotid artery stenting (CAS) is recommended. Patients who present with fixed neurologic deficits of more than 6 hours duration should be considered for CEA once their condition has been stabilized. CEA should be performed within 2 weeks of the neurologic event.
- The use of a patch angioplasty repair technique is associated with a reduction in risk of stroke of any type and stroke or death during the perioperative period. Patching is also associated with a decreased rate of perioperative arterial occlusion and recurrent stenosis.
- Plaque characteristics associated with a higher risk for stroke include hypoechogenicity on ultrasound, plaque heterogenicity, luminal irregularity, and ulceration.

INTRODUCTION

Stroke is the fourth leading cause of death in the United States.[1] It is also the number one cause of long-term disability. According to population-based studies, the incidence of carotid stenosis increases with age from 0.2% in men younger than 50 years to 7.5% in octogenarian men. In women, the incidence of moderate carotid stenosis ranges from 0% to 5%.[2]

Division of Vascular Surgery, Feinberg School of Medicine, Northwestern University, 676 North Saint Clair Street, Suite 650, Chicago, IL 60611, USA
* Corresponding author.
E-mail address: herodrig@nmh.org

Surg Clin N Am 93 (2013) 813–832
http://dx.doi.org/10.1016/j.suc.2013.05.004
0039-6109/13/$ – see front matter © 2013 Elsevier Inc. All rights reserved.

PATHOPHYSIOLOGY
Plaque Location

Most carotid occlusive disease occurs at the carotid bifurcation. This area of the vasculature represents a unique configuration where the area of the vessels at the bifurcation increases rather than decreases because of the presence of the carotid bulb. This change in caliber, along with the flow divider at the carotid bifurcation, creates a pattern of turbulent flow and areas of variable shear stress along the walls of the carotid vessels. Carotid plaque is consistently found along the outer wall of the internal carotid artery (ICA), opposite the flow divider, which corresponds to an area of low shear stress (**Fig. 1**)[3] and is often at the level of the C4 vertebrae.

Plaque Pathology

Carotid plaques are not unlike other atherosclerotic plaques in the body. The plaques start as fibrointimal thickening and progress to become symptomatic in a variety of ways.[4] Studies relating pathologic findings with symptoms have demonstrated that intraplaque hemorrhage, thrombus formation, and ulceration are consistent with a vulnerable plaque that may cause symptoms. Symptomatic plaques are more likely to have gross ulceration or rupture, thinning of the fibrous cap, intraplaque fibrin, as well as intraplaque hemorrhage. Most plaque ruptures occur at the midpoint of the plaque rather than at the edges or shoulders.[5] Emboligenic potential and symptomatic

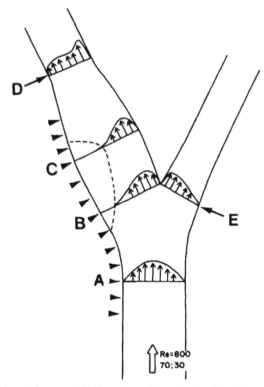

Fig. 1. Flow dynamics at the carotid bifurcation. (*From* Zarins CK, Giddens DP, Bharadvaj BK, et al. Carotid bifurcation atherosclerosis; quantitative correlation of plaque localization with flow velocity profiles and wall shear stress. Circ Res 1983;53:502–14; with permission.)

status have been correlated with hypoechoic and homogenic patterns on duplex ultrasonography.[6–8]

DIAGNOSIS OF CAROTID STENOSIS
Duplex Criteria

Duplex criteria for diagnosis of carotid stenosis were standardized in 1987 by Dr Strandness at the University of Washington. This first set of criteria, known as the University of Washington criteria, stratified carotid stenosis into 5 categories using both duplex and B mode evaluation. These criteria are shown in **Table 1**.

A limitation of the University of Washington criteria is that the category of 50% to 79% is too broad in terms of diagnosis. For asymptomatic patients, the difference between 50% and 60% stenosis can change the recommended treatment. The Society of Radiologists in Ultrasound created a consensus document incorporating additional duplex criteria including the ICA/common carotid artery (CCA) ratio to better stratify to the 50% to 79% group, which is shown in **Table 2**.

Besides being highly operator dependent, other limitations of duplex ultrasound are its inability to accurately determine velocities in the presence of heavily calcified plaque due to artifact created by shadowing and in the setting of contralateral carotid occlusion. It is often the only imaging needed before proceeding to CEA. Some indications for additional imaging include heavily calcified plaque, inability to visualize color flow filling from wall to wall in the distal ICA, and atypical symptoms.

Computed Tomography Angiography

Computed tomography (CT) angiography is a noninvasive alternative to conventional carotid angiography. It has been shown to correlate accurately with carotid angiography in terms of determining the degree of carotid stenosis.[9] It also provides additional information regarding the carotid wall architecture, including presence of calcification and thrombus as well as the level of the carotid bifurcation compared with bony landmarks, which may aid in operative planning.

Magnetic Resonance Angiography

Magnetic resonance angiography (MRA) is another option for preoperative cross-sectional imaging for carotid stenosis. In a systematic review of published studies on duplex ultrasound and MRA using digital subtraction angiography as the gold standard, MRA was found to be both sensitive and specific at detecting carotid stenosis and in fact was found to be more discriminatory than duplex ultrasound at detecting stenosis between 70% and 99%.[10]

Table 1			
Strandness criteria for the diagnosis of carotid stenosis using Doppler ultrasound			
Stenosis (%)	**PSV (cm/s)**	**EDV (cm/s)**	**Plaque Character**
0	<125	—	None
1–15	<125	—	Minimal
16–49	<125	—	Moderate
50–79	>125	—	Prominent
80–99	>125	>140	Severe

Abbreviations: EDV, end diastolic velocity; PSV, peak systolic velocity.

Table 2
Consensus criteria for the diagnosis of carotid stenosis using Doppler ultrasound

Stenosis (%)	Primary Parameters		Additional Parameters	
	ICA PSV (cm/s)	Plaque Estimate	ICA/CCA PSV Ratio	ICA EDV (cm/s)
Normal	<125	None	<2.0	<40
<50	<125	<50	<2.0	<40
50–69	125–230	>50	2.0–4.0	40–100
>70	>230	>50	>4.0	>100
Near occlusion	High, low, ND	Visible	Variable	Variable
Total occlusion	Not detectable	Visible, no detectable lumen	NA	NA

Abbreviations: EDV, end diastolic velocity; NA, not applicable; ND, not detectable; PSV, peak systolic velocity.

ASYMPTOMATIC CAROTID DISEASE: ASYMPTOMATIC CAROTID ARTERY STENOSIS TRIAL

The Endarterectomy for Asymptomatic Carotid Artery Stenosis, or ACAS, trial was a multicenter, randomized trial conducted in 39 medical centers in the United States and Canada. There were 1662 patients with asymptomatic carotid artery stenosis of greater than 60% randomized to medical therapy or CEA. The results demonstrated a 5-year stroke risk of 11% in patients randomized to medical therapy compared with 5.1% in patients randomized to surgical therapy, demonstrating a benefit to CEA for asymptomatic patients. When broken down by gender, women had a higher perioperative stroke rate than men (3.6% vs 1.7%) and less of a benefit from surgical therapy. This study demonstrated CEA to be associated with an absolute risk reduction of 6% and a relative risk reduction of 53%. The perioperative stroke rate was 2.3%. This study demonstrated clearly that there is a benefit for the surgical treatment of asymptomatic carotid stenosis of 60% or more if the perioperative stroke rate can be kept less than 2.3%. This benefit is modest and was not substantiated in women.[11]

Asymptomatic Carotid Surgery Trial

Similarly, the Asymptomatic Carotid Surgery Trial was a multicenter randomized trial of 126 centers from 30 different countries. Asymptomatic patients younger than 75 years with more than 70% stenosis by duplex were randomized to immediate CEA versus deferral of CEA until a clear indication existed. The results of this trial conducted in Europe were strikingly similar to the results of ACAS with a 5-year risk of stroke of 6.1% for patients treated with immediate CEA versus 11.8% for those in the control group. The 30-day perioperative stroke rate in the surgical arm was 3.1%.[12]

Recent Data Regarding Asymptomatic Carotid Disease

With improvements in medical therapy for carotid occlusive disease such as the addition of statins and plavix, some feel a need for updated data on asymptomatic carotid disease. To compare the effects of improved medical therapy, Spence and colleagues[13] reviewed data on 468 patients with asymptomatic, high-grade carotid stenosis, 199 treated before 2003 and 269 after 2003. The latter group received an intensified medical regimen aimed to achieve a better control of plasma lipids. The outcomes of the study were microemboli detected by transcranial Doppler (TCD), plaque progression by ultrasound, and cardiovascular event rates. Plaque progression in the first year of follow-up decreased significantly, and cardiovascular events and microemboli on TCD markedly declined with more intensive medical therapy (17.6% had stroke, death, myocardial infarction (MI) or CEA for symptoms before 2003, vs 5.6% since 2003).

An interesting study addressing the issue of asymptomatic carotid disease in high-risk patients was reported by Erzurum and colleagues.[14] This study was a retrospective one of 196 asymptomatic veterans with carotid stenosis greater than 80%. One hundred thirty-seven patients underwent CEA, 21 refused surgical intervention, and 36 were not offered surgical intervention based on comorbid conditions. The conditions were advanced malignant disease, severe cardiac disease, severe dementia, and otherwise frail medical condition. The group of patients that refused surgical intervention had a significantly higher rate of neurologic events. Nevertheless, the nonoperative group (those patients not offered surgical intervention because of severe comorbidities) had similar rates of neurologic events compared with the surgical group. The comorbid group also had a significantly decreased rate of survival compared with either of the other groups. The conclusion of this study was that nonoperative management of carotid stenosis is reasonable in patients who have a limited life expectancy related to other medical comorbidities.

ASYMPTOMATIC CAROTID STENOSIS: CONCLUSIONS

The role of CEA in the management of asymptomatic patients with carotid stenosis should be individualized. Recent evidence suggests that improvements in the medical management of atherosclerosis has translated in improvement in stroke risk of both medically and surgically treated patients.

The following are the recommendations of the Society for Vascular Surgery (SVS) regarding the role of CEA in the management of asymptomatic carotid disease:

Neurologically asymptomatic patients with >60% stenosis should be considered for CEA provided that the patient has a 3–5 year life expectancy and perioperative stroke and death rates can be <3% (grade 1A evidence). Neurologically asymptomatic patients deemed "high risk" for CEA should be considered for primary medical management. CEA can be considered in these patients only with evidence that perioperative morbidity and mortality is 3% or less. Carotid Artery Stenting (CAS) should not be performed in these patients except as part of an ongoing clinical trial (grade 1, level of evidence B).[15,16]

SYMPTOMATIC CAROTID DISEASE
North American Symptomatic Carotid Endarterectomy Trial

The first major randomized trial in patients with symptomatic carotid artery stenosis was the North American Symptomatic Carotid Endarterectomy Trial (NASCET). It involved 50 medical centers and 659 patients with carotid stenosis 70% to 99% randomized to medical or surgical treatment. The risk of ipsilateral stroke at 24 months was 26% in patients treated with medical management compared with 9% in patients treated with surgery. There was a 5.8% rate of perioperative stroke and death.

Another arm of the study randomized patients with moderate carotid stenosis. This study involved 2226 patients grouped by 50% to 69% stenosis and less than 50% stenosis followed over an average of 5 years. The 5-year rate of stroke in the 50% to 69% patients with stenosis was 22.2% in patients treated medically compared with 15.7% in patients treated surgically. In patients with less than 50% stenosis, the 5-year rate of stroke was 18.7% in patients treated medically compared with 14.9% in patients treated surgically. The overall recommendations from this trial were that all patients with severe carotid stenosis who were symptomatic benefited from CEA. Patients with moderate carotid stenosis (50%–69%) had a modest benefit from CEA, and patients with less than 50% stenosis did not clearly benefit from CEA.[17]

The SVS guidelines recommend optimal medical therapy for neurologically symptomatic patients with stenosis less than 50%, as there are no data to support CAS or CEA in this patient group. For patients with symptomatic carotid stenosis greater than 50%, CEA or CAS is recommended. CEA is preferred for patients older than 70 years with long, preocclusive lesions. CAS is preferred over CEA in patients with hostile necks, high bifurcations, and prior cranial nerve deficits or in those with severe coronary artery disease (CAD), congestive heart failure, or chronic obstructive pulmonary disease.[15]

Timing to Intervention

In an analysis of pooled data from randomized control trials, Rothwell and Warlow[18] found that CEA after transient ischemic attack (TIA) is most beneficial during the first 2 weeks. Twenty-five percent of strokes are preceded by a TIA, and 45% of the TIAs occur the week prior.[19] Based on these and other observations, CEA should not be delayed following TIA; it should be performed within 2 weeks.

For many years, traditional teaching suggested delaying CEA after stroke for 6 weeks to avoid cerebral hyperperfusion or conversion to hemorrhagic stroke. Current evidence does not support this approach. This concept is clearly stated in the SVS guidelines for the management of extracranial carotid disease: "Patients who presented with fixed neurologic deficits of more than 6 hours duration should be considered for CEA once their condition has been stabilized. CEA should be performed within 2 weeks of the neurologic event."[15] Individual situations in which delaying CEA may be prudent include those with a high risk of conversion to hemorrhagic stroke. These include patients with altered level of consciousness or large size of stroke as evidenced by cerebral imaging.

CEA and Coronary Artery Bypass Graft

Because of the similarity in risk factors, patients with carotid disease often have concomitant CAD. In general, patients with symptomatic carotid stenosis should undergo CEA before or combined with coronary artery bypass graft (CABG). Alternatively, in selected centers with adequate experience, CAS before CABG is performed as long as antiplatelet therapy is continued around the time of CABG. For asymptomatic high-grade bilateral stenosis, CEA or combined procedure should be considered, with CEA done on the higher degree of stenosis or the dominant hemisphere.

The recommendations for asymptomatic unilateral disease are less clear. Unilateral, high-grade carotid stenosis can be treated before, concomitant with, or after CABG. A randomized trial out of Italy examined 185 patients with asymptomatic carotid disease undergoing CABG. They were randomized to CEA or combined procedure or CEA following CABG. The CABG first group was found to have a significantly greater number of 90-day stroke 8.8% versus 1%.[20] The extremely low rate of perioperative stroke observed in combined CEA/CABG in this trial is in contradiction with the accumulated worldwide experience regarding combined CEA/CABG. A much larger multicentric study, the coronary artery bypass graft surgery in patients with asymptomatic carotid stenosis (CABACS) trial, started enrolling patients in 2010, comparing CABG alone to combined CABG/CEA. Until the results of such trials are available, it seems prudent to individualize decisions regarding the management of asymptomatic patients with high-grade carotid stenosis undergoing CABG, with most patients not requiring carotid intervention.

TECHNICAL ASPECTS OF CAROTID ENDARTERECTOMY
Patch Angioplasty Repair

Well-established data comparing carotid patch angioplasty with primary repair have demonstrated decreased rates of restenosis when patch angioplasty repair is used. A Cochran review analyzing 13 randomized trials and more than 2000 patients showed that the use of patch angioplasty was associated with a reduction in risk of stroke of any type and stroke or death during the perioperative period. Patching is also associated with a decreased rate of perioperative arterial occlusion and recurrent stenosis both within the perioperative period and at 1 year of follow-up.[21]

Eversion Endarterectomy

Eversion CEA is an alternative to traditional endarterectomy that does not require the use of alternative material (vein or prosthetic graft) for a patch. Outcomes of eversion endarterectomy have been compared with traditional CEA with primary repair and patch angioplasty in several randomized trials. Pooled results show no significant difference between rates of perioperative stroke and death (1.7% for eversion and 2.6% for patch angioplasty). Nevertheless, eversion endarterectomy was associated with a significantly lower rate of restenosis (2.5% for eversion vs 5.2% for patch angioplasty).[22] Based on these data, patch angioplasty or eversion CEA is recommended rather than primary closure to reduce the early and late complications of CEA.[15]

CEREBRAL MONITORING
Routine Shunting

Routine shunting affords excellent results and relieves the effects of carotid clamping on cerebral blood flow. There have been no data to show an increase in thromboembolic events or traumatic complications. Stroke rates with routine shunting were found to be 0.7% to 3.6%.[23,24] The main advantage of routine shunting is that when it is needed, the results of shunting are better with routine users rather than with selective users.

Selective Shunting

To perform selective shunting, some type of cerebral monitoring is needed to determine the need for shunt. One option includes performing the procedure under local anesthesia with the patient awake.[25] Other options for patients under general anesthesia include electroencephalographic monitoring (looking for a 50% amplitude and slowing of alpha and beta frequencies), carotid stump pressures (typical cutoff of 40 mm Hg), TCD, and somatosensory evoked potential (SSEP), which can be technically challenging but has good results in retrospective reviews. Selective shunting using these various methods resulted in perioperative stroke rates of 1.6% for EEG, 4.8% for TCD, 1.6% for stump pressure, 1.8% for SSEP, and 1.1% for local anesthesia.[24]

In terms of randomized trials, shunting compared with no shunting yielded stroke rates of 3.4% with shunting compared with 4.5% with no shunting.[22] Shunting compared with selective shunting had a 0% stroke rate for routine shunting compared with 2% for selective shunting.[26] Stump pressure alone compared with stump pressure + EEG had a 2.9% rate of stroke versus 4.5%, respectively.[24] In conclusion, either routine or selective shunting is effective. Stump pressure, EEG, and SSEP are all acceptable ways of determining the need for selective shunting in the right hands.

Type of Anesthesia

CEA can be performed under moderate sedation with local anesthesia, which has the advantage of allowing neurologic function intraoperatively. The general anaesthesia versus local anaesthesia for carotid surgery (GALA) trial is a randomized clinical trial comparing general anesthesia with local anesthesia for CEA. The primary outcome of 30 day death, stroke, or MI was 4.8% for general anesthesia and 4.5% for local anesthesia, which was not significantly different.[25]

Completion Studies

Intraoperative completion studies can be used to rule out technical imperfections in the repair that are potential sources of perioperative stroke. Duplex ultrasound (**Fig. 2**) and cerebral angiogram are commonly used completion studies following carotid endarterectomy. When compared on their diagnostic value at detecting both major and minor intraoperative defects, they were found to have a similar sensitivity of 100% at detecting major defects, but duplex ultrasound had a better sensitivity of 87% versus 59% for angiography at detecting minor defects.[27] In a review of comparative studies on completion imaging, a significant difference was not demonstrated between types of studies or with no studies at all.[28] If a completion study is desired, both duplex ultrasound and angiogram are adequately sensitive, with the advantage of being less invasive.

High Bifurcation

Exposure of the internal carotid can be difficult in the setting of a high carotid bifurcation if there is distal internal carotid disease extending about the level of C2. There are a variety of techniques to allow for additional distal exposure beyond the traditional incision. The standard approach often allows for exposure up to the level of the distal third of the second cervical vertebra. One of the first steps is to ligate the posterior belly of the digastric muscle, which can extend the exposure to the level of the center of the first vertebra. The next step involves anterior subluxation of the mandible, which

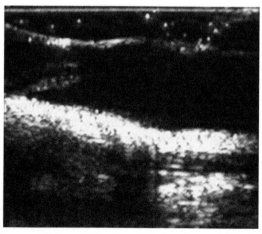

Fig. 2. Carotid duplex completion study after CEA showing an intimal flap.

allows the exposure to extend to the first cervical vertebra. An additional step that can be taken is styloidectomy, which often gains an additional 5 mm of exposure.[29] Nasotracheal intubation can improve exposure, especially when combined with mandibular subluxation.[30] An alternative approach to exposure is the retrojugular approach. This technique involves a similar skin incision along the border of the sternocleidomastoid, but the internal jugular vein is retracted medially, while the sternoclediomastoid is retracted laterally. This technique exposes the ICA in a more anterior and superficial plane. This technique is protective of the hypoglossal nerve, as it often gets swept medially with the internal jugular vein. Distal exposure is gained by further mobilizing the internal jugular vein and separating the hypoglossal nerve and vagus nerve to expose the internal jugular underneath.[31]

COMPLICATIONS OF CEA
Perioperative Stroke Management

The potential causes of perioperative stroke are arterial thrombosis, embolization, and cerebral ischemia during clamping, and intracerebral hemorrhage. The goal of management in perioperative stroke is early recognition and immediate therapy to maximize the changes of recovering neurologic function.

Intraoperative Stroke

If a new focal neurologic deficit is noted intraoperatively, or in the operating room immediately after the patient awakens from anesthesia, the artery should be re-explored immediately to check for thrombosis. The incision should be reopened and ICA palpated for a pulse as well as using Doppler to check the flow. If flow is present, the next step involves duplex ultrasound or angiogram to identify any technically correctable problems such as a local flap. If the artery must be reopened, clamping of the ICA should be avoided, which prevents further embolization and allows backflow to clear distal ICA thrombus. If no flow is present, balloon catheters are used to perform thrombectomy, but there is a risk of a carotid artery-cavernous sinus fistula, and care must be taken with balloon catheters in the distal ICA.

Postoperative Stroke

When a patient awakens with a normal neurologic examination and develops a new focal deficit, the first step is still to prove that the ICA is patent, which is done either by duplex ultrasound or by returning to the operating room for angiogram. CT is another option with the advantage of ruling out intracerebral hemorrhage but can cause delay in intervention, and timing is crucial because most neurologic deficits are reversible if flow is restored within 1 to 2 hours. If thrombosis is present, similar steps should be taken as described earlier. If the vessel is patent, head CT should be performed to rule out cerebral hemorrhage, followed by carotid angiography to evaluate for a technical defect or intracerebral embolus. Mechanical thrombectomy has been described of the distal ICA with a 60% to 70% recanalization rate and improved neurologic outcome in those patients that were recanalized.[32,33] Intra-arterial thrombolysis for distal embolization has been described after intracranial hemorrhage is ruled out, although this carries a significant risk of hemorrhage and should be used only in select patients.[34]

Hyperperfusion Syndrome

Hyperperfusion syndrome is a rare postoperative complication that manifests as postoperative headache, with potential seizure and intracranial hemorrhage. The incidence is rare, with reports ranging from 0.2% to 3%. It peaks in the range of postoperative day 2 to 7. The mechanism is thought to be due to loss of autoregulation of cerebral perfusion pressure due to chronically low pressure in the cerebral bed.[35] Transcranial duplex has been used to monitor increased regional cerebral blood flow in intracerebral arterial beds, and an increase of 100% has been shown to correlate with an increased risk of hyperperfusion syndrome.[36] Although rare, a high suspicion to monitor patients for hyperperfusion syndrome should be present when evaluating patients postoperatively because of the risk of intracerebral hemorrhage, which is frequently fatal.

Cranial Nerve Injuries

Given the dissection required to perform CEA, cranial nerve injuries are one of the most common complications related to the procedure. Nerves at risk of being injured are the greater auricular nerve, hypoglossal, marginal mandibular branch of the facial nerve, superior laryngeal nerve, glossopharyngeal nerve, and the recurrent laryngeal nerve. In the literature, rates of cranial nerve injuries range from 5.5% to 23%.[37–40] In the absence of a complete nerve transaction, most deficits are transient and resolve within 4 to 6 weeks. In the setting of bilateral procedures, bilateral nerve injuries are life threatening, causing airway obstruction, potentially requiring tracheostomy. **Table 3** summarizes the anatomy and functional deficit related to some of the more common cranial nerve injuries.

Patch Infection

Deep surgical site infection following CEA is rare but is one of the most feared complications following CEA (**Fig. 3**). The incidence is low at 0.25% to 0.5% and tends to be higher when prosthetic material is used. The manifestation of patch infection can range from asymptomatic pseudoaneurysm to patch rupture and carotid blow out. The principles of managing patch infections involve removing all infected material, removing all prosthetic material, reconstructing the carotid artery, and covering the defect with viable tissue. When there is suspicion for a patch infection, preoperative imaging can help plan operative washout and repair. Options for a suitable conduit to repair the arterial defect include the superficial femoral artery, cryopreserved arterial conduit, or the great saphenous vein. Arterial conduit is preferred in the setting of infection because of the risk of thin-walled venous degeneration. When superficial femoral artery (SFA) is the planned conduit, preoperative duplex is recommended to evaluate the conduit. Often a large defect is present in the neck at the end of reconstruction, and if there is not adequate tissue coverage of the arterial repair, muscle

Table 3 Cranial nerve injuries		
Cranial Nerve	**Anatomy**	**Deficit**
Vagus	Between IJV and carotid	Ipsilateral VC paralysis
Hypoglossal	Anterior to ICA (lateral to medial) gives off ansa	Ipsilateral tongue deviation
Marginal mandibular branch of facial	Deep to platysma, angle of mandible	Paralysis ipsilateral orbicularis orbi
Facial	Base of styloid into parotid	Facial paralysis
Glossopharyngeal	Follows stylopharyngeal muscle anterior to ICA	Dysphagia, aspiration

Abbreviaitons: IJV, internal jugular vein; VC, vocal cord.

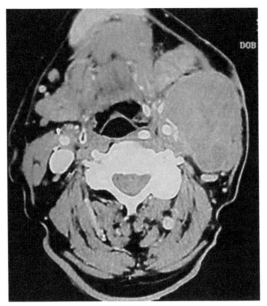

Fig. 3. CT scan showing a large fluid collection immediately adjacent to an endarterectomized carotid artery repaired with a prosthetic patch.

flap reconstruction may be required. Common options for muscle flap coverage include sternocleidomastoid flap or pectoralis major.[41]

CAROTID ARTERY STENTING

CAS has emerged as a viable option for the management of carotid occlusive disease. A myriad of data in the form of retrospective studies, registries, and randomized trials have compared this minimally invasive option to CEA.

Randomized Trials

Carotid revascularization endarterectomy versus stenting trial

The carotid revascularization endarterectomy versus stenting trial (CREST) study was a National Institutes of Health–sponsored randomized multicentric trial comparing CAS with CEA.[42] It involved patients with standard risk with either symptomatic disease and greater than 50% stenosis or asymptomatic disease with greater than 60% stenosis.

Outcomes were MI, stroke, or death within 30 days or ipsilateral stroke over a 4-year follow-up period. Rates of early (30 day) MI, stroke, or death were not significantly different between CAS (5.2%) and CEA (4.5%) nor were ipsilateral 4-year stroke rates, which were 7.2% for CAS and 6.8% for CEA. When 30-day stroke and MI were separated, CAS had a higher rate of perioperative stroke 4.1% versus 2.3%, whereas CEA had a higher rate of MI 2.3% versus 1.1% (**Table 4**). To determine the impact of this finding, longitudinal random effect growth curve models and the SF-36 physical and mental health scales were used. The results of this analysis showed that major or minor stroke had a more significant impact on physical and mental health than MI (**Fig. 4**). When stratified by indication for treatment, patients who were symptomatic had a significantly increased rate of 30-day stroke, death,

Table 4 Overall CREST outcomes	CAS (%)	CEA (%)
30-d Stroke, death, MI	5.2	4.5
+ Ipsilateral stroke 4 y	7.2	6.8
30-d stroke	4.1	2.3
30-d MI	1.1	2.3

or MI with CAS (6.0% vs 3.2%), whereas asymptomatic patients had similar rates (**Table 5**).

Several other randomized trials have been performed. The Endarterectomy versus Angioplasty in Patients with Symptomatic Severe Carotid Stenosis (EVA-3S) trial was a randomized clinical trial in Europe comparing CAS with CEA in symptomatic patients with stenosis greater than 60%. The 30-day rate of disabling stroke and death was 1.5% following CEA and 3.4% following CAS with a relative risk of 2.2 with CAS. Local complications were more common following CAS, and systemic complications and cranial nerve injuries were more common following CEA.[43] The Stent-Protected Angioplasty versus Carotid Endarterectomy (SPACE) trial randomized patients with symptomatic carotid stenosis greater than 70% to CAS versus CEA. The 2-year rate of ipsilateral or periprocedural stroke or death did not differ significantly between to 2 treatment strategies 9.5% for CAS versus 8.8% for CEA.[44] The International Carotid Stenting Study (ICSS) is another randomized trial comparing symptomatic patients with carotid stenosis greater than 50%. The outcome in the published interim

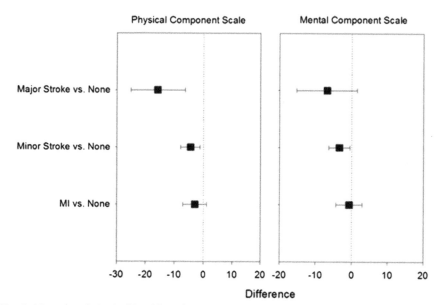

Fig. 4. Mental and physical health scales in CREST. (*From* Brott TG, Hobson RW II, Howard G, et al. Stenting versus endarterectomy for treatment of carotid-artery stenosis (supplement). N Engl J Med 2010;363:11–23; with permission. Copyright © 2010, Massachusetts Medical Society.)

Table 5		
CREST periprocedural outcomes by symptomatic status: Stroke and death rates		
Symptom Status	CAS (%)	CEA (%)
Symptomatic	6.0	3.2
Asymptomatic	2.5	1.4

analysis was 120-day stroke, death, or procedural MI. According to the interim analysis, CEA had lower rates of stroke, death, or periprocedural MI at 5.4% compared with 8.5% for CAS. Three-year analysis is pending.[45]

Summary Data

A meta-analysis was performed by Murad and colleagues[46] on randomized trials for carotid endarterectomy versus stenting and the conclusion was that CAS increases the risk of perioperative stroke, while CEA increases the risk of perioperative MI.

From the large body of evidence accumulated that has compared these 2 options for the treatment of carotid disease, several observations can be made. First, it is clear that operator experience influences the outcomes of both CEA and CAS. As evidenced by the results of the CREST trial, in properly selected patients treated by truly experienced physicians, the results of both CAS and CEA are well within the complications thresholds suggested in current guidelines for both symptomatic and asymptomatic patients.[42] Second, CEA is associated with lower rates of periprocedural strokes and CAS with lower rates of MI. With this in view, it seems that the 2 therapies can be selectively used in a complementary rather than competitive fashion. For example, patients with hostile necks and those at high risk for perioperative cardiac events who require carotid revascularization benefit from CAS. On the other hand, the lower perioperative event rate associated with CEA offers a clear advantage to patients with high potential for embolism. Several of the guidelines proposed by the SVS for the management of carotid disease reflect these considerations.[15]

Specific Considerations Regarding CAS

Age greater than 80 years
Data were analyzed on the CREST lead-in phase and stratified by age groups of 60 to 69, 70 to 79, and greater than 80 years. The rate of perioperative stroke and death increased by age group, and an increased proportion (12.1%) of patients older than 80 years were found to have perioperative stroke or death, suggesting that CAS is riskier in older patients.[47] Another nonrandomized study, the Carotid RX ACCULINK/ RX CCUNET post approval trials to uncover unanticipated or rate events (CAPTURE-2) postapproval study, compared outcomes on patients younger and older than 80 years. Death/stroke rates were found to be significantly higher in octogenarians (4.5%) compared with younger patients (3.0%).[48] Reasons why octogenarians may have increased risk of stroke with CAS likely relate to the fact that older patients tend to have extensive atherosclerotic disease, more tortuous vessels, or calcified and shaggy aortic arches, increasing the risk of embolization during instrumentation.

Aortic arch type
Aortic arch type is classified by the origin of the major branches relative to the curvature of the arch. When evaluating a patient for carotid stenting, the type of aortic arch can determine the technical difficulty and may correlate with the periprocedural risk for stroke. To classify the type of arch, a horizontal line is drawn along the outer and inner

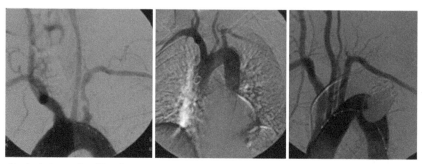

Fig. 5. Arch-type classification.

curvature of the aortic arch. Type I arches have the vessel of interest originate at or above the horizontal plane of the outer curvature of the arch. Type II arches have the vessels originate between the horizontal planes of the inner and outer curvatures of the aortic arch, and in type III arches, the vessel lies below the plane of the inner curvature (**Fig. 5**).

Open-cell versus closed-cell stents

There are different configurations of stents available for CAS. Closed-cell stents have a smaller free stent area and aligned annular rings, which could theoretically allow less microembolization at the time of placement. Open-cell stents have better flexibility and adaptability in tortuous vessels. Timaran and colleagues[49] compared closed-cell versus open-cell stenting to determine if there was a difference in subclinical embolization between the stent configurations. Subclinical embolization was detected by both TCD intraoperative and diffusion-weighted magnetic resonance imaging (DW-MRI) in the postoperative period. The results demonstrated similar rates of subclinical embolization as detected by both TCD and DW-MRI, demonstrating that one type of stent is not superior to the other with regards to cerebral embolization.

Cerebral protection devices

Cerebral protection devices were developed to decrease the risk of distal embolization during carotid stent placement. At present, the standard of care for placement

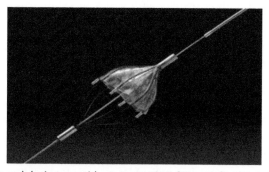

Fig. 6. Distal filter used during carotid artery stenting. (*From* Colombo A, Iakovou I. The balance of evidence for carotid artery stenting with cerebral protection. Controversies and Consensus in Imaging and Intervention 2004;2:19–22.)

of carotid stent requires use of a cerebral protection device. The options for cerebral protection devices include a distal filter, a flow reversal system with proximal occlusion, and a distal occlusion balloon.

Distal filters are the most commonly used devices (**Fig. 6**). They open like an umbrella to capture debris during the CAS procedure. The advantages include the maintenance of antegrade cerebral blood flow and the ability to perform angiography throughout the procedure. The disadvantages are the need to cross the lesion before deployment of the protective filter, as well as the risk that the filter may become occluded with debris, requiring prompt removal.

Flow reversal is an alternative cerebral protection method (**Fig. 7**). It involves proximal occlusion of the CCA and external carotid artery by compliant balloons. Flow reversal is then maintained from the ICA by either shunting through a side arm of the introducer into the femoral vein or active syringe aspiration after the stenting and ballooning phases, which are performed with blocked flow. The main advantage is that the lesion is not crossed before cerebral protection is established. Disadvantages include the requirement of larger introducers and may be technically more demanding.

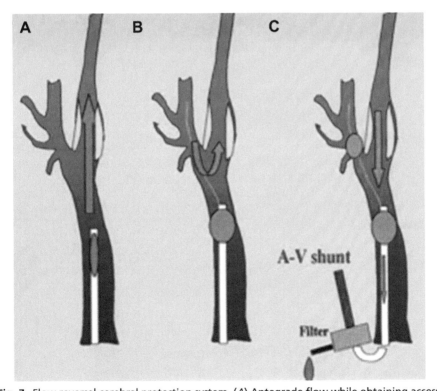

Fig. 7. Flow reversal cerebral protection system. (*A*) Antegrade flow while obtaining access. (*B*) Proximal occlusion balloon with maintained prograde flow via the external carotid. (*C*) Reversal of flow established in the internal carotid artery after occlusion of the external carotid. (*From* Parodi JC, La Mura R, Ferreira LM, et al. Initial evaluation of carotid angioplasty and stenting with three different cerebral protection devices. J Vasc Surg 2000;32(6):1127–36; with permission.)

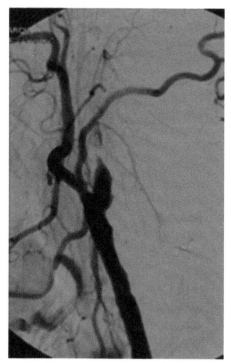

Fig. 8. Distal occlusion balloon.

Distal occlusion balloons were the original protection devices, which are established by occluding the distal ICA with a balloon and flushing and suctioning after stent deployment; this is the simplest form of distal protection, but it does require crossing the lesion before establishing protection, and there is a risk of distal spasm of occlusion of the ICA with a balloon (**Fig. 8**).

Plaque morphology

As discussed earlier, rupture-prone plaques tend to have a large lipid core, thin fibrous cap, few smooth muscle cells, and many macrophages. The use of duplex ultrasound preoperatively to determine characteristics of carotid plaques that increase the risk of

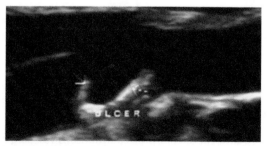

Fig. 9. Ulcerated plaque on duplex ultrasound.

embolization has been studied. Polak and colleagues[50] demonstrated an association between ipsilateral stroke and patients who had hypoechoic plaques on duplex ultrasound.

Biasi and colleagues[51] used the gray scale median (GSM), which is a reproducible measure of plaque echogenicity to study the effect of plaque echogenicity on risk of stroke in carotid stent patients. They found that a GSM greater than 25 was an independent risk factor for stroke in patients receiving CAS. Other features of carotid plaques associated with increased risk of embolization include plaque heterogenicity, luminal irregularity, and ulceration (**Fig. 9**).

SUMMARY

Carotid disease is a major contributor to stroke, one of the leading causes of death and disability in the United States. Clinically significant stenosis can be detected by duplex ultrasound using well-established criteria. In addition to optimal medical management, surgical and endovascular revascularizations of carotid disease have been demonstrated to be effective interventions that reduce the risk of stroke in properly selected patients.

REFERENCES

1. Minino AM, Murphy SL, Xu J, et al. Deaths: final data for 2008. Natl Vital Stat Rep 2011;59(10):1–126. Available at: http://www.cdc.gov. Accessed October 1, 2012.
2. de Weerd M, Greving JP, Hedblad B, et al. Prevalence of asymptomatic carotid artery stenosis in the general population: an individual participant data meta-analysis. Stroke 2010;41(6):1294–7.
3. Zarins CK, Giddens DP, Bharadvaj BK, et al. Carotid bifurcation atherosclerosis; quantitative correlation of plaque localization with flow velocity profiles and wall shear stress. Circ Res 1983;53:502–14.
4. Imparto AM, Riles TS, Gorstein F. The carotid bifurcation plaque: pathologic findings associated with cerebral ischemia. Stroke 1979;10:238–45.
5. Carr S, Farb A, Pearce WH, et al. Atherosclerotic plaque rupture in symptomatic carotid stenosis. J Vasc Surg 1996;23:755–66.
6. Tegos TJ, Stavropoulos P, Sabetai MM, et al. Determinants of carotid plaque instability: echoicity versus heterogeneity. Eur J Vasc Endovasc Surg 2001; 22(1):22–30.
7. Taylor DC, Strandness DE Jr. Carotid artery duplex scanning. J Clin Ultrasound 1987;15(9):635–44.
8. Grant EG, Benson CB, Moneta GL, et al. Carotid artery stenosis: grayscale and Doppler ultrasound diagnosis - Society of Radiologist in Ultrasound Consensus Conference. Ultrasound Q 2003;19(4):190–8.
9. Dillon EH, van Leeuwen MS, Fernandez MA, et al. CT angiography: application to the evaluation of carotid artery stenosis. Radiology 1993;189:211–9.
10. Nederkoom PJ, van der Graaf Y, Myriam Hunik MG. Duplex ultrasound and magnetic resonance angiography compared with digital subtraction angiography in carotid artery stenosis. Stroke 2003;34:1324–31.
11. Walker MD, Marler JR, Goldstein M, et al. Endarterectomy for asymptomatic carotid artery stenosis. JAMA 1995;273(18):1421–8.
12. Halliday A, Mansfield A, Marro J, et al. Prevention of disabling and fatal strokes by successful carotid endarterectomy in patients without recent neurological symptoms: randomized controlled trial. Lancet 2004;363(9420):1491–502.

13. Spence JD, Coates V, Li H, et al. Effects of intensive medical therapy on micro-emboli and cardiovascular risk in asymptomatic carotid stenosis. Arch Neurol 2010;67(2):180–6.
14. Erzurum VZ, Littooy FN, Steffen G, et al. Outcome of nonoperative management of asymptomatic high-grade carotid stenosis. J Vasc Surg 2002;3(4):663–7.
15. Ricotta JJ, AbuRahma A, Ascher E, et al. Updated Society of Vascular Surgery guidelines for management of extracranial carotid disease. J Vasc Surg 2011; 54:e1–31.
16. Beneficial effect of carotid endarterectomy in symptomatic patients with high-grade carotid stenosis. North American Symptomatic Carotid Endarterectomy Trial Collaborators. N Engl J Med 1991;325:445–53.
17. Rothwell PM, Eliasziw M, Gutnikov SA, et al. Analysis of pooled data from the randomized controlled trials of endarterectomy for symptomatic carotid stenosis. Lancet 2003;361:107–61.
18. Rothwell RM, Warlow CP. Timing of TIAs preceding stroke: time window for prevention is very short. Neurology 2005;64:817–20.
19. Illuminati G, Ricco JB, Calio F, et al. Short-term results of a randomized trial examining timing of carotid endarterectomy in patients with severe asymptomatic unilateral carotid stenosis undergoing coronary artery bypass grafting. J Vasc Surg 2011;54:993–6.
20. Bond R, Rerkasem K, Naylor AR, et al. Systematic review of randomized controlled trials of patch angioplasty versus primary closure and different types of patch materials during carotid endarterctomy. J Vasc Surg 2004;40(5):1126–35.
21. Cao P, De Rango P, Zannetti S, et al. Eversion versus conventional carotid endarterectomy for preventing stroke. Cochrane Database Syst Rev 2000;(4): CD001921.
22. Hamdan AD, Pomposelli FB Jr, Gibbons GW, et al. Perioperative strokes after 1001 consecutive carotid endarterectomy procedures without an electroencephalogram: incidence, mechanism, and recovery. Arch Surg 1999;134(4): 412–5.
23. Aburahma AF, Mousa AY, Stone PA. Shunting during carotid endarterectomy. J Vasc Surg 2011;54(5):1502–10.
24. Lewis SC, Warlow CP, Bodenham AR, et al. General anaesthesia versus local anaesthesia for carotid surgery (GALA): a multicenter, randomized controlled trial. Lancet 2008;372(9656):2132–42.
25. AbuRahma AF, Stone PA, Haas SM, et al. Prospective randomized trial of routine versus selective shunting in carotid endarterectomy based on stump pressure. J Vasc Surg 2010;51:1133–8.
26. Valenti D, Gaggiano A, Bernardi G, et al. Intra-operartive assessment of technical defects after carotid endarterectomy: a comparison between angiography and colour duplex scan. Cardiovasc Surg 2003;11(1):26–9.
27. Rockman CB, Halm EA. Intraoperative imaging: does it really improve perioperative outcomes of carotid endarterectomy. Semin Vasc Surg 2007;20(4):236–43.
28. Mock CN, Lilly MP, McRae RG, et al. Selection of the approach to the distal internal carotid artery from the second cervical vertebra to the base of the skull. J Vasc Surg 1991;13(6):846–53.
29. Sionian GT, Pappas PJ, Padberg FT Jr, et al. Mandibular subluxation for distal internal carotid exposure: technical considerations. J Vasc Surg 1999;30(6): 1116–20.
30. Menon NJ, Krijgsman B, Sciacca L, et al. The retrojugular approach to carotid endarterectomy - a safer technique? Eur J Vasc Endovasc Surg 2005;29(6):608–10.

31. Flint AC, Duckwiler GR, Budzik RF, et al. Mechanical thrombectomy of intracranial internal carotid occlusion: pooled results of the MERCI and Multi MERCI part I trials. Stroke 2007;38(4):1274–80.

32. Imai K, Mori T, Izumotoa H, et al. Clot removal therapy by aspiration and extraction for acute embolic carotid occlusion. AJNR Am J Neuroradiol 2006;27(7): 1521–7.

33. Perler BA, Murphy K, Sternbach Y, et al. Immediate postoperative thrombolytic therapy: an aggressive strategy for neurologic salvage when cerebral thromboembolism complicates carotid endarterectomy. J Vasc Surg 2000;31(5): 1033–7.

34. Wagner WH, Cossman DV, Farber A, et al. Hyperperfusion syndrome after carotid endarterectomy. Ann Vasc Surg 2005;19(4):479–86.

35. Dalman JE, Beenakkers IC, Moll FL, et al. Transcranial Doppler monitoring during carotid endarterectomy helps to identify patients at risk of postoperative hyperperfusion. Eur J Vasc Endovasc Surg 1999;18:222–7.

36. Forssell C, Takolander R, Berggvist D, et al. Cranial nerve injuries associated with carotid endarterectomy. A prospective study. Acta Chir Scand 1985; 151(7):595–8.

37. Schauber MD, Fontenelle LJ, Solomon JW, et al. Cranial/cervical nerve dysfunction after carotid endarterectomy. J Vasc Surg 1997;25(3):481–7.

38. Cunningham EJ, Bond R, Mayberg MR, et al. Risk of persistent cranial nerve injury after carotid endarterectomy. J Neurosurg 2004;101(3):445–8.

39. Verta MJ Jr, Applebaum EL, McClusky DA, et al. Cranial nerve injuring during carotid endarterectomy. Ann Surg 1977;185(2):192–5.

40. Naughton PA, Garcia-Toca M, Rodriguez HE, et al. Carotid artery reconstruction for infected carotid patches. Eur J Vasc Endovasc Surg 2010;40:492–8.

41. Brott TG, Hobson RW II, Howard G, et al. Stenting versus endarterectomy for treatment of carotid artery stenosis. N Engl J Med 2010;363:11–23.

42. Yadav JS, Wholey MH, Kuntz RE, et al. Protected carotid artery stenting versus endarterectomy in high risk patients. N Engl J Med 2004;351:1493–501.

43. Mas JL, Chatellier G, Beyssen B, et al. Endarterectomy versus stenting in patients with symptomatic severe carotid stenosis. N Engl J Med 2006;355: 1660–71.

44. Eckstein HH, Ringleb P, Allenberg JR, et al. Results of the stent-protected angioplasty versus carotid endarterectomy (SPACE) study to treat symptomatic stenosis at 2 years: a multinational prospective, randomized trial. Lancet Neurol 2008;7(10):893–902.

45. Dobson EJ, Featherstone RL, Bonati LH, et al. Carotid artery stenting compared with endarterectomy in patients with symptomatic carotid stenosis (International Carotid Stenting Study): an interim analysis of a randomized controlled trial. Lancet 2010;375(9717):985–7.

46. Murad MH, Shahrour A, Shah ND, et al. A systematic review and meta-analysis of randomized trials of carotid endarterectomy vs stenting. J Vasc Surg 2011; 53(3):792–7.

47. Hobson RW II, Howard VJ, Roubin GS, et al. Carotid artery stenting is associated with increased complications in octogenarians: 30-day stroke and death rates in the CREST lead-in phase. J Vasc Surg 2004;40(6):1106–11.

48. Chaturvedi S, Matsumura JS, Gray W, et al. Carotid artery stenting in octogenarians: periprocedural stroke risk predictor analysis from multicenter carotid ACCULINK/ACCUNET post approval trial to uncover rare events (CAPTURE 2) clinical trial. Stroke 2010;41(4):757–64.

49. Timaran CH, Rosero EB, Higuera A, et al. Randomized clinical trial of open-cell vs closed-cell stents for carotid stenting and effects of stent design on cerebral embolization. J Vasc Surg 2011;54(5):1310–6.e1.

50. Polak JF, Shemanski L, O'Leary DH, et al. Hypoechoic plaque at US of the carotid artery: an independent risk factor for incident stroke in adults aged 65 years of older: Cardiovascular Health Study. Radiology 1998;208(3):649–54.

51. Biasi GM, Froio A, Diethrich EB, et al. Carotid plaque echolucency increases the risk of stroke in carotid stenting: the imaging in carotid angioplasty and risk of stroke (ICAROS) study. Circulation 2004;110(6):756–62.

Nonarteriosclerotic Vascular Disease

William Wu, MD, Rabih A. Chaer, MD*

KEYWORDS

- Thromboangiitis obliterans • Takayasu autoimmune arteritis • Giant cell arteritis
- Polyarteritis nodosa • Kawasaki disease • Small-vessel vasculitides
- Radiation arteritis • Raynaud phenomenon

KEY POINTS

- Thromboangiitis obliterans, or Buerger disease, is a chronic nonatherosclerotic endarteritis manifesting as inflammation and thrombosis of distal extremity small and medium-sized arteries resulting in relapsing episodes of distal extremity ischemia.
- Takayasu arteritis is a rare syndrome characterized by inflammation of the aortic arch, pulmonary, coronary, and cerebral vessels predominantly presenting with cerebrovascular symptoms, myocardial ischemia, or upper extremity claudication in young, often female, patients.
- Kawasaki disease is a small- and medium-vessel acute systemic vasculitis of young children, with morbidity and mortality stemming from coronary artery aneurysms.
- Microscopic polyangiitis, Churg-Strauss syndrome, and Wegener granulomatosis are systemic small-vessel vasculitides, affecting arterioles, capillary beds and venules, and each presenting with variable effects on the pulmonary, renal and gastrointestinal systems.

THROMBOANGIITIS OBLITERANS (BUERGER DISEASE)

Thromboangiitis obliterans (TAO), or Buerger disease, is a chronic nonatherosclerotic endarteritis manifesting as inflammation and thrombosis of distal extremity small and medium-sized arteries, resulting in relapsing episodes of distal extremity ischemia. It can often lead to digital and limb amputations. Since being described as a distinct entity by Leo Buerger in 1908, the evolving understanding of this disease has ascribed immunologic, genetic, and environmental factors to its cause.[1]

Pathogenesis

Buerger disease has a well-established association with smoking, and there is increasing evidence to suggest an immune-mediated vessel injury from tobacco

Division of Vascular Surgery, University of Pittsburgh Medical Center, 200 Lothrop Street, Pittsburgh, PA 15213, USA
* Corresponding author. Division of Vascular Surgery, University of Pittsburgh Medical Center, 200 Lothrop Street, Suite A1011, Pittsburgh, PA 15213.
E-mail address: chaerra@upmc.edu

Surg Clin N Am 93 (2013) 833–875
http://dx.doi.org/10.1016/j.suc.2013.04.003
0039-6109/13/$ – see front matter © 2013 Elsevier Inc. All rights reserved.

exposure. Both smokers and patients with TAO show increased levels of tobacco glycoprotein compared with nonsmokers, and it has been shown that patients with the disease have increased urinary levels of a tobacco metabolite.[2,3] Chewing tobacco may also trigger exacerbations of the disease.[4] Cellular immunity likely plays a role, because endothelial deposition of circulating complexes has been described in this population.[5] In addition, humoral immunity seems to play a role in TAO, because anti-endothelial antibodies, anticollagen antibodies, cytoplasmic antineutrophil cytoplasmic antibodies (c-ANCA), perinuclear antineutrophil cytoplasmic antibodies (p-ANCA) as well as anticardiolipin antibodies have been identified in patients with TAO.[6–9] More recently, endothelial injury with associated antiendothelial cell antibodies has been shown in patients with Buerger disease in clinically unaffected vasculature.[10] There is increasing evidence of a genetic component to the disease, because patients with certain HLA haplotypes have a predisposition to Buerger disease.[2,11,12] The result is a usually episodic acute endarteritis, leading to arterial and venous thrombosis.

Clinical Presentation

The classic presentation is that of distal limb ischemia and digital gangrene in the male smoker in his 30s to 40s, although an increase in women has been described and has been attributed to increased prevalence of female smokers.[11] Although the disease usually manifests as acute ischemia in vessels distal to the popliteal and brachial arteries, involvement of proximal limb, mesenteric, cerebral, coronary, and pulmonary vasculature has been described.[13,14] Patients present with exacerbations of ischemic limb pain and acute ischemia on a background of claudication, resulting in multiple minor and major amputations. Superficial thrombophlebitis and Raynaud syndrome may be found in up to 50% of patients with TAO.[15,16]

Diagnosis

A thorough history and physical examination should be the cornerstone of establishing or, more frequently, excluding a diagnosis of Buerger disease. Patients tend to be young, nondiabetic, and nonhypertensive smokers presenting with palpable proximal pulses but distal limb ischemia without significant atherosclerosis risk factors or history of trauma. Recurrence of disease correlating with failed attempt at smoking cessation may also be a strong diagnostic indicator.

Imaging studies

Noninvasive vascular testing with 4-limb digital plethysmography can confirm the degree of limb ischemia, and if the diagnosis remains unclear or the symptoms severe or limb-threatening, diagnostic arteriography may reveal segmental, abrupt arterial occlusion distal to normal-appearing vessels; infrageniculate vessels may be symmetrically diseased, with characteristic corkscrew collaterals (**Fig. 1**).[17]

Diagnostic criteria systems

Several systems of diagnostic criteria have been developed for TAO, extending the traditional 1983 Shionoya criteria, by which the following 5 findings are necessary for diagnosis: (1) smoking history, (2) onset before age 50 years, (3) infrapopliteal arterial occlusive lesions, (4) either upper limb involvement or phlebitis migrans, and (5) absence of atherosclerotic risk factors other than smoking.[18–20] Mills and Porter developed a set of criteria that include noninvasive vascular testing, and the Japanese Ministry of Health and Welfare Criteria mandates both noninvasive and angiographic findings.[15,21,22] Regardless, it is widely accepted that atherosclerosis and vasculitides of other causes as well as traumatic and embolic causes must be excluded to diagnose Buerger disease. Mills suggests as part of the diagnostic workup to consider a

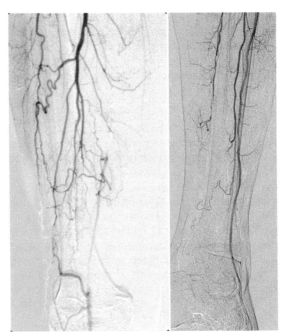

Fig. 1. (*Left*) A 60 year-old man with claudication. Angiography shows corkscrew collaterals at the level of the thigh. (*Right*) A 53-year-old man with a history of digital amputations presenting with acute limb ischemia. Angiography shows corkscrew collaterals of the tibial vessels.

complete blood count, liver function panel, metabolic panel and lipid panel as a metabolic baseline, erythrocyte sedimentation rate (ESR) to rule out necrotizing arteritis, antinuclear antibodies and rheumatoid factor to evaluate for autoimmune vasculitis, anticentromere antibodies to screen for CREST syndrome, Scl-70 to screen for scleroderma, VDRL (Venereal Disease Research Laboratory) test to rule out syphilitic vasculitis, and a hypercoagulation screen (protein C, S, and antithrombin III levels, antiphospholipid antibody and factor V Leiden).[21] Any history of intravenous (IV) drug abuse should also be carefully considered and a drug screen performed in these cases.[10] Surgical biopsy of affected tissue may be confirmative, but usually unnecessary.

Treatment

Risk factor reduction
It has long been observed that abstinence from tobacco remains the most effective means of preventing exacerbations and progression of ischemia and gangrene. Patients should be firmly counseled that recidivism will likely lead to minor and major amputation. It has also been recently suggested that substitution of chewing tobacco for smoking is insufficient to prevent disease progression and amputation.[4]

Medical management
The prostacyclin analogue iloprost may offer some symptomatic relief as well as improving ulcer healing.[21,23,24] A prospective study of 133 randomized patients with TAO compared iloprost with low-dose aspirin and showed higher rates of complete

ischemic symptom resolution in the iloprost arm (63% vs 28% in the aspirin arm) as well as higher rates of complete ulcer healing (35% in iloprost arm vs 13% in aspirin arm).[23] Bone marrow transplant as a means of stimulating angiogenesis to augment collateral circulation has been met with mixed results.[10,24–26] Local wound care and management of infection and thrombophlebitis should be addressed in a standard manner.

Surgical management

Therapeutic angiogenesis was first described by Ilizarov in 1992[27] through the use of horizontal distraction tibial osteotomy as a means of stimulating neoangiogenesis in patients with TAO with grade III to IV ischemia. A 10-year experience in surgical management of patients with Buerger disease by a group from Turkey[28] performing 161 sympathectomies and 19 bypasses showed 57.9% secondary bypass patency at 5.4 years and an overall 95.6% limb salvage rate within that time frame. This group published similar results in a different 216 patient cohort 11 years earlier.[28] Although bypass is challenging because of lack of healthy distal targets, a recent study from an interventional cardiology group in Italy used endovascular recanalization of tibial and pedal arteries in 17 consecutive patients with Buerger disease presenting with Rutherford grade 3 to 5 critical limb ischemia, showing 100% 23-month amputation-free survival.[29] Technical success was achieved in 19 of 20 limbs treated (95%), with a 100% limb salvage rate and clinical improvement in 16 of 19 limbs (84%) at a mean 23-month follow-up.[29] One study reported successful catheter-directed thrombolysis with concomitant antiinflammatory infusion in 13 patients with grade III to IV arterial insufficiency.[30] Despite more than 100 years of study in the diagnosis and treatment of this disease, amputation rate remains as high as 20% in North America; however, mortality has remained stable.[14]

VASCULITIDES

Takayasu Autoimmune Arteritis (a Large-Vessel Giant Cell Arteritis)

Takayasu arteritis (TA) is a rare syndrome characterized by inflammation of the aortic arch, pulmonary, coronary, and cerebral vessels, predominantly presenting as stroke, transient ischemic attack (TIA), myocardial infarction (MI), and upper extremity claudication in women in their 20s to 40s.[31] The pulseless disease was first described in 1830, and was later named after Mikito Takayasu, a Japanese ophthalmologist, in 1908.[31,32]

Pathogenesis

There is increasing evidence to suggest that the histologic panarteritis characteristic of TA is primarily a cell-mediated autoimmune phenomenon, with cellular infiltration of macrophages and CD4+ and CD8+ T cells.[33,34] More recently, adaptive and innate immunity have also been ascribed a role in its pathogenesis.[35] The vasa vasorum are first affected, leading to inflammatory infiltration of the adventitia, with subsequent involvement of the media and intima.[36,37] Acute disease may lead to intimal thrombosis and stenosis. As the inflammation subsides, fibrosis may develop in an irregular skip lesion pattern, with different areas of the affected vessel in different stages of inflammation and resolution.[36] Stenotic lesions similar to those in atherosclerotic disease often subsequently develop, albeit with significant medial destruction and fibrosis and periadventitial fibrosis.[37,38] In addition, acute disease may lead to luminal thrombosis. Pathologic examination has shown inflammation and destruction of arterial smooth muscle and elastic media, which may lead to aneurysmal degeneration.[31,39]

Clinical presentation

The natural history of TA is characterized by a background of chronic, vague constitutional symptoms (eg, myalgias, fevers), with the development of an acute inflammatory phase with subsequent occlusive cerebrovascular (cerebrovascular accident or TIA), coronary (MI), upper extremity, or mesenteric symptoms. In addition, the thoracic or abdominal aorta may be affected by dissection or aneurysmal degeneration.[40] The trajectory of symptoms can vary between patients, with as many as one-third to one-half presenting acutely without preceding constitutional symptoms.[17,41] A phase characterized by fibrosis and degeneration after an inflammatory phase leads to occlusive and occasional aneurysmal disease, with different phenotypic propensities in different geographic regions.[42–45] Takayasu disease in Japan usually presents with ischemic disease of the aortic arch vessels, whereas patients in Korea, India, and Thailand more frequently present with renovascular hypertension.[45,46] Women are more often affected than men (1.6:1 to 8:1), and Asian (particularly Japanese) and Latin American populations are more often affected compared with Western populations.[31,42,47–51] A retrospective study of 75 patients at the Cleveland Clinic found a pulse asymmetry in an extremity as the initial presentation in 57% of patients, with limb blood pressure discrepancy in 53% and a bruit in 53%.[52] There are several classifications of the anatomic distribution of disease in TA. The original Ueno classification system described disease of the arch and arch vessels (type I), descending thoracic and abdominal aorta and their branches (type II), a combination of arch and descending aorta and their branches (type III), with a later modification by Lupi-Herrera adding a type IV for pulmonary arterial involvement (**Table 1**).[53,54]

Diagnosis

The inconsistent and variable presentation of TA and the relative rarity of the disease may delay diagnosis.[55] These patients may present with a background of constitutional symptoms, abdominal pain, and anorexia, with refractory hypertension (from renal stenosis and aortic coarctation) and an acute episode of cerebrovascular (particularly visual) or coronary insult or upper extremity claudication in an otherwise young and healthy patient.[17] The 1990 American College of Rheumatology (ACR) criteria, based on studies of North American patients with TA, was found to have a 90.5% sensitivity and 97.8% specificity when patients met at least 3 of 6 criteria (**Table 2**).[56] A 20-year prospective study at the National Institutes of Health found that ESR was increased in 72% of patients with active disease compared with 44% in patients in remission.[41] The study also found that vasculitis was identified in only 44% of surgical specimens (from the aortic arch, renal arteries, and femoral arteries), with operations performed during disease inactivity (**Fig. 2**).[41]

Table 1 Classification of TA with prevalence (Lupi-Herrera modification of original 1967 Ueno classification)		
Type	**Anatomic Areas Affected**	**Prevalence (%)**
I	Arch and its branches	8.4
II	Descending aorta and its branches	11.2
III	Arch and descending aorta and branches	65.4
IV	Pulmonary artery involvement	15

Data from Lupi-Herrera E, Sanchez-Torres G, Marcushamer J, et al. Takayasu's arteritis. Clinical study of 107 cases. Am Heart J 1977;93(1):94–103.

Table 2	
American College of Rheumatology diagnostic criteria for Takayasu Arteritis (1990)	
Criteria (3 of 6 Required to Make Diagnosis)	
Age at disease onset	Symptoms or signs of TA before 40 years of age
Claudication	Upper or lower extremity fatigue with exercise
Diminished brachial pulse	Unilateral or bilateral diminished brachial pulse on examination
Asymmetric brachial blood pressure (BP)	>10 mm Hg difference between brachial systolic BP
Bruit	Audible over aorta or either subclavian artery
Angiographic abnormalities	Narrowing or occlusion of aorta, aortic branches or large arteries in upper extremities, usually focal or segmental. Must not be secondary to atherosclerosis, fibromuscular dysplasia, or other causes

From Arend WP, Michel BA, Bloch DA, et al. The American College of Rheumatology 1990 criteria for the classification of Takayasu arteritis. Arthritis Rheum 1990;33(8):1129–34.

Imaging studies Arteriography, computed tomography angiography (CTA) and, increasingly, magnetic resonance angiography (MRA) and duplex ultrasonography should be targeted to the anatomic area of clinical suspicion.[57–60] CTA and MRA may show aortic wall thickening in TA; as the disease progresses, angiography identifies luminal stenosis, occlusion, or aneurysmal changes.[61]

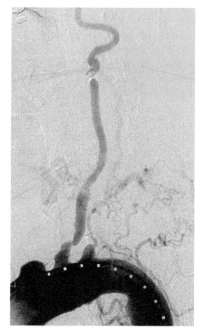

Fig. 2. A 50-year-old woman with TA presenting with symptomatic left carotid stenosis and history of stroke. The innominate and left subclavian arteries are occluded.

Treatment

Medical management

Immunosuppression in the form of corticosteroids (CS) is the mainstay of treatment in the acute phase, and recent evidence has shown that agents such as azathioprine, mycophenolate mofetil, and methotrexate may also be useful in inducing remission.[62] Even with adjunctive immunosuppressive agents, steroid-free remission has been shown to be limited; in a retrospective study from the Cleveland Clinic, only 28% of 75 patients were able to be steroid-free for more than 6 months.[52] Multiple trials are under way to determine the role of the anti–tumor necrosis factor α (anti-TNF-α) in treating TA, with promising results in sustaining steroid-free remission.[62,63]

Surgical management

Surgical treatment depends on whether the patient develops aneurysmal or ischemic disease. Timing of surgical intervention has been shown to be important, because long-term patency tends to be higher when surgery is performed with the disease in a quiescent phase.[64,65] A recent single-institution retrospective review over 16 years found that 10% of patients with TA with supra-aortic arterial disease required surgical intervention, and that surgical bypass had superior primary patency compared with endovascular intervention (87% vs 47%, with stenosis defined as a 50% or greater lesion) at median 23-month follow-up.[66] A retrospective study at the Cleveland Clinic examined 75 patients treated for TA.[52] Of the 20 patients treated with percutaneous angioplasty (PTA), 18 were successfully treated, with recurrent stenosis in 14 of the 18 (78%) at 3 years. Of the 44 surgical bypasses performed in 17 patients, 36% developed recurrent stenosis in 3 years, and all but 1 of the recurrences required reintervention. A cohort of 60 patients with TA was also studied at the National Institutes of Health between 1970 and 1990.[41] Fifty bypass procedures were performed in 23 patients and 20 percutaneous angioplasties were performed on 11 patients. Of those receiving surgical bypass, a 28% restenosis or occlusion rate was noted at 5.3 years. In contrast, in the group treated with endovascular interventions, there was a 44% restenosis or occlusion rate within the same time frame, again highlighting the high recurrence rate of all types of interventions, albeit with an increased durability of surgical revascularization (**Tables 3** and **4**).

In response to the Cleveland Clinic's 2007 study, which found a high (78%) restenosis rate in the PTA group (10 treated with stents, 10 with angioplasty alone), a more recent study at the Cleveland Clinic retrospectively reviewed 4 patients with TA, each with more than 1 vascular bed treated with covered stents.[68] The study showed improved patency, with no restenosis at 4 years. The group postulates that excluding the intimal surface of the diseased vessel with a covered stent may mitigate the inflammation and restenosis.[68] A study published in 2011 from the University of Southern California analyzed 40 patients with TA who underwent a total of 60 bypasses and 4 percutaneous interventions.[67] At a mean follow-up of 6.4 years, 16 patients (40%) required additional intervention. Twelve had developed either recurrence or progression in the treated vascular bed, and 13 had developed disease in a different vascular bed, requiring treatment. The results of the study emphasized the importance of lifelong surveillance for patients with TA requiring surgical intervention.

Mortality and morbidity

There is considerable geographic variation in long-term (10-year) mortality, ranging from 80% in India to 97% in North America and Japan.[42,52,69–71] Fifteen-year follow-up of a Japanese cohort has shown that mortality has improved from 80%

Table 3
Open surgical bypass for TA, selected studies

Reference	Number of Procedures/ Patients	Follow-Up (Y, Mean)	Restenosis/ Occlusion (%)	Perioperative Morbidity (% of Procedures)	Perioperative Mortality (N)
Kerr et al,[41] 1994[a]	50/23	5.3	28[b]	30[c]	0
Maksimowicz-McKinnon et al,[52] 2007[d]	44/17[e]	3	36[f]	N/A[g]	2 (early)
Ham et al,[67] 2011[h]	55/31	6.4	32	N/A	N/A
Kim et al,[66] 2012[i]	20/15	3.3	13[j]	26[k]	1 (>30 d)

Abbreviation: N/A, not applicable.
  [a] 12 common carotid, 10 axillosubclavian, 7 iliofemoral, 7 renal, 6 coronary bypasses.
  [b] Author describes 24% restenosis, 4% thrombosis.
  [c] Complications in 14/39 (36%) of synthetic graft bypasses, 1/11 (9%) of autologous bypasses.
  [d] Aneurysmal disease: 7 aortic root, 1 descending aorta, 1 axillary; stenotic disease: 7 carotid, 3 axillary, 5 subclavian, 12 coronary, 2 mesenteric, 5 renal, 1 iliofemoral.
  [e] 46% of open surgical procedures followed failed intervention.
  [f] Author describes 36% restenosis/occlusion.
  [g] Author describes 2 perioperative deaths but does not describe perioperative complications.
  [h] Author describes 31 renal revascularization procedures, 7 aortobi-iliac/femoral bypasses, 3 infrarenal aortic replacements, 1 aortoaortic bypass, 1 ascending aortic replacement, 7 aortocarotid bypasses, 1 femoroaxillary bypass (cerebrovascular), 4 upper extremity bypasses. 5 nephrectomies were not included in this table. Total mortality and morbidity were not discussed.
  [i] 19 aortic arch vessel bypasses, 2 with coronary bypass, 1 with arch replacement, 1 with aortic valve replacement.
  [j] 1 restenosis and 2 occlusions developed in 24 arteries.
  [k] 2 patients with cerebral hyperperfusion and hemorrhage, 1 patient with cardiac tamponade, 1 patient with hemodynamically unstable bradycardia.

Table 4
Endovascular interventions for TA, selected studies

Reference	Number of Procedures/ Patients	Follow-up (Y, Mean)	Restenosis/ Occlusion (%)
Kerr et al,[41] 1994[a]	20/11	5.3	44[b]
Maksimowicz-McKinnon et al,[52] 2007[c]	20/20	3	78[d]
Ham et al,[67] 2011[e]	4/4	6.4	75
Kim et al,[66] 2012[f]	15/10	3.3	53

  [a] 8 subclavian, 7 renal, 4 iliofemoral, 1 thoracic aorta.
  [b] Restenosis occurred at 3.5–13.6 months. 33% success at reintervention.
  [c] Stenotic vessels treated: 1 abdominal aorta, 2 carotid, 2 axillary, 4 subclavian, 1 coronary, 8 renal, 2 iliofemoral; 10 with stents. Author does not specify which lesions were treated with stent versus percutaneous transluminal angioplasty (PTA).
  [d] 14 of 18 initially successful PTA procedures developed restenosis; 13 of these required reintervention.
  [e] 4 renal PTAs were performed, 3 of which required additional procedures.
  [f] 1 carotid PTA, 4 subclavian PTA, 1 external carotid PTA, 1 vertebral PTA, 3 carotid stents, 2 successful subclavian stents, 2 failed subclavian stents, 1 vertebral stent.

between 1957 and 1975 to 96% between 1976 and 1990.[72] In that study, subgroup analysis showed that 15-year survival was significantly reduced with age (58% for >35 years vs 93% for ≤35 years), presence of complicated disease (66% vs 96% without complications), and progressive course of disease (68% vs 93% with a stable course). Morbidity may be significant, because up to two-thirds may struggle with activities of daily living and one-fourth may be unable to work.[52]

Giant Cell Arteritis (a Large Vessel Arteritis)

Giant cell arteritis (GCA), is a systemic granulomatous large-vessel vasculitis preferentially affecting the extracranial carotid arteries. When the disease affects the temporal arteries, it is called temporal arteritis; however, the two are often used interchangeably. It is also known as Horton disease.[73] GCA and Takayasu arteritis may exist as different phenotypic expressions along the spectrum of a single disease process.[74,75] However, GCA presents with a different epidemiologic pattern, usually affecting Caucasians and women in their fifth decade or later.[17,76] Aortic and branch vessel disease is present in both patients with Giant cell arteritis and Takayasu arteritis.

Pathogenesis

The cause of disease is not completely understood but there likely exists a combination of environmental, infectious, and genetic factors.[76] Like in TA, an inflammatory infiltrate of macrophages and T lymphocytes results in a panarteritis.[77] There is also a component of neoangiogenesis and proliferation of vasa vasorum, which contributes to the proinflammatory state and intimal hyperplasia.[77,78] The sequence of inflammation and injury leads to intimal proliferation and occlusion, although medial destruction caused by matrix metalloproteinase proteolysis may result in stenotic lesions or aneurysmal disease after vascular remodeling.[77,79] On pathologic examination, the presence of giant cells is pathognomonic, found in approximately 50% of cases, but this finding is not required to make the diagnosis.[39,76]

Clinical presentation

Similar to TA, GCA may have a variable clinical presentation. Patients may report a history of vague constitutional symptoms, which may include fever, myalgia, headache, weight loss, and diplopia or loss of visual acuity.[80] Polymyalgia rheumatica (PMR) has been shown to have an association with as many as 50% of patients with GCA, whereas 15% of patients with PMR have GCA.[81–83] Although temporal artery inflammation is the classic presentation, extracranial disease is becoming increasingly appreciated and may manifest as aortic arch or abdominal aortic aneurysmal disease (in up to 10% to 50% of cases) or stenotic disease of the axillary or subclavian arteries.[84–86] Although 75% of cases of GCA may be associated with extracranial disease, most of these cases may be clinically silent, as symptomatic disease was described in only 27% of all patients with GCA in a population study.[80,86] Symptomatic aortic disease presents in up to 10% to 15% of patients with GCA, and rupture may occur in up to one-third of this subset.[87–89]

Diagnostic Workup

Clinical diagnosis

An elderly patient presenting with new-onset headaches, visual changes, or jaw claudication in the background of constitutional symptoms such as fevers and myalgia merits evaluation for GCA.[17] There is a well-described association between PMR and GCA. A thorough history and physical examination, including ophthalmologic evaluation and extremity pulse examination, are vital. There are several possible mechanisms explaining the visual changes in GCA in addition to ischemic optic neuritis, which include retinal artery occlusion and retrobulbar neuritis; overall visual disturbances may occur in up to 50% of these patients.[17,90] The presence of 3 or more of the ACR criteria has a 94% sensitivity and 91% specificity (**Box 1**).[91]

Temporal artery biopsy

Temporal artery biopsy, although specific, is frequently unnecessary, particularly considering that it often does not change the course of management.[92] A 2002 meta-analysis of 21 studies[93] showed that 39% of temporal artery biopsies were positive while a normal ESR conveying a likelihood ratio (LR) of 0.2. That study showed that jaw claudication and diplopia carried a positive LR (4.2 and 3.4, respectively), as did temporal artery beading (4.6), prominence (4.3), and tenderness (2.6). Still, some argue that the ACR criteria without biopsy are only 75% sensitive.[94] Patients in whom the diagnosis is equivocal or the treatment may be intolerable may warrant a temporal artery biopsy. There has been much interest in determining the minimum length of artery needed. Multiple studies have suggested that a biopsy length of 1 cm may be sufficient.[95–97] Although a study from Johns Hopkins University showed that bilateral temporal artery biopsy has been shown to increase diagnostic yield by only 3%, a more recent study of 127 patients found a 13% increase in sensitivity with bilateral specimens.[98,99] One study[100] reported that histologically-proven GCA is more likely to be found in patients of greater age (77 vs 69 years old) or with a higher ESR (60 vs 40 mm/h). Treatment should not be delayed in waiting for a temporal artery biopsy, because the pathologic changes have been found to persist even 1 to 2 weeks after treatment initiation.[101] Of patients who receive temporal artery biopsies and do not respond to treatment, alternative diagnoses such as diabetes or neoplasms must be considered.[102]

Imaging studies

A study from Greece in 2006[103] reported the presence of temporal artery halo on ultrasonography to yield 82% sensitivity and 92% specificity if unilateral and 100% if

---

Box 1
ACR 1990 Criteria for GCA[a]

1. Age at disease onset 50 years or older

   Development of symptoms or findings beginning at age 50 years or older

2. New headache

   New onset of or new type of localized pain in the head

3. Temporal artery abnormality

   Temporal artery tenderness to palpation or decreased pulsation, unrelated to arteriosclerosis of cervical arteries

4. Increased ESR

   ESR 50 mm/h or greater by the Westergren method

5. Abnormal artery biopsy

   Biopsy specimen with artery showing vasculitis characterized by a predominance of mononuclear cell infiltration or granulomatous inflammation, usually with multinucleated giant cells

[a] The presence of 3 criteria are required to make the diagnosis.
From Hunder GG, Bloch DA, Michel BA, et al. The American College of Rheumatology 1990 criteria for the classification of giant cell arteritis. Arthritis Rheum 1990;33(8):1122–8.

bilateral, suggesting an attractive alternative to biopsy. [18F]fluorodeoxyglucose (FDG)-positron emission tomography (PET) has been shown to be a useful tool in the diagnosis and workup of GCA. One study found PET to have 56% sensitivity, 98% specificity, 93% positive predictive value, and 80% negative predictive value in diagnosing GCA or PMR.[104] However, a recent study found that the diagnostic accuracy of PET decreased from 93% to 65% after initiation of CS or immunosuppressive therapy.[105] Contrast-enhanced magnetic resonance imaging (MRI) showing mural inflammation and thickening of temporal arteries has been shown to be 81% sensitive and 97% specific.[106] MRI may also identify thickening of the occipital and cervical arteries, suggestive of inflammation.[107] PET may also be used to monitor post-treatment disease activity.[108,109]

Extracranial evaluation

Once a patient has been diagnosed with GCA, screening for extracranial disease may be prudent, considering that most extracranial disease may be clinically silent.[80,86] MRA and 18-FDG PET have been shown to have a role in screening for this group of patients, with PET more likely to show active inflammation and ability to differentiate from atherosclerotic changes compared with MRA.[80,110,111] Ultrasonography may also be a useful modality in screening for extracranial disease.[110,112,113] CTA was shown to be less effective than duplex in evaluating aneurysmal disease in these patients.[114] The importance of surveillance is becoming increasingly recognized, because aortitis in this population may carry an increased risk for mortality and stroke.[111,115]

Treatment

Medical management

CS play a primary role in the treatment of GCA and should be initiated as soon as the clinical diagnosis is made. The ACR has recommended a starting dose of 40 to 60 mg daily until symptom resolution and ESR normalization (usually around 4 weeks), then over the next 6 months tapered to 10 mg daily.[84,116] A lower maintenance dose should be continued thereafter for up to 2 years. Steroids may induce remission in up to 75% of patients, with intravenous CS induction potentially shortening time to remission.[117] Adjunctive treatment with methotrexate may reduce symptom recurrence compared with CS treatment alone.[118,119] Treatment should be initiated early to prevent vision loss, with parenteral CS potentially more effective than enteral in the setting of acute vision loss.[90,120] Only 5% to 7% of patients recover visual acuity, even with prompt treatment.[90] Use of low-dose aspirin may be considered as a preventive measure.[84]

Surgical management

Surgical treatment is usually reserved for management of aortic aneurysmal disease, clinically significant stenosis or occlusion of extracranial vessels that has failed CS treatment.[84] Data supporting surgical or endovascular treatment of GCA is limited primarily to case reports and small series. Carotid to axillary and brachial bypass has been described effectively treating subclavian occlusion after failure of medical management.[73,121] A single-center experience from Germany described 8 patients with GCA with various occlusive arterial lesions (including arch, extremity, and renal vessels) treated with PTA or stent and reported 67.6% primary patency and 74.4% secondary patency at a mean follow-up of 12 months.[122]

Polyarteritis Nodosa (a Medium-Vessel Arteritis)

Polyarteritis nodosa (PAN) is an uncommon systemic inflammatory syndrome characterized by necrotizing arteritis resulting in focal aneurysmal degeneration, particularly affecting the visceral, renal, and soft tissue vasculature. Kussmaul and Maier first described the entity in 1866.[123] The formal distinction between PAN and microscopic polyangiitis (MPA) was made at the Chapel Hill Consensus Conference in 1994.[124]

Pathogenesis and epidemiology

PAN is a rare disorder that affects men more often than women and occurs primarily in patients in their 40s to 60s.[125] PAN can be idiopathic, secondary to viral infection, or associated with a neoplastic process, each with a different natural history. Most cases are idiopathic. Hepatitis B virus (HBV), hepatitis C virus, and human immunodeficiency virus have each been implicated in the pathogenesis of the infectious form, which accounts for one-third of all cases.[126–128] The incidence of PAN has decreased as hepatitis vaccination has become more common.[129] It is suspected that viral antigens trigger the complement cascade, resulting in the neutrophil and lymphocyte-rich infiltrate within the arterial media as well as eventual fibrosis, thrombosis, or aneurysmal degeneration.[76]

Clinical presentation

Although our understanding of the pathogenesis is limited, different subtypes of clinical presentation have been well described, which include a generalized systemic form and a cutaneous form. Although constitutional symptoms, such as fever, myalgias, and weight loss, are found in up to 93% of cases, end-organ dysfunction as a result of malperfusion is the most profound and disabling manifestation of the disease.[130] Organ ischemia is usually the result of visceral microaneurysmal disease, and associated arterial branch occlusion, with one or both present in up to 40% to 90% of patients with PAN.[131,132] The kidneys are most commonly affected, with up to 66% of patients with renal microaneurysms, often presenting with areas of renal cortical infarction.[130] Hypertension, as a result of renal injury, presents in up to 35% of cases.[130] Renal biopsy typically shows histologic evidence of PAN in up to 70% of cases.[130] Abdominal pain is found in up to 36% of cases, and is attributed to mesenteric arterial branch occlusion more often than aneurysmal rupture.[130] There have been numerous case reports of neuro-ophthalmologic disease as the presenting symptom of PAN.[133,134] Neurologic symptoms are common, found in up to 79% of cases, particularly in the form of peripheral neuropathy.[130] Cutaneous involvement, such as purpura, urticaria, tender subcutaneous nodules, or ulcerating livedo reticularis, is found in up to 50% of cases.[130,135,136]

Diagnosis

The 1990 ACR guidelines require at least 3 of 10 criteria to diagnose PAN, with an 82.2% sensitivity and 86.6% specificity (**Table 5**).[137] Because of the difficulty in reproducing the sensitivity and specificity originally stated, the ACR diagnostic guidelines were called into question.[138–140] In 2008, an updated set of diagnostic criteria was proposed based on the French Vasculitis Study Group (FVSG) database, with HBV positivity, arteriographic abnormalities, and neuropathy as positive predictors and ANCA positivity, asthma, upper aerodigestive signs, cryoglobulin positivity, and glomerulopathy as negative predictors.[141] Combined, a sensitivity of 70.6% and specificity of 92.3% for all PAN cases and 76.6% and 88.9% for HBV-negative PAN has been reported.[141] A study from Colombia[142] evaluated patients who were biopsied to evaluate for suspected vasculitis, and of 165,556 biopsy specimens, only 0.18% were positive. Of the positive specimens, 65% were obtained from skin, 12% from amputated extremities, and 8% from muscle. This finding reinforces the fact that a thorough history and physical examination coupled with a high degree of clinical suspicion are critical in making the diagnosis, with or without a biopsy. The involvement of the vascular surgeon is likely to be in patients with end-organ damage with either symptomatic or incidentally discovered visceral aneurysms, or renal failure.

Table 5
ACR criteria for the classification of PAN

Criterion (3 or More Are Necessary)	Definition
Weight loss ≥4 kg	Loss of ≥4 kg of body weight since the illness began, not caused by dieting or other factors
Livedo reticularis	Mottled reticular pattern over the skin in portions of the extremities or torso
Testicular pain or tenderness	Pain or tenderness of the testicles not caused by infection, trauma, or other causes
Myalgias, weakness, or leg tenderness	Diffuse myalgias (excluding shoulder and hip girdle), weakness of muscles, or tenderness of leg muscles
Mononeuropathy or polyneuropathy	Development of mononeuropathy, multiple mononeuropathies, or polyneuropathy
Diastolic BP >90 mm Hg	Development of hypertension with the diastolic BP >90 mm Hg
Increased blood urea nitrogen (BUN) or creatinine	BUN >40 mg/dL (14.3 mmol/L) or creatinine >1.5 mg/dL (114 μmol/L), not caused by dehydration or obstruction
Hepatitis B virus	Presence of hepatitis B surface antigen or antibody in serum
Arteriographic abnormality	Arteriogram showing aneurysms or occlusions of the visceral arteries, not caused by arteriosclerosis, fibromuscular dysplasia, or other noninflammatory causes
Biopsy of small or medium-sized artery containing polymorphonuclear lymphocytes	Histologic changes showing the presence of granulocytes or granulocytes and mononuclear leukocytes in the artery wall

From Lightfoot RW Jr, Michel BA, Bloch DA, et al. The American College of Rheumatology 1990 criteria for the classification of polyarteritis nodosa. Arthritis Rheum 1990;33(8):1088–93.

Radiographic findings Angiography has a sensitivity of 89% and specificity of 90% in diagnosing PAN, as determined in a study of 156 patients who had received traditional angiography with suspected vasculitis.[143] The study found a positive predictive value of only 55% but a negative predictive value of 98%. An observational study from the Mayo Clinic examined 56 patients with PAN with angiography and found that 48% had aneurysmal lesions, 12% had ectatic lesions, and 98% of patients had either stenosis or occlusion, including all but one of the patients with aneurysmal or ectatic disease.[132] A total of 39% had occlusive lesions without aneurysms. CTA may show these lesions equally well, with multidetector whole-body computed tomography (CT) as a proposed solution to identify multifocal lesions (**Fig. 3**).[144,145]

Treatment

Medical management
Treatment strategy for PAN has evolved with our understanding of its different causes. A flare of PAN should be treated with pulse intravenous CS (ie, 15 mg/kg methylprednisolone daily for 1–3 days), followed with a high-dose regimen of CS for 2 to 3 weeks (ie, 1 mg/kg daily).[146,147] Plasmapheresis should be subsequently used to remove circulating immune complexes if the patient has HBV-associated PAN.[76,148–152] Hepatitis infection should be treated with antiviral agents, such as lamivudine for HBV.

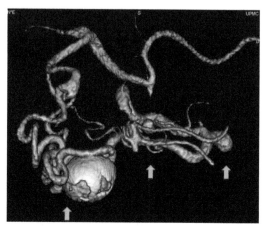

Fig. 3. A three-dimensional reconstruction from CTA performed on a 50-year-old woman presenting with abdominal pain with suspected PAN. There are multiple visceral aneurysms (*arrows*).

Even with appropriate treatment, relapse after medical management may be as high as 20% to 40%.[147,153]

The use of adjunctive immunomodulating agents such as cyclophosphamide or azathioprine has been critically investigated for decades and has generated a significant amount of often-conflicting data. In a 1979 study,[154] the addition of the cytotoxin cyclophosphamide to CS was shown to improve prognosis in relapsing cases of vasculitis. In contrast, in 1980, Cohen[155] found no difference in outcomes when cyclophosphamide was added to CS in patients with polyarteritis.

A prospective study in 1991 compared patients with PAN treated with corticosteroids and plasmapheresis with CS, plasmapheresis, and cyclophosphamide, and found no difference in 10-year survival (72% and 75%, respectively).[156] However, the cyclophosphamide arm did have lower disease relapse. Nevertheless, cyclophosphamide has been associated with multiple complications including hemorrhagic cystitis, bone marrow suppression, and even bladder and hematologic malignancies.[157,158] In an effort to study the prognostic factors for PAN (and other vasculitides) in light of the increasing number of potentially morbid treatment modalities, the FVSG developed the Five Factor Score (FFS).[146] Through multivariate analysis, it was shown that the presence of certain factors could predict mortality: a serum creatinine level greater than 1.58 g/dL, proteinuria level greater than 1 g daily, gastrointestinal bleeding (or infarction, perforation, or pancreatitis), central nervous system involvement, or cardiomyopathy. Each of these factors is given a point and the total is the FFS. A 46% 5-year mortality was observed in patients with an FFS of 2 and 12% mortality in patients with a score of 0.[146,153] The scoring system introduced the concept of severity-targeted treatment as well as the concept of vasculitides of different severities having different natural histories and responses to treatment.

In an analysis of 4 prospective trials totaling 278 patients, it was shown that the addition of cyclophosphamide to CS significantly prolonged estimated survival in patients with FFS 2 or greater, to approximately 70% compared with 55% at 60 months.[159] In contrast, patients with an FFS of 0 or 1 showed no difference in mortality with the addition of cyclophosphamide to their CS regimens. CS alone maintained remission in only 40% of cases of PAN with FFS of 0, and either azathioprine or cyclophosphamide was effective in treating relapses or CS-resistant disease.[147]

A French multicenter prospective randomized trial treated 58 low-prognostic-risk (ie, without severe end-organ damage) patients with PAN with CS alone, finding that 22% of them had developed recurrence at a mean follow-up of 62 months.[147] This group was then treated with adjunctive immunosuppressants, randomized to either azathioprine or cyclophosphamide.[147] After a mean follow-up of 56 months, similar rates of sustained remission were achieved (4 of 9 patients treated with azathioprine and 5 of 10 patients treated with cyclophosphamide). In general, it seems that initial disease severity mirrors mortality and warrants more aggressive treatment.[159]

Surgical management

Surgical treatment of PAN is rarely necessary, and generally has been limited to the treatment of visceral aneurysms and their associated complications. A retrospective study from the Mayo Clinic compared 15 patients who underwent revascularization for chronic occlusive mesenteric vasculitis (4 with PAN) with 163 patients who were revascularized for atherosclerotic mesenteric ischemia and found similar freedom from symptoms (83% and 75%, respectively) and primary graft patency (83% vs 84%) at 22 months; however, the results did not reach statistical significance.[160] Acute mesenteric ischemia usually results in intestinal infarction, with its attendant high morbidity and mortality.[161,162] A retrospective study by the FVSG found 132 of 348 (38%) patients with PAN who presented with gastrointestinal symptoms, including abdominal pain (36%), bleeding (3%), and perforation (4%). Of the patients with gastrointestinal symptoms, 38 (14%) required surgery.[130] A percutaneous approach to treating visceral arterial disease caused by vasculitis is being increasingly described. There have been many reports of successful endovascular coil embolization of ruptured or bleeding hepatic artery aneurysms.[163–166] Massive gastrointestinal bleeding controlled with endovascular glue embolization has also been described.[167] A case report of bilateral cavernous internal carotid artery aneurysms attributed to PAN was treated successfully with endovascular stent and coil embolization.[168]

Kawasaki Disease (a Medium-Vessel Arteritis)

Kawasaki disease (KD) is a small-vessel and medium-vessel acute systemic vasculitis of young children, affecting multiple organs. The morbidity and mortality of the disease primarily stems from coronary artery aneurysms.[169] It was first described by Tomisaku Kawasaki in 1974 and is now the leading cause of acquired pediatric heart disease in North America and Japan.[170]

Pathogenesis and epidemiology

KD mainly affects children aged 6 months to 5 years, and patients with Asian descent have a strong predisposition over Caucasians.[171,172] The cause of KD is unclear, with an infectious cause long suspected and suggested by the IgA response and intracytoplasmic inclusion bodies that have been shown in KD.[173] Although multiple infectious agents have been implicated, including rotavirus, measles, *Pneumococcus*, and *Meningococcus* infection, investigations have failed to definitively identify any of these as a causative agent.[174–176] More recently, attention has turned toward an immunogenic cause of KD, with the presence of a genetic predisposition. Patients with active KD develop an IgA B-cell and CD8+ T-cell response with an initial neutrophil, then mononuclear and lymphocytic infiltrate.[177] This inflammatory cascade triggers enzymatic injury to the internal elastic lamina.[177–179] Although KD is characterized by a systemic vasculitis, the coronary arteries seem most prominently affected.[177] Matrix metalloproteinase remodeling develops over weeks to months, with intimal hyperplasia and neoangiogenesis, resulting in arterial fibrosis, stenosis, occlusion, and aneurysmal degeneration.[177] The epidemiologic patterns of KD suggest an underlying genetic predisposition that may allow the development of clinically significant disease. Along with other loci of susceptibility, ITPKC, a negative regulator of T-cell activation, is a gene polymorphism that has been associated with the development of KD.[180,181]

Clinical presentation

KD primarily affects children younger than 5 years, and presents as an acute febrile illness, followed by bilateral nonpurulent conjunctivitis, oromucosal inflammation, strawberry tongue, peripheral rash and, least commonly, cervical lymphadenopathy.[177] The febrile illness may be accompanied by arthralgia, gastrointestinal distress, or irreconcilability.[177] Development of coronary aneurysms, occurring in up to 15% to 25% of untreated patients, usually presents as an MI but may also manifest as sudden death, heart failure, or valvular insufficiency.[177] A retrospective review from Japan of 1100 patients with KD undergoing coronary catheterization found 262 to have coronary lesions, 165 patients with aneurysmal or dilated coronaries (15% of all patients), occlusion in 20 (2%), segmental stenosis in 15 (1%), and localized stenosis in 62 patients (6%).[182] Although uncommon, KD may present in adults with similar mucocutaneous symptoms, but more frequently with cervical lymphadenopathy (93% vs 15% in children), hepatitis (65% vs 10%), and arthralgia (61% vs 24%–38%).[183]

Diagnosis

If clinical features raise suspicion for KD, C-reactive protein (CRP) level and ESR should be obtained, and if abnormally high (CRP >3.0 mg/dL or ESR >40 mm/h), albumin, hemoglobin/hematocrit, alanine aminotransferase (ALT), platelets, white blood cell count and urine analysis should be added (**Table 6**).[177] If 3 or more of these supplemental laboratory tests meet diagnostic criteria, antiplatelet treatment should be initiated and transthoracic echocardiography performed. Even if 2 or fewer of the additional testing criteria are met, the patient should still undergo echocardiography to evaluate for coronary disease.[177] Echocardiography provides valuable anastomotic information, including coronary artery diameters.[184] The Japanese Ministry of Health criteria[177] defined a coronary artery diameter as abnormal if it was greater than 3 mm in a child younger than 5 years and greater than 4 mm in a child 5 years or older. However, a later study from Children's Hospital in Boston[185] found those criteria to misclassify certain patients' coronary dimensions as normal, and suggested a body-surface-area adjustment. MRA and ultrafast CT may also be used as a noninvasive means to assess proximal coronary anatomy.[186–190] Coronary catheterization and angiography provide the highest level of detail, showing stenoses, occlusions, and

Table 6	
Additional laboratory tests for KD if CRP or ESR is increased	
Albumin (g/dL)	≤3.0
Hemoglobin/hematocrit	Low for age
ALT	Increased for age
Platelets after 7 d (/mm^3)	≥450,000
White blood cells (/mm^3)	≥15,000
Urine white blood cells (cells/high-power field)	≥10

From Newburger JW, Takahashi M, Gerber MA, et al. Diagnosis, treatment, and long-term management of Kawasaki disease: a statement for health professionals from the Committee on Rheumatic Fever, Endocarditis and Kawasaki Disease, Council on Cardiovascular Disease in the Young, American Heart Association. Circulation 2004;110(17):2748.

formation of collaterals, and may be necessary in planning treatment.[177] Noninvasive imaging, including echocardiography, can also provide information regarding the presence of myocarditis, pericardial effusion, and aortic root dilatation.[177]

A more recent concept is incomplete KD, which is defined by a fever of 5 days or longer, and 2 to 3 clinical criteria, without an alternative explanation for the symptoms.[191] The implication of incomplete KD and how it applies to both the pediatric and adult population remains to be defined.

Treatment

Treatment guidelines for KD from the American Heart Association published in 1994[177] indicate treatment modalities based on severity of coronary artery involvement (**Table 7**).

Medical management

Once the diagnosis is made, the patient should be started on high-dose aspirin therapy (80–100 mg/kg/d, divided up into 4 doses).[177] The dose is decreased to 3 to 5 mg/kg daily once the patient has been afebrile for 48 to 72 hours. Concomitant IV immunoglobulin (IVIG) infusion, with an initial 2-g/kg dose, should be administered within the first 7 to 10 days of illness.[192] Patients at risk for Reye syndrome can be given clopidogrel rather than aspirin. It has been shown that, unlike IVIG, aspirin does not decrease the risk of aneurysm formation.[193–196] Even with timely treatment, up to 5% of patients may still develop coronary aneurysms, although most of these are transient.[197] Of the 10% of patients who do not initially respond to aspirin and IVIG, a second round of IVIG or a course of pulse CS has been shown to be of benefit.[198,199] It has been suggested that abciximab (an antiplatelet GPIIb/IIIa inhibitor) may induce aneurysmal remodeling and regression, although its effectiveness has not yet been proven.[200] Other promising agents include infliximab (an anti-TNF-α monoclonal antibody) and cyclophosphamide, although controlled studies are lacking.[199,201] An acute MI in the setting of KD may be an indication for intracoronary thrombolysis for coronary thrombosis, with subsequent warfarin therapy.[202]

Surgical management

Coronary angiography is indicated for coronary aneurysmal disease coupled with other tests suggesting myocardial ischemia (See **Table 7**).[177] Revascularization of obstructive coronary lesions may be achieved with traditional bypass or percutaneous intervention. Surgical revascularization has had better success than percutaneous intervention; a Japanese survey study evaluating 244 patients with KD who had undergone coronary artery bypass graft had patency rates at 5 and 10 years of 82% and 78% with arterial conduit and 63% and 36% with venous conduit.[203] A follow-up study[204] showed that 87% and 44% 20-year patency rates were achieved with internal mammary and saphenous vein conduit, respectively.

Small-Vessel Vasculitides (MPA, Churg-Strauss Syndrome, Wegener Granulomatosis)

MPA, Churg-Strauss syndrome (CSS) and Wegener granulomatosis (WG) are systemic inflammatory syndromes that affect vessels smaller than arteries, including arterioles, capillary beds, and venules.[205] Patients affected with these rare disorders are generally ANCA-positive and may present with a wide spectrum of clinical disease, frequently with pulmonary disease or renal dysfunction.[205,206]

History

Although Kussmaul and Maier first described periarteritis nodosa in 1866, it was not until the 1950s when appreciation for the spectrum of distinct small-vessel diseases

Table 7
American Heart Association treatment guidelines for KD

Risk Level	Extent of Disease	Medical Therapy	Follow-Up and Diagnostic Testing	Invasive Testing
I	No coronary artery changes at any stage of illness	None beyond first 6–8 wk	CV risk assessment, counseling at 5-y intervals	None
II	Transient coronary artery ectasia disappears within first 6–8 wk	None beyond first 6–8 wk	CV risk assessment, counseling at 5-y intervals	None
III	One small to medium-sized coronary artery aneurysm per major coronary artery	Low-dose aspirin (3–5 mg/kg daily) until aneurysm regression documented	Annual cardiology follow-up with echocardiogram and EKG, combined with CV risk assessment, counseling; stress test or myocardial perfusion scan every other year	Angiography if noninvasive tests suggest ischemia
IV	≥1 large or giant coronary artery aneurysm or multiple or complex aneurysms in the same coronary artery; no obstruction	Long-term antiplatelet (aspirin) therapy and coumadin (goal international normalized ratio 2–2.5) and LMWH (goal anti-Xa level 0.5–1 U/mL)	Echocardiogram and EKG every 6 mo; stress test or myocardial perfusion scan annually	First angiography at 6–12 mo after diagnosis or sooner if clinically indicated; repeat angiography if any clinical, laboratory or noninvasive tests suggest ischemia
V	Coronary arterial obstruction	Long-term low-dose aspirin; coumadin or LMWH if giant aneurysm persists; consider β-blockers to reduce myocardial oxygen consumption	Echocardiogram and EKG every 6 mo; stress test or myocardial perfusion scan annually	Angiography recommended to assess therapeutic options

Abbreviations: CV, cardiovascular; EKG, electrocardiography; LMWH, low-molecular-weight heparin.

Adapted from Newburger JW, Takahashi M, Gerber MA, et al. Diagnosis, treatment, and long-term management of Kawasaki disease: a statement for health professionals from the Committee on Rheumatic Fever, Endocarditis and Kawasaki Disease, Council on Cardiovascular Disease in the Young, American Heart Association. Circulation 2004;110(17):2764.

began to be developed.[123,207–210] In 1931, Klinger first described an inflammatory syndrome, which was eventually named after the observations of Wegener published in 1939.[211,212] Churg and Strauss[213] in 1951 described a group of patients with necrotizing vasculitis, eosinophilia, asthma, and necrotizing glomerulonephritis. It was not until the 1994 international consensus conference at Chapel Hill that MPA was formally recognized as an entity distinct from PAN.[124]

Pathogenesis

WG and CSS each are associated with a systemic necrotizing granulomatous inflammation of small vessels, whereas the vasculitis of MPA is nongranulomatous. Although the complete cause of the small-vessel vasculitides is not fully understood, the effects of ANCA play a critical role in the pathobiology and pathophysiology. Most patients with WG carry proteinase-3 (PR3)–specific ANCA, whereas the disease of patients with MPA and CSS is characterized by myeloperoxidase-specific ANCA.[214] There is evidence that circulating ANCA complexes trigger neutrophil activation and subsequent vascular damage from proteolysis and generation of reactive oxygen intermediates.[215,216] In addition to the inflammatory autoimmune effects of the ANCAs, there are genetic susceptibilities to each of these diseases, with certain HLA subtypes associated with each, and α_1-antitrypsin deficiency associated with WG.[95,217–221] There is also evidence that environmental toxins, particularly crystalline silica exposure, are associated with each of these vasculitides.[138,222–224] Although numerous studies exist, there is a lack of strong evidence for a causative role of medications or infectious agents in the small-vessel vasculitides.[206] Each of these disorders is likely influenced by multiple causes.

Epidemiology and clinical presentation

WG and MPA tend to affect adults in their 50s to 70s, whereas CSS presents in younger patients, aged in their 30s to 40s.[225–228] Like most of the vasculitides discussed here, the small-vessel diseases also present with constitutional symptoms, such as fever, malaise, and myalgias. However, underscoring the systemic effects on small vessels, musculoskeletal (arthralgias), cutaneous (purpura), gastrointestinal (abdominal pain), or neurologic (peripheral neuropathy) symptoms may be a part of the clinical constellation as well.[205] Perhaps the best-described signs and symptoms is the manner in which these 3 disorders affect the lungs and kidneys. Each of the 3 disorders affects the lungs, but each in a different manner. Alveolar hemorrhage is present in each, but whereas patients with MPA develop interstitial lung disease, patients with WG and CSS develop pulmonary parenchymal nodules and masses (attributable to granulomatous inflammation).[206] The acute inflammatory phase may evolve into parenchymal fibrosis or sclerosis or bronchitis obliterans.[229] Crescentic glomerulonephritis is characteristic in the small-vessel vasculitides, more frequently in MPA and WG than in CSS, and may be associated with frequency of ANCA positivity.[205,230] CSS generally presents in 3 stages: first with asthma and airway hypersensitivity, which may precede further disease progression by years, then a phase with characteristic eosinophilic tissue infiltration, which may or may not include necrotizing granulomata, then the development of small-vessel vasculitic changes.[206,231] The overall natural history of CSS seems to have 2 phenotypic presentations, depending on ANCA positivity. Whereas ANCA-positive CSS is characterized by glomerulonephritis, mononeuritis multiplex, and alveolar hemorrhage (traits consistent with small-vessel vasculitides), ANCA-negative CSS is characterized by heart and nonalveolar lung involvement.[230,232]

Diagnosis

There is no consensus on a standard diagnostic workup to differentiate between the small-vessel vasculitides. The systemic nature of inflammation in each of the 3 disorders may cause multiorgan disease; therefore, there is often a significant degree of overlap with many of the symptoms. A thorough history and physical examination must be correlated with laboratory and histopathologic findings when appropriate. Initial laboratory studies may include ANCA, antinuclear antibodies, complement, cryoglobulins, fecal blood, antibodies to hepatitis B and C, rheumatoid factor, azotemia, and a urinalysis to evaluate for hematuria and proteinuria.[205] Chest and sinus radiographs and CT scans may reveal the sequelae of pulmonary disease. Electromyography may identify peripheral neuropathy. Evidence of conditions that are known to cause vasculitis, such as drug hypersensitivity, infection, rheumatoid arthritis, systemic lupus erythematosus, cancer, and inflammatory bowel disease should be ruled out if there is clinical ambiguity.[205] Biopsy of skin, muscle, lung, or nerve may aid the diagnosis. Expected findings include a neutrophil-rich infiltrate in biopsy of skin lesions that have appeared in the past 24 to 48 hours, or crescentic pauci-immune glomerulonephritis on percutaneous renal biopsy.[205] In patients presenting with neuropathy, a superficial peroneal nerve biopsy may show a perineural arteritis; simultaneous peroneus brevis muscle biopsy may increase the diagnostic sensitivity (**Table 8**).[240]

Treatment

Treatment is primarily medical, with CS used for induction, maintenance, and relapse treatment. Corticosteroids, methotrexate, mycophenolate mofetil, and rituximab have each been shown to have a role as adjuvant treatment.[214,241,242] Concomitant alveolar hemorrhage with renal failure carries a mortality as high as 50% in ANCA-positive vasculitides.[243–245] Plasmapheresis in addition to CS has been shown to improve recovery of renal function in ANCA-positive vasculitides presenting with renal failure, with one study showing 75% freedom from dialysis at 2 years.[150,243,246] Plasmapheresis has also been shown to improve patient survival.[150,243,245–248] As a group, the small-vessel vasculitides show a 70% to 92% remission rate with CS treatment, with relapse risk correlating with PR3-antibody positivity and presence of lung disease.[249] Infection prophylaxis is an important consideration in the context of the immunosuppressive effects of these treatment regimens. Lung transplant has been described to treat life-threatening alveolar hemorrhage and respiratory failure.[250]

Treatment of microscopic polyarteritis

Without treatment, MPA (in a study before the distinction of MPA and PAN) carries a poor prognosis, with 5-year survival of 15% or less.[251,252] A study of 107 ANCA-positive patients (mostly with MPA)[236] showed an 8.7 relative risk of death at 2.5 years

Table 8
Differential diagnostic features of small-vessel vasculitides

Feature	MPA	WG	CSS
Signs and symptoms of small-vessel vasculitis[a]	+	+	+
IgA-dominant immune deposits	−	−	−
Cryoglobulins in blood and vessels	−	−	−
ANCA in blood	+ (50%–80%)	+ (85%)	+ (50%–70%)
Necrotizing granulomas	−	+	+
Asthma and eosinophilia	− (rare)	− (rare)	+
Pulmonary involvement	50%–70%	85%	40%–70%
Glomerulonephritis	90%	80%	10%–25%
Gastrointestinal involvement	30%	<5%	30%–50%

[a] All of these small-vessel vasculitides can manifest any or all of the shared features of small-vessel vasculitides, such as purpura, nephritis, abdominal pain, peripheral neuropathy, myalgias, and arthralgias. Each is distinguished by the presence and absence of certain specific features.
Data from Refs.[153,205,231,233–239]

in patients presenting with alveolar hemorrhage and a 5.6 times decrease in mortality in patients treated with cyclophosphamide in addition to CS for initial therapy compared with CS alone. In a cohort study from 1996,[253] remission rate of MPA (combined with patients with necrotizing glomerulonephritis) was shown to be higher (85 vs 56%) with dual treatment with CS and cyclophosphamide as primary therapy. Of the 77% of the MPA subset responding to initial treatment, relapse at 15 months was 32%. One study[247] also reported on 5 patients with MPA who received plasmapheresis in addition to CS and cyclophosphamide (CYC). Average pretreatment creatinine was 5.6 g/dL, and 4 of 5 were dialysis-free and attained remission after treatment.[247]

Treatment of WG

A prospective, single-center trial randomized 32 patients with WG to 2 groups: CS and CYC alone, and CS with CYC and plasmapheresis.[254] The study showed a 94% 1-year survival and a 56% 5-year survival, without a difference between the 2 groups. Freedom from dialysis was higher in the plasmapheresis group, and significant when initial serum creatinine was 2.85 mg/dL or greater. Methotrexate has also been shown to help attain remission in WG.[214] In an observational study, 7 patients with WG with alveolar hemorrhage and an average pretreatment creatinine of 4.7 mg/dL underwent plasmapheresis after CS and CYC.[247] Five of the 7 attained disease remission (3 complete and 2 partial) and freedom from dialysis; the 2 patients who did not reach remission continued to be hemodialysis dependent. Pulmonary findings regressed in all patients. Relapse risk in WG may be higher than in MPA or CSS, correlating with its higher rate of PR3-ANCA positivity and increased incidence of pulmonary involvement.[249]

Treatment of CSS

Over the past 3 decades, the FVSG has established a multinational database that has generated valuable evidence regarding the management of vasculitides. A prospective randomized trial of 71 patients with PAN or CSS showed that the addition of cyclophosphamide to CS and plasmapheresis decreased recurrence, but did not change 10-year survival (72%, compared with 75%); however, all patients received plasma exchange in addition to CS.[156] The FFS was originally developed to examine prognostic factors in patients with PAN and CSS, identifying increasing mortality in patients with 2 or more factors (53% mortality at 6 years) compared with 1 (31%) and the best prognosis in patients without any factors (14%) (see section on PAN treatment).[146]

RADIATION ARTERITIS

The injurious effect of radiation on soft tissue has been recognized since 1899, when Gassman described endothelial injury and proliferation in small vessels, leading to luminal narrowing.[255] As the use of radiotherapy continues to grow, a phenomenon that is increasingly recognized is the resultant arterial injury and occlusive disease in medium and large vessels.

Pathogenesis

Ionizing radiation damages radiosensitive endothelial cells, leading to intimal inflammation, fibrin deposition, and proliferation.[256] Medial fibrosis caused by injury to vasa vasorum develops in the weeks after the more immediate intimal changes.[256,257] The resultant lesion is radiographically and grossly similar to an atherosclerotic lesion, albeit with adjacent nonirradiated vessels spared.[256,258] However, there is a histopathologic difference between radiation-induced and atherosclerotic lesions.[259,260] The perivascular fibrosis that develops over decades is believed to limit the formation of effective collaterals.[261] As little as 20 to 80 Gy may produce a luminal narrowing, and 39.5 to 80 Gy may be sufficient to produce a lesion in the iliofemoral system.[262,263]

Clinical Presentation

The natural history of radiation arteritis (RA) of larger vessels spans at least 2 to 3 decades, with development of mural thrombosis within the first 5 years, fibrotic lesions in the first decade after exposure, and a later more extensive fibrosis resembling atherosclerosis after the second or third decade.[257] Because the head/neck and pelvis are areas where radiosensitive malignancies frequently develop, the carotid and iliofemoral arterial beds are commonly affected by radiation therapy. The pattern of disease in these beds seems to be dependent on what areas are irradiated. Radiation exposure has been shown to increase significant (>70%) carotid artery stenoses 5-fold (22% vs 4% of age-matched and risk-matched controls) and these lesions are twice as likely as nonradiation associated lesions to be associated with neurologic deficits (80% of these lesions were symptomatic).[264,265] In addition, upper extremity ischemia from axillosubclavian arterial stenosis may result from external-beam radiation therapy for breast cancer or axillary lymphoma.[266,267] Aortoiliac and femoral disease results from pelvic irradiation and either presents as de novo isolated stenotic lesions and lower extremity ischemia over the span of 1 to 2 decades, or as an exacerbation of existing atherosclerotic disease.[161,268] Rarely, RA lesions may develop aneurysmal degeneration, and this has been described in the carotid as well as femoral beds.[269–271]

Diagnosis

A detailed history and physical examination combined with judicious use of imaging studies are necessary to identify RA. Underlying atherosclerotic disease may confound the picture, particularly in elderly patients. An acute exacerbation of ischemic disease in a previously irradiated area should also generate suspicion. Angiography and CTA are expected to show a region of arterial disease that appears atherosclerotic in a previously irradiated field, but with normal or less-affected adjacent vessels (**Fig. 4**).

Treatment

In general, whether patients with RA present with thromboembolic, occlusive, or aneurysmal disease, the treatment should be tailored to the lesion and the area affected.[270] The evidence describing treatment of RA lesions is varied but most has focused on carotid lesions. It has been suggested that radiation-associated arterial lesions represent a clinicopathologic entity distinct from atherosclerosis; histopathologic studies have shown a difference between RA-associated and atherosclerotic carotid plaques.[260] The Mayo Clinic performed a retrospective review[272] of 60 patients treated for radiation-induced carotid artery stenosis (33 with stenting with embolic protection and 27 with open repair) and found similar freedom from restenosis (80% surgery vs 72% stenting) but higher survival at 7 years (75% vs 29%) in the surgery group. Indications for treatment in patients undergoing surgery or stenting were similar; in the operative group, 16 patients (44%) had asymptomatic lesions with greater than 80% stenosis and 20 (56%) had symptomatic stenosis greater than 50%, compared with 18 (49%) asymptomatic patients and 19 (51%) symptomatic patients in the stenting group. In the open repair group, 36 lesions were treated, 29 (80%) of which were amenable to carotid endarterectomy (CEA), 5 (14%) required interposition, and 2 (6%) were treated with bypass. At 30 days, there was 1 stroke (3%) in the operative group and 2 strokes (6%) in the carotid artery stenting (CAS) group, and no periprocedural

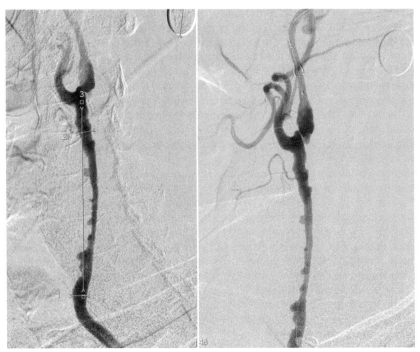

Fig. 4. A 61-year-old man being followed for bilateral carotid stenosis 10 years after radiation therapy for squamous cell carcinoma of the tongue. Angiography shows long segments of severe stenosis.

mortality in either. There were 2 MIs (6%), 6 cranial nerve injuries (17%), and 3 wound complications (8%) in the operative group and none of these complications in the stenting group. A recent meta-analysis from the Netherlands[273] examined the outcomes of 533 radiation-associated carotid lesions that were treated (361 CAS and 172 CEA) and reported comparable cardiovascular adverse event rates (3.9% for CAS vs 3.5% for CEA). The long-term restenosis rate (an average 5.4 per 100 person-years) and cerebrovascular event rate (4.9 per 100 person-years) were higher in the endovascular group compared with the surgical group (2.8 restenoses per 100 person-years and 2.8 cerebrovascular events per 100 person-years).[273]

There is some disparity in the outcomes of endovascular stenting for radiation-associated carotid disease compared with the outcomes of stenting for atherosclerotic disease. A recent study[274] compared results of carotid stenting in 28 patients who had received cervical radiation therapy with 182 patients who had not and found no difference in the rates of 30-day composite stroke/MI or 12-month freedom from restenosis. Other studies have evaluated outcomes at a longer follow-up period and found different results. A prospective study from the University of Rochester[275] stud-. ied 150 patients undergoing CAS (127 for atherosclerotic disease and 23 for RA) and found no difference in 3-year mortality but a significantly lower primary patency rate (20% vs 74% at 3 years) as well as lower overall patency rate (91% vs 100% at 3 years) in the carotid stenting group. In addition, the Eastern Virginia Medical School group[276] retrospectively found a significantly higher rate of restenosis at 2 years with carotid stenting versus open repair in anatomically high-risk lesions associated with radiation injury.

Alternatively, open carotid surgery may be feasible in this group of patients with acceptable results, but because of the significant perivascular fibrosis, loss of tissue planes, and adventitial and medial damage, the vessel wall is often not amenable to a patch repair, at times necessitating bypass or interposition.[277,278] There may be more fibrosis and fragility of the irradiated carotid artery wall, but the degree of inflammation may be less, because the lesion has developed over decades.[260] If necessary, the use of autologous conduit should be considered because of risk of infection in irradiated fields. Nevertheless, despite the negative perception of open carotid surgery in irradiated fields, the perioperative morbidity and mortality of open surgery for radiation-associated carotid lesions has been comparable with nonirradiated atherosclerotic lesions.[277,278]

Regarding extremity occlusive disease, there have been case reports of upper and lower extremity surgical revascularization for radiation-induced arterial lesions, with varying degrees of success.[279–281] Baerlocher and colleagues[282] found that radiation-associated iliac lesions have a tendency toward high elastic recoil and may require high inflation pressures in stent deployment. Claudication or critical limb ischemia are the main indications for treatment of axillosubclavian ischemic or occlusive disease associated with RA. Bypass surgery may be more straightforward than interposition, considering that the latter may require more dissection around the brachial plexus in an irradiated field. The use of ipsilateral or contralateral carotid inflow and vein bypass has been shown to be successful in that setting.[267] In general, for axillosubclavian and iliofemoral disease associated with RA, extra-anatomic tunneling, and use of autologous conduit may be prudent to avoid extensive dissection and long-term risk of infection in irradiated fields. There have been case reports on axillosubclavian stenting in the setting of radiation-associated occlusive disease with technical success.[283,284] One center stented 2 patients with severe upper extremity claudication with clinical improvement and long-term freedom from symptoms, one at 10-month follow-up and the other at 18-month follow-up.[283]

RAYNAUD PHENOMENON

Raynaud phenomenon (RP) is a vasospastic disorder, triggered by decreased temperature or emotion, manifesting as acral discoloration and paresthesias. Primary RP lacks a known cause, whereas secondary RP is associated with rheumatologic, hematologic, and occlusive disorders, namely systemic sclerosis (**Table 9**).[285] Because of different pathoetiologic mechanisms, the 2 show different clinical behavior (**Fig. 5**).

Pathogenesis and Epidemiology

The syndrome is named after Maurice Raynaud, who first described the phenomenon in the 1860s.[286] It is a relatively common disorder, affecting 3% to 5% of the general population.[287] Primary RP is believed to be a benign, reversible vasospastic process. The homeostasis between vasospasm and vasodilatation, through deranged neuroregulation and circulating mediator imbalance, is biased toward vasospasm.[288–290] A deficiency in the circulating vasodilator calcitonin gene-related neuropeptide, and an upregulation in α_2-adrenoreceptor activation are the putative mechanisms that lead to vasospasm in primary RP.[288,291] Secondary RP is believed to include a fixed structural component of disease and is associated with vascular endothelial disease.[292,293] Both primary and secondary RP have been shown to be associated with increased platelet activation, particularly the GPIIb/IIIa receptor.[294,295] Patients with RP show an abnormal tendency toward cold-induced vasospasm and impaired

Table 9
Conditions associated with secondary RP

Rheumatologic	Hematologic	Occlusive Arterial Disease
Systemic sclerosis (90% of these patients have RP)	Polycythemia rubra vera	External neurovascular compression, carpal tunnel syndrome
Mixed connective tissue disease (85%)	Leukemia	Thoracic outlet syndrome
Systemic lupus erythematosus (40%)	Thrombocytosis	Thrombosis
Dermatomyositis or polymyositis (25%)	Cold agglutinin diseases (*Mycoplasma* infections)	Buerger disease
Rheumatoid arthritis (10%)	Paraproteinemias	Embolization
Sjögren syndrome	Protein C or S deficiency, antithrombin III deficiency	Arteriosclerosis
Vasculitides	Factor V Leiden mutation Hepatitis B and C (associated with cryoglubulinemia)	

Adapted from Goundry B, Bell L, Langtree M, et al. Diagnosis and management of Raynaud's phenomenon. BMJ 2012;344:e289.

vasodilatory effect in response to warmth.[292,296] A third type of RP has been associated with hand-arm vibration (also known as vibration-white-finger) syndrome.

Clinical Presentation

RP is characterized by digital, nose, or ear discoloration preceded by temperature drop or emotional stress. The color change has been described as triphasic, with an initial phase of vasoconstriction resulting in pallor, subsequent cyanosis, and pain caused by transient ischemic changes, then rubor and a burning sensation associated with reperfusion.[285] In patients with secondary RP, critical digital ischemia may be more likely to result in gangrene and tissue loss.[285]

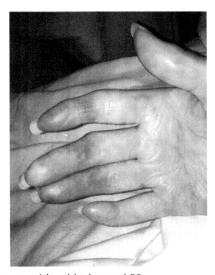

Fig. 5. A 42-year-old woman with cold-triggered RP.

Diagnosis

A detailed history in a patient reporting acral color change or neurologic symptoms is the mainstay in the diagnosis of RP. A symptom journal may be useful in documenting and capturing symptoms. Secondary triggers must be elucidated, which include tobacco exposure, cocaine, β-blockers, clonidine, chemotherapy, sympathomimetics, and unopposed exposure to estrogen.[285] Evaluating for systemic disorders has natural implications. In particular, carefully assessing for skin changes, sclerodactyly, digital ulceration, pigmentation changes, or rash may help identify systemic sclerosis or another rheumatologic disorder.[285] If clinical suspicion exists, further investigation for rheumatologic or systemic disorders may be warranted, including laboratory tests and imaging. Unilateral symptoms may suggest a thoracic outlet syndrome, which warrants a screening chest radiograph to evaluate for cervical rib.[285] There is no consensus on a gold-standard diagnostic test for RP. A cold-provocation test, performed by measuring digital pressures before and after submersion of the patient's hand in 15°C water for 5 minutes, may be helpful. A pressure difference of greater than 30 mm Hg as well as a digital brachial index of less than 0.7 are suggestive of the diagnosis.[297,298] Correlation with digital plethysmography, laser Doppler perfusion studies, or video capillaroscopy with temperature-provocation studies may also aid in diagnosis.[299,300] Also suggestive of the diagnosis is the need for more than 20 minutes to rewarming in a cold-stimulation test, compared with less than 15 minutes in unaffected patients.[285] In cases in which workers using power tools present with a history consistent with vibration-triggered acrocyanosis and symptoms, careful documentation and diagnostic workup are critical, because they may affect worker's compensation and disability claims.[301,302]

Treatment

Medical management

The patient should be counseled and advised to avoid triggers if possible; for instance, keeping ones hands and feet warm during cold weather months. Failing this, the mainstay of treatment of uncomplicated RP is with pharmacologic vasodilation.[303] Nifedipine has been shown to reduce severity and frequency of attacks, and may be better tolerated in a sustained-release formulation.[304,305] Most of the studies performed used fixed dosing of nifedipine, between 10 and 20 mg orally 3 times daily or 50 mg daily of an extended-release formulation.[304] Similarly, angiotensin II receptor blockade with losartan has been shown to decrease frequency and severity of RP exacerbations.[306] Other pharmacologic interventions include IV iloprost, a prostacyclin analogue, which may aid in the healing of digital ulceration.[307] In addition, phosphodiesterase inhibitors, through limited studies, have been suggested to help alleviate the symptoms of both primary and secondary RP, and may help heal digital ulcers.[308–310] Topical nitrates have also recently been shown to have benefit in alleviation of an acute RP attack.[311,312]

Surgical management

Indications for surgical treatment of RP are limited to amputation and debridement for gangrene or ischemic infection, and more rarely, sympathectomy or arteriolysis.[313] A recently published literature review[314] over the past 30 years has shown that thoracic sympathectomy, which can be performed thoracoscopically, improves symptoms in both primary and secondary RP, with a 92% (primary RP) and 89% (secondary RP) improvement of upper extremity symptoms with a 58% and 89% long-term benefit, respectively. Another study[315] showed long-term symptomatic and objective (using laser Doppler perfusion) improvement after thoracic sympathectomy with 28% return of symptoms at 5 years. A case series of 6 patients[315] showed that peripheral sympathectomy was able to salvage 12 of the 14 chronically ischemic digits after failure of medical management. Another case series found 5 of 6 patients with scleroderma to have sustained improved quality of life and decreased symptoms at 5 years after palmar sympathectomy in combination with radial and ulnar arteriolysis.[316] The role of arteriolysis has been described in a report of 22 digits in 7 patients with painful chronic digital vasospasm who were treated with microsurgical arteriolysis alone and had sustained decreased pain in all digits and complete resolution in 19 digits.[317]

Although the key therapy remains in preventive and medical interventions, the role of surgery is focused on the management of persistent symptoms or complications, and the choice of therapy should be based on local availability and expertise.

REFERENCES

1. Buerger L. Thromboangiitis obliterans: a study of the vascular lesions leading to presenile spontaneous gangrene. Am J Med Sci 1908;136:567–80.
2. Papa M, Bass A, Adar R, et al. Autoimmune mechanisms in thromboangiitis obliterans (Buerger's disease): the role of tobacco antigen and the major histocompatibility complex. Surgery 1992;111(5):527–31.
3. Matsushita M, Shionoya S, Matsumoto T. Urinary cotinine measurement in patients with Buerger's disease–effects of active and passive smoking on the disease process. J Vasc Surg 1991;14(1):53–8.
4. Lawrence PF, Lund OI, Jimenez JC, et al. Substitution of smokeless tobacco for cigarettes in Buerger's disease does not prevent limb loss. J Vasc Surg 2008; 48(1):210–2.
5. Lee T, Seo JW, Sumpio BE, et al. Immunobiologic analysis of arterial tissue in Buerger's disease. Eur J Vasc Endovasc Surg 2003;25(5):451–7.
6. Eichhorn J, Sima D, Lindschau C, et al. Antiendothelial cell antibodies in thromboangiitis obliterans. Am J Med Sci 1998;315(1):17–23.
7. Kobayashi M, Ito M, Nakagawa A, et al. Immunohistochemical analysis of arterial wall cellular infiltration in Buerger's disease (endarteritis obliterans). J Vasc Surg 1999;29(3):451–8.
8. Adar R, Papa MZ, Halpern Z, et al. Cellular sensitivity to collagen in thromboangiitis obliterans. N Engl J Med 1983;308(19):1113–6.
9. Spittell JA. Thromboangiitis obliterans–an autoimmune disorder? N Engl J Med 1983;308(19):1157–8.
10. Olin JW, Shih A. Thromboangiitis obliterans (Buerger's disease). Curr Opin Rheumatol 2006;18(1):18–24.
11. Cutler DA, Runge MS. 86 years of Buerger's disease–what have we learned? Am J Med Sci 1995;309(2):74–5.
12. Numano F, Sasazuki T, Koyama T, et al. HLA in Buerger's disease. Exp Clin Immunogenet 1986;3(4):195–200.
13. Hurelbrink CB, Barnett Y, Buckland ME, et al. Revisiting cerebral thromboangiitis obliterans. J Neurol Sci 2012;317(1–2):141–5.
14. Mills JL. Buerger's disease: current status. Vasc Med 1994;5:139–50.
15. Mills JL, Porter JM. Buerger's disease (thromboangiitis obliterans). Ann Vasc Surg 1991;5(6):570–2.
16. Olin JW. Thromboangiitis obliterans (Buerger's disease). N Engl J Med 2000; 343(12):864–9.
17. Landry GJ, Edwards JM. Nonatherosclerotic vascular disease. In: Moore WS, editor. Vascular and endovascular surgery. Philadelphia: Saunders; 2006. p. 107–39.
18. Shionoya S. What is Buerger's disease? World J Surg 1983;7(4):544–51.

19. Shionoya S. Buerger's disease (thromboangiitis obliterans). In: Rutherford RB, editor. Vascular surgery. 3rd edition. Philadelphia: WB Saunders; 1989. p. 207–17.

20. Shionoya S. Diagnostic criteria of Buerger's disease. Int J Cardiol 1998; 66(Suppl 1):S243–5 [discussion: S247].

21. Mills JL Sr. Buerger's disease in the 21st century: diagnosis, clinical features, and therapy. Semin Vasc Surg 2003;16(3):179–89.

22. Mills JL, Porter JM. Buerger's disease: a review and update. Semin Vasc Surg 1993;6(1):14–23.

23. Fiessinger JN, Schafer M. Trial of iloprost versus aspirin treatment for critical limb ischaemia of thromboangiitis obliterans. The TAO Study. Lancet 1990; 335(8689):555–7.

24. Puechal X, Fiessinger JN. Thromboangiitis obliterans or Buerger's disease: challenges for the rheumatologist. Rheumatology (Oxford) 2007;46(2):192–9.

25. Durdu S, Akar AR, Arat M, et al. Autologous bone-marrow mononuclear cell implantation for patients with Rutherford grade II-III thromboangiitis obliterans. J Vasc Surg 2006;44(4):732–9.

26. Miyamoto K, Nishigami K, Nagaya N, et al. Unblinded pilot study of autologous transplantation of bone marrow mononuclear cells in patients with thromboangiitis obliterans. Circulation 2006;114(24):2679–84.

27. Ilizarov GA. The tension-stress effect on the genesis and growth of tissues. Transosseous osteosynthesis: theoretical and clinical aspects of the regeneration and growth of tissue. Berlin: Springer; 1992.

28. Bozkurt AK, Besirli K, Koksal C, et al. Surgical treatment of Buerger's disease. Vascular 2004;12(3):192–7.

29. Graziani L, Morelli L, Parini F, et al. Clinical outcome after extended endovascular recanalization in Buerger's disease in 20 consecutive cases. Ann Vasc Surg 2012;26(3):387–95.

30. Gervaziev VB, Kolobova OI. Intraarterial thrombolytic therapy in obliterative thromboangiitis of the lower extremities. Khirurgiia (Mosk) 1993;2:26–32 [in Russian].

31. Numano F, Okawara M, Inomata H, et al. Takayasu's arteritis. Lancet 2000; 356(9234):1023–5.

32. Takayasu M. A case with unusual changes of the central vessels in the retina. Acta Soc Ophthalmol Jpn 1908;12:554–5.

33. Noguchi S, Numano F, Gravanis MB, et al. Increased levels of soluble forms of adhesion molecules in Takayasu arteritis. Int J Cardiol 1998;66(Suppl 1):S23–33 [discussion: S35–6].

34. Numano F. Takayasu's arteritis: clinical aspects. In: Hoffman GS, Weyand CM, Langford CA, et al, editors. Inflammatory diseases of blood vessels. New York: Marcel Dekker; 2002. p. 455.

35. Arnauda L, Haroche J, Mathian A, et al. Pathogenesis of Takayasu's arteritis: a 2011 update. Autoimmun Rev 2011;11(1):61–7.

36. Hottchi M. Pathological study on Takayasu arteritis. Heart Vessels Suppl 1992;7: 11–7.

37. Numano F, Kishi Y, Tanaka A, et al. Inflammation and atherosclerosis. Atherosclerotic lesions in Takayasu arteritis. Ann N Y Acad Sci 2000;902:65–76.

38. Hodgins GW, Dutton JW. Subclavian and carotid angioplasties for Takayasu's arteritis. J Can Assoc Radiol 1982;33(3):205–7.

39. Jacobs MR, Allen NB. Giant cell arteritis. In: Churg AC, J, editors. Systemic vasculitides. New York: Igaku-Shoin; 1991. p. 143–58.

40. Kerr GS. Takayasu's arteritis. Rheum Dis Clin North Am 1995;21(4):1041–58.
41. Kerr GS, Hallahan CW, Giordano J, et al. Takayasu arteritis. Ann Intern Med 1994;120(11):919–29.
42. Jain S, Kumari S, Ganguly NK, et al. Current status of Takayasu arteritis in India. Int J Cardiol 1996;54(Suppl):S111–6.
43. Robbs JV, Abdool-Carrim AT, Kadwa AM. Arterial reconstruction for non-specific arteritis (Takayasu's disease): medium to long term results. Eur J Vasc Surg 1994;8(4):401–7.
44. Suwanwela N, Piyachon C. Takayasu arteritis in Thailand: clinical and imaging features. Int J Cardiol 1996;54(Suppl):S117–34.
45. Yajima M, Numano F, Park YB, et al. Comparative studies of patients with Takayasu arteritis in Japan, Korea and India–comparison of clinical manifestations, angiography and HLA-B antigen. Jpn Circ J 1994;58(1):9–14.
46. Numano F, Kobayashi Y. Takayasu arteritis–beyond pulselessness. Intern Med 1999;38(3):226–32.
47. Koide K. Takayasu arteritis in Japan. Heart Vessels Suppl 1992;7:48–54.
48. Kumar S, Subramanyan R, Mandalam KR, et al. Aneurysmal form of aortoarteritis (Takayasu's disease): analysis of thirty cases. Clin Radiol 1990;42(5):342–7.
49. Numano F, Kobayashi Y, Maruyama Y, et al. Takayasu arteritis: clinical characteristics and the role of genetic factors in its pathogenesis. Vasc Med 1996;1(3):227–33.
50. Sharma BK, Jain S. A possible role of sex in determining distribution of lesions in Takayasu arteritis. Int J Cardiol 1998;66:S81–4.
51. Zheng D, Fan D, Liu L. Takayasu arteritis in China: a report of 530 cases. Heart Vessels Suppl 1992;7:32–6.
52. Maksimowicz-McKinnon KC, Clark TM, Hoffman GS. Limitations of therapy and a guarded prognosis in an American cohort of Takayasu arteritis patients. Arthritis Rheum 2007;56(3):1000–9.
53. Lupi-Herrera E, Sanchez-Torres G, Marcushamer J, et al. Takayasu's arteritis. Clinical study of 107 cases. Am Heart J 1977;93(1):94–103.
54. Ueno A, Awane Y, Wakabayashi A, et al. Successfully operated obliterative brachiocephalic arteritis (Takayasu) associated with the elongated coarctation. Jpn Heart J 1967;8(5):538–44.
55. Sharma BK, Siveski-Iliskovic N, Singal PK. Takayasu arteritis may be underdiagnosed in North America. Can J Cardiol 1995;11(4):311–6.
56. Arend WP, Michel BA, Bloch DA, et al. The American College of Rheumatology 1990 criteria for the classification of Takayasu arteritis. Arthritis Rheum 1990;33(8):1129–34.
57. Mavrogeni S, Dimitroulas T, Chatziioannou SN, et al. The role of multimodality imaging in the evaluation of Takayasu arteritis. Semin Arthritis Rheum 2013;42(4):401–12.
58. Park JH, Chung JW, Lee KW, et al. CT angiography of Takayasu's arteritis: comparison with conventional angiography. J Vasc Interv Radiol 1997;8:393–400.
59. Sharma S, Rajani M, Talwar KK. Angiographic morphology in nonspecific aortoarteritis (Takayasu's arteritis): a study of 126 patients from north India. Cardiovasc Intervent Radiol 1992;15(3):160–5.
60. Sun Y, Yip PK, Jeng JS, et al. Ultrasonographic study and long-term follow-up of Takayasu's arteritis. Stroke 1996;27(12):2178–82.
61. Matsunaga N, Hayashi K, Sakamoto I, et al. Takayasu arteritis: protean radiologic manifestations and diagnosis. Radiographics 1997;17(3):579–94.

62. Liang P, Hoffman GS. Advances in the medical and surgical treatment of Takayasu arteritis. Curr Opin Rheumatol 2005;17(1):16–24.
63. Comarmond C, Plaisier E, Dahan K, et al. Anti TNF-alpha in refractory Takayasu's arteritis: cases series and review of the literature. Autoimmun Rev 2012; 11(9):678–84.
64. Fields CE, Bower TC, Cooper LT, et al. Takayasu's arteritis: operative results and influence of disease activity. J Vasc Surg 2006;43(1):64–71.
65. Weaver FA, Yellin AE, Campen DH, et al. Surgical procedures in the management of Takayasu's arteritis. J Vasc Surg 1990;12(4):429–37 [discussion: 438–9].
66. Kim YW, Kim DI, Park YJ, et al. Surgical bypass vs endovascular treatment for patients with supra-aortic arterial occlusive disease due to Takayasu arteritis. J Vasc Surg 2012;55(3):693–700.
67. Ham SW, Kumar SR, Rowe VL, et al. Disease progression after initial surgical intervention for Takayasu arteritis. J Vasc Surg 2011;54(5):1345–51.
68. Qureshi MA, Martin Z, Greenberg RK. Endovascular management of patients with Takayasu arteritis: stents versus stent grafts. Semin Vasc Surg 2011; 24(1):44–52.
69. Hall S, Barr W, Lie JT, et al. Takayasu arteritis. A study of 32 North American patients. Medicine (Baltimore) 1985;64:89–99.
70. Mason JC. Takayasu arteritis–advances in diagnosis and management. Nat Rev Rheumatol 2010;6(7):406–15.
71. Subramanyan R, Joy J, Balakrishnan KG. Natural history of aortoarteritis (Takayasu's disease). Circulation 1989;80(3):429–37.
72. Ishikawa K, Maetani S. Long-term outcome for 120 Japanese patients with Takayasu's disease. Clinical and statistical analyses of related prognostic factors. Circulation 1994;90(4):1855–60.
73. Van Damme H, Fourny J, Zicot M, et al. Giant cell arteritis (Horton's disease) of the axillary artery–case reports. Angiology 1989;40(6):593–601.
74. Chaigne-Delalande S, de Menthon M, Lazaro E, et al. Giant-cell arteritis and Takayasu arteritis: epidemiological, diagnostic and treatment aspects. Presse Med 2012;41(10):955–65 [in French].
75. Sheps SG, McDuffie FC. Vasculitis. In: Juergens JL, JA, Gairbaim JF, editors. Peripheral vascular disease. Philadelphia: WB Saunders; 1980. p. 493–553.
76. Warrington KJ, Cooper LT Jr. Vasculitis and other arteriopathies. In: Cronewett JK, Johnston KW, editors. Rutherford's vascular surgery. 7th edition. Philadelphia: Saunders; 2010. p. 1156–67.
77. Ly KH, Regent A, Tamby MC, et al. Pathogenesis of giant cell arteritis: more than just an inflammatory condition? Autoimmun Rev 2010;9(10):635–45.
78. Kaiser M, Younge B, Bjornsson J, et al. Formation of new vasa vasorum in vasculitis. Production of angiogenic cytokines by multinucleated giant cells. Am J Pathol 1999;155(3):765–74.
79. Weyand CM, Goronzy JJ. Pathogenic mechanisms in giant cell arteritis. Cleve Clin J Med 2002;69(Suppl 2):SII28–32.
80. Janssen SP, Comans EH, Voskuyl AE, et al. Giant cell arteritis: heterogeneity in clinical presentation and imaging results. J Vasc Surg 2008;48(4):1025–31.
81. Brooks RC, McGee SR. Diagnostic dilemmas in polymyalgia rheumatica. Arch Intern Med 1997;157(2):162–8.
82. Myklebust G, Gran JT. A prospective study of 287 patients with polymyalgia rheumatica and temporal arteritis: clinical and laboratory manifestations at onset of disease and at the time of diagnosis. Br J Rheumatol 1996;35(11):1161–8.

83. Salvarani C, Cantini F, Boiardi L, et al. Polymyalgia rheumatica and giant-cell arteritis. N Engl J Med 2002;347(4):261–71.
84. Assie C, Marie I. Giant cell arteritis-related upper/lower limb vasculitis. Presse Med 2011;40(2):151–61 [in French].
85. Bongartz T, Matteson EL. Large-vessel involvement in giant cell arteritis. Curr Opin Rheumatol 2006;18(1):10–7.
86. Nuenninghoff DM, Hunder GG, Christianson TJ, et al. Incidence and predictors of large-artery complication (aortic aneurysm, aortic dissection, and/or large-artery stenosis) in patients with giant cell arteritis: a population-based study over 50 years. Arthritis Rheum 2003;48(12):3522–31.
87. Brack A, Martinez-Taboada V, Stanson A, et al. Disease pattern in cranial and large-vessel giant cell arteritis. Arthritis Rheum 1999;42(2):311–7.
88. Evans JM, Bowles CA, Bjornsson J, et al. Thoracic aortic aneurysm and rupture in giant cell arteritis. A descriptive study of 41 cases. Arthritis Rheum 1994; 37(10):1539–47.
89. Evans JM, O'Fallon WM, Hunder GG. Increased incidence of aortic aneurysm and dissection in giant cell (temporal) arteritis. A population-based study. Ann Intern Med 1995;122(7):502–7.
90. Hayreh SS, Zimmerman B, Kardon RH. Visual improvement with corticosteroid therapy in giant cell arteritis. Report of a large study and review of literature. Acta Ophthalmol Scand 2002;80(4):355–67.
91. Hunder GG, Bloch DA, Michel BA, et al. The American College of Rheumatology 1990 criteria for the classification of giant cell arteritis. Arthritis Rheum 1990; 33(8):1122–8.
92. Quinn EM, Kearney DE, Kelly J, et al. Temporal artery biopsy is not required in all cases of suspected giant cell arteritis. Ann Vasc Surg 2012;26(5):649–54.
93. Smetana GW, Shmerling RH. Does this patient have temporal arteritis? JAMA 2002;287(1):92–101.
94. Murchison AP, Gilbert ME, Bilyk JR, et al. Validity of the American College of Rheumatology criteria for the diagnosis of giant cell arteritis. Am J Ophthalmol 2012;154(4):722–9.
95. Mahr AD, Neogi T, Merkel PA. Epidemiology of Wegener's granulomatosis: lessons from descriptive studies and analyses of genetic and environmental risk determinants. Clin Exp Rheumatol 2006;24(2 Suppl 41):S82–91.
96. Taylor-Gjevre R, Vo M, Shukla D, et al. Temporal artery biopsy for giant cell arteritis. J Rheumatol 2005;32(7):1279–82.
97. Ypsilantis E, Courtney ED, Chopra N, et al. Importance of specimen length during temporal artery biopsy. Br J Surg 2011;98(11):1556–60.
98. Boyev LR, Miller NR, Green WR. Efficacy of unilateral versus bilateral temporal artery biopsies for the diagnosis of giant cell arteritis. Am J Ophthalmol 1999; 128(2):211–5.
99. Breuer GS, Nesher G, Nesher R. Rate of discordant findings in bilateral temporal artery biopsy to diagnose giant cell arteritis. J Rheumatol 2009;36(4): 794–6.
100. Saedon H, Saedon M, Goodyear S, et al. Temporal artery biopsy for giant cell arteritis: retrospective audit. JRSM Short Rep 2012;3(10):73.
101. Achkar AA, Lie JT, Hunder GG, et al. How does previous corticosteroid treatment affect the biopsy findings in giant cell (temporal) arteritis? Ann Intern Med 1994;120(12):987–92.
102. Roth AM, Milsow L, Keltner JL. The ultimate diagnoses of patients undergoing temporal artery biopsies. Arch Ophthalmol 1984;102(6):901–3.

103. Karahaliou M, Vaiopoulos G, Papaspyrou S, et al. Colour duplex sonography of temporal arteries before decision for biopsy: a prospective study in 55 patients with suspected giant cell arteritis. Arthritis Res Ther 2006;8(4):R116.

104. Blockmans D, Stroobants S, Maes A, et al. Positron emission tomography in giant cell arteritis and polymyalgia rheumatica: evidence for inflammation of the aortic arch. Am J Med 2000;108(3):246–9.

105. Fuchs M, Briel M, Daikeler T, et al. The impact of 18F-FDG PET on the management of patients with suspected large vessel vasculitis. Eur J Nucl Med Mol Imaging 2012;39(2):344–53.

106. Bley TA, Uhl M, Carew J, et al. Diagnostic value of high-resolution MR imaging in giant cell arteritis. AJNR Am J Neuroradiol 2007;28(9):1722–7.

107. Bley TA, Uhl M, Venhoff N, et al. 3-T MRI reveals cranial and thoracic inflammatory changes in giant cell arteritis. Clin Rheumatol 2007;26(3):448–50.

108. Balink H, Houtman PM, Collins J. 18F-FDG PET versus PET/CT as a diagnostic procedure for clinical suspicion of large vessel vasculitis. Clin Rheumatol 2011; 30(8):1139–41.

109. Meller J, Strutz F, Siefker U, et al. Early diagnosis and follow-up of aortitis with [(18)F]FDG PET and MRI. Eur J Nucl Med Mol Imaging 2003;30(5):730–6.

110. Forster S, Tato F, Weiss M, et al. Patterns of extracranial involvement in newly diagnosed giant cell arteritis assessed by physical examination, colour coded duplex sonography and FDG-PET. Vasa 2011;40(3):219–27.

111. Martinez-Valle F, Solans-Laque R, Bosch-Gil J, et al. Aortic involvement in giant cell arteritis. Autoimmun Rev 2010;9(7):521–4.

112. Borchers AT, Gershwin ME. Giant cell arteritis: a review of classification, pathophysiology, geoepidemiology and treatment. Autoimmun Rev 2012;11(6–7):A544–54.

113. Schmidt WA, Blockmans D. Use of ultrasonography and positron emission tomography in the diagnosis and assessment of large-vessel vasculitis. Curr Opin Rheumatol 2005;17(1):9–15.

114. Agard C, Said L, Ponge T, et al. Abdominal aortic involvement in active giant cell (temporal) arteritis: a study of 20 patients by Doppler ultrasonography and computed tomographic angiography. Presse Med 2009;38(1):11–9 [in French].

115. Espitia O, Neel A, Leux C, et al. Giant cell arteritis with or without aortitis at diagnosis. A retrospective study of 22 patients with longterm followup. J Rheumatol 2012;39(11):2157–62.

116. Meskimen S, Cook TD, Blake RL Jr. Management of giant cell arteritis and polymyalgia rheumatica. Am Fam Physician 2000;61(7):2061–8, 2073.

117. Proven A, Gabriel SE, Orces C, et al. Glucocorticoid therapy in giant cell arteritis: duration and adverse outcomes. Arthritis Rheum 2003;49(5):703–8.

118. Jover JA, Hernandez-Garcia C, Morado IC, et al. Combined treatment of giant-cell arteritis with methotrexate and prednisone. A randomized, double-blind, placebo-controlled trial. Ann Intern Med 2001;134(2):106–14.

119. Mahr AD, Jover JA, Spiera RF, et al. Adjunctive methotrexate for treatment of giant cell arteritis: an individual patient data meta-analysis. Arthritis Rheum 2007; 56(8):2789–97.

120. Chan CC, Paine M, O'Day J. Steroid management in giant cell arteritis. Br J Ophthalmol 2001;85(9):1061–4.

121. AbuRrahma AF, Thaxton L. Temporal arteritis: diagnostic and therapeutic considerations. Am Surg 1996;62(6):449–51.

122. Both M, Jahnke T, Reinhold-Keller E, et al. Percutaneous management of occlusive arterial disease associated with vasculitis: a single center experience. Cardiovasc Intervent Radiol 2003;26(1):19–26.

123. Kussmaul A, Maier R. Ueber eine bisher nicht beschriebene eigenthümliche Arterienerkrankung (Periarteritis nodosa), die mit Morbus Brightii und rapid fortschreitender allgemeiner Muskellähmung einhergeht. Dtsch Arch Klin Med 1866;1:484–518 [in German].

124. Jennette JC, Falk RJ, Andrassy K, et al. Nomenclature of systemic vasculitides. Proposal of an international consensus conference. Arthritis Rheum 1994;37(2): 187–92.

125. Guillevin L, Le Thi Huong D, Godeau P, et al. Clinical findings and prognosis of polyarteritis nodosa and Churg-Strauss angiitis: a study in 165 patients. Br J Rheumatol 1988;27(4):258–64.

126. Calabrese LH. Vasculitis and infection with the human immunodeficiency virus. Rheum Dis Clin North Am 1991;17(1):131–47.

127. Guillevin L, Lhote F, Cohen P, et al. Polyarteritis nodosa related to hepatitis B virus. A prospective study with long-term observation of 41 patients. Medicine (Baltimore) 1995;74(5):238–53.

128. Saadoun D, Terrier B, Semoun O, et al. Hepatitis C virus-associated polyarteritis nodosa. Arthritis Care Res 2011;63(3):427–35.

129. Guillevin L, Mahr A, Callard P, et al. Hepatitis B virus-associated polyarteritis nodosa: clinical characteristics, outcome, and impact of treatment in 115 patients. Medicine (Baltimore) 2005;84(5):313–22.

130. Pagnoux C, Seror R, Henegar C, et al. Clinical features and outcomes in 348 patients with polyarteritis nodosa: a systematic retrospective study of patients diagnosed between 1963 and 2005 and entered into the French Vasculitis Study Group Database. Arthritis Rheum 2010;62(2):616–26.

131. Ewald EA, Griffin D, McCune WJ. Correlation of angiographic abnormalities with disease manifestations and disease severity in polyarteritis nodosa. J Rheumatol 1987;14(5):952–6.

132. Stanson AW, Friese JL, Johnson CM, et al. Polyarteritis nodosa: spectrum of angiographic findings. Radiographics 2001;21(1):151–9.

133. Golnik KC. Neuro-ophthalmologic manifestations of systemic disease: rheumatologic/inflammatory. Ophthalmol Clin North Am 2004;17(3):389–96, vi.

134. Schroeder W, Kunert H, Muller-Jensen A. Early neuro-ophthalmological symptoms of periarteritis nodosa. A case report (author's transl). Klin Monbl Augenheilkd 1976;168(6):794–8 [in German].

135. Daoud MS, Hutton KP, Gibson LE. Cutaneous periarteritis nodosa: a clinicopathological study of 79 cases. Br J Dermatol 1997;136(5):706–13.

136. Kluger N, Pagnoux C, Guillevin L, et al. Comparison of cutaneous manifestations in systemic polyarteritis nodosa and microscopic polyangiitis. Br J Dermatol 2008;159(3):615–20.

137. Lightfoot RW Jr, Michel BA, Bloch DA, et al. The American College of Rheumatology 1990 criteria for the classification of polyarteritis nodosa. Arthritis Rheum 1990;33(8):1088–93.

138. Lane SE, Watts RA, Barker TH, et al. Evaluation of the Sorensen diagnostic criteria in the classification of systemic vasculitis. Rheumatology (Oxford) 2002;41(10):1138–41.

139. Rao JK, Allen NB, Pincus T. Limitations of the 1990 American College of Rheumatology classification criteria in the diagnosis of vasculitis. Ann Intern Med 1998;129(5):345–52.

140. Sorensen SF, Slot O, Tvede N, et al. A prospective study of vasculitis patients collected in a five year period: evaluation of the Chapel Hill nomenclature. Ann Rheum Dis 2000;59(6):478–82.

141. Henegar C, Pagnoux C, Puéchal X, et al. A paradigm of diagnostic criteria for polyarteritis nodosa: analysis of a series of 949 patients with vasculitides. Arthritis Rheum 2008;58(5):1528–38.

142. Patarroyo PA, Restrepo JF, Rojas SA, et al. Are classification criteria for vasculitis useful in clinical practice? Observations and lessons from Colombia. J Autoimmune Dis 2009;6:1.

143. Hekali P, Kajander H, Pajari R, et al. Diagnostic significance of angiographically observed visceral aneurysms with regard to polyarteritis nodosa. Acta Radiol 1991;32(2):143–8.

144. Kato T, Fujii K, Ishii E, et al. A case of polyarteritis nodosa with lesions of the superior mesenteric artery illustrating the diagnostic usefulness of three-dimensional computed tomographic angiography. Clin Rheumatol 2005;24(6): 628–31.

145. Tsai WL, Tsai IC, Lee T, et al. Polyarteritis nodosa: MDCT as a "one-stop shop" modality for whole-body arterial evaluation. Cardiovasc Intervent Radiol 2008; 31(Suppl 2):S26–9.

146. Guillevin L, Lhote F, Gayraud M, et al. Prognostic factors in polyarteritis nodosa and Churg-Strauss syndrome. A prospective study in 342 patients. Medicine (Baltimore) 1996;75(1):17–28.

147. Ribi C, Cohen P, Pagnoux C, et al. Treatment of polyarteritis nodosa and microscopic polyangiitis without poor-prognosis factors: a prospective randomized study of one hundred twenty-four patients. Arthritis Rheum 2010; 62(4):1186–97.

148. Guillevin L, Fain O, Lhote F, et al. Lack of superiority of steroids plus plasma exchange to steroids alone in the treatment of polyarteritis nodosa and Churg-Strauss syndrome. A prospective, randomized trial in 78 patients. Arthritis Rheum 1992;35(2):208–15.

149. Guillevin L, Lhote F. Treatment of polyarteritis nodosa and Churg-Strauss syndrome: indications of plasma exchanges. Transfus Sci 1994;15(4):371–88.

150. Jayne DR, Gaskin G, Rasmussen N, et al. Randomized trial of plasma exchange or high-dosage methylprednisolone as adjunctive therapy for severe renal vasculitis. J Am Soc Nephrol 2007;18(7):2180–8.

151. Lhote F, Cohen P, Guillevin L. Polyarteritis nodosa, microscopic polyangiitis and Churg-Strauss syndrome. Lupus 1998;7(4):238–58.

152. Pusey CD, Rees AJ, Evans DJ, et al. Plasma exchange in focal necrotizing glomerulonephritis without anti-GBM antibodies. Kidney Int 1991;40(4): 757–63.

153. Langford CA. Treatment of polyarteritis nodosa, microscopic polyangiitis, and Churg-Strauss syndrome: where do we stand? Arthritis Rheum 2001;44(3): 508–12.

154. Fauci AS, Katz P, Haynes BF, et al. Cyclophosphamide therapy of severe systemic necrotizing vasculitis. N Engl J Med 1979;301(5):235–8.

155. Cohen RD, Conn DL, Ilstrup DM. Clinical features, prognosis, and response to treatment in polyarteritis. Mayo Clin Proc 1980;55(3):146–55.

156. Guillevin L, Jarrousse B, Lok C, et al. Longterm followup after treatment of polyarteritis nodosa and Churg-Strauss angiitis with comparison of steroids, plasma exchange and cyclophosphamide to steroids and plasma exchange. A prospective randomized trial of 71 patients. The Cooperative Study Group for Polyarteritis Nodosa. J Rheumatol 1991;18(4):567–74.

157. Hoffman GS, Kerr GS, Leavitt RY, et al. Wegener granulomatosis: an analysis of 158 patients. Ann Intern Med 1992;116(6):488–98.

158. Talar-Williams C, Hijazi YM, Walther MM, et al. Cyclophosphamide-induced cystitis and bladder cancer in patients with Wegener granulomatosis. Ann Intern Med 1996;124(5):477–84.

159. Gayraud M, Guillevin L, le Toumelin P, et al. Long-term followup of polyarteritis nodosa, microscopic polyangiitis, and Churg-Strauss syndrome: analysis of four prospective trials including 278 patients. Arthritis Rheum 2001;44(3):666–75.

160. Rits Y, Oderich GS, Bower TC, et al. Interventions for mesenteric vasculitis. J Vasc Surg 2010;51(2):392–400.e2.

161. Nylander G, Pettersson F, Swedenborg J. Localized arterial occlusions in patients treated with pelvic field radiation for cancer. Cancer 1978;41(6):2158–61.

162. Wood MK, Read DR, Kraft AR, et al. A rare cause of ischemic colitis: polyarteritis nodosa. Dis Colon Rectum 1979;22(6):428–33.

163. Donmez H, Men S, Dilli A, et al. Giant gastroduodenal artery pseudoaneurysm due to polyarteritis nodosa as a cause of obstructive jaundice: imaging findings and coil embolization results. Cardiovasc Intervent Radiol 2005;28(6):850–3.

164. Hidalgo J, Crego M, Montlleo M, et al. Embolization of a bleeding aneurysm in a patient with spontaneous perirenal haematoma due to polyarteritis nodosa. Arch Esp Urol 2005;58(7):694–7.

165. Nakashima M, Suzuki K, Okada M, et al. Successful coil embolization of a ruptured hepatic aneurysm in a patient with polyarteritis nodosa accompanied by angioimmunoblastic T cell lymphoma. Clin Rheumatol 2007;26(8):1362–4.

166. Park SS, Kim BU, Han HS, et al. Hemobilia from ruptured hepatic artery aneurysm in polyarteritis nodosa. Korean J Intern Med 2006;21(1):79–82.

167. Koc O, Ozbek O, Gumus S, et al. Endovascular management of massive gastrointestinal bleeding associated with polyarteritis nodosa. J Vasc Interv Radiol 2009;20(2):277–9.

168. Oh MS, Kim MH, Chu MK, et al. Polyarteritis nodosa presenting with bilateral cavernous internal carotid artery aneurysms. Neurology 2008;70(5):405.

169. Amano S, Hazama F, Kubagawa H, et al. General pathology of Kawasaki disease. On the morphological alterations corresponding to the clinical manifestations. Acta Pathol Jpn 1980;30(5):681–94.

170. Burns JC, Kushner HI, Bastian JF, et al. Kawasaki disease: a brief history. Pediatrics 2000;106(2):E27.

171. Holman RC, Curns AT, Belay ED, et al. Kawasaki syndrome hospitalizations in the United States, 1997 and 2000. Pediatrics 2003;112(3 Pt 1):495–501.

172. Nakamura Y, Yashiro M, Uehara R, et al. Epidemiologic features of Kawasaki disease in Japan: results from the nationwide survey in 2005-2006. J Epidemiol 2008;18(4):167–72.

173. Rowley AH, Shulman ST. Pathogenesis and management of Kawasaki disease. Expert Rev Anti Infect Ther 2010;8(2):197–203.

174. Pitzer VE, Burgner D, Viboud C, et al. Modelling seasonal variations in the age and incidence of Kawasaki disease to explore possible infectious aetiologies. Proc Biol Sci 2012;279(1739):2736–43.

175. Takahashi K, Oharaseki T, Yokouchi Y. Pathogenesis of Kawasaki disease. Clin Exp Immunol 2011;164(Suppl 1):20–2.

176. Vitale EA, La Torre F, Calcagno G, et al. *Mycoplasma pneumoniae*: a possible trigger of Kawasaki disease or a mere coincidental association? Report of the first four Italian cases. Minerva Pediatr 2010;62(6):605–7.

177. Newburger JW, Takahashi M, Gerber MA, et al. Diagnosis, treatment, and long-term management of Kawasaki disease: a statement for health professionals

from the Committee on Rheumatic Fever, Endocarditis and Kawasaki Disease, Council on Cardiovascular Disease in the Young, American Heart Association. Circulation 2004;110(17):2747–71.

178. Brown TJ, Crawford SE, Cornwall ML, et al. CD8 T lymphocytes and macrophages infiltrate coronary artery aneurysms in acute Kawasaki disease. J Infect Dis 2001;184(7):940–3.

179. Takeshita S, Tokutomi T, Kawase H, et al. Elevated serum levels of matrix metalloproteinase-9 (MMP-9) in Kawasaki disease. Clin Exp Immunol 2001; 125(2):340–4.

180. Burgner D, Davila S, Breunis WB, et al. A genome-wide association study identifies novel and functionally related susceptibility loci for Kawasaki disease. PLoS Genet 2009;5(1):e1000319.

181. Onouchi Y, Gunji T, Burns JC, et al. ITPKC functional polymorphism associated with Kawasaki disease susceptibility and formation of coronary artery aneurysms. Nat Genet 2008;40(1):35–42.

182. Suzuki A, Kamiya T, Kuwahara N, et al. Coronary arterial lesions of Kawasaki disease: cardiac catheterization findings of 1100 cases. Pediatr Cardiol 1986;7(1): 3–9.

183. Wolff AE, Hansen KE, Zakowski L. Acute Kawasaki disease: not just for kids. J Gen Intern Med 2007;22(5):681–4.

184. Research Committee on Kawasaki Disease. Report of Subcommittee on Standardization of Diagnostic Criteria and Reporting of Coronary Artery Lesions in Kawasaki Disease. Tokyo: 1984.

185. de Zorzi A, Colan SD, Gauvreau K, et al. Coronary artery dimensions may be misclassified as normal in Kawasaki disease. J Pediatr 1998;133(2):254–8.

186. Danias PG, Stuber M, Botnar RM, et al. Coronary MR angiography clinical applications and potential for imaging coronary artery disease. Magn Reson Imaging Clin N Am 2003;11(1):81–99.

187. Duerinckx A, Troutman B, Allada V, et al. Coronary MR angiography in Kawasaki disease. Am J Roentgenol 1997;168(117):114–6.

188. Frey EE, Matherne GP, Mahoney LT, et al. Coronary artery aneurysms due to Kawasaki disease: diagnosis with ultrafast CT. Radiology 1988;167(3):725–6.

189. Greil GF, Stuber M, Botnar RM, et al. Coronary magnetic resonance angiography in adolescents and young adults with Kawasaki disease. Circulation 2002;105(8):908–11.

190. Sakuma H, Goto M, Nomura Y, et al. Three-dimensional coronary magnetic resonance angiography with injection of extracellular contrast medium. Invest Radiol 1999;34(8):503–8.

191. Gomard-Mennesson E, Landron C, Dauphin C, et al. Kawasaki disease in adults: report of 10 cases. Medicine (Baltimore) 2010;89(3):149–58.

192. Dajani AS, Taubert KA, Gerber MA, et al. Diagnosis and therapy of Kawasaki disease in children. Circulation 1993;87(5):1776–80.

193. Durongpisitkul K, Gururaj VJ, Park JM, et al. The prevention of coronary artery aneurysm in Kawasaki disease: a meta-analysis on the efficacy of aspirin and immunoglobulin treatment. Pediatrics 1995;96(6):1057–61.

194. Furusho K, Kamiya T, Nakano H, et al. High-dose intravenous gammaglobulin for Kawasaki disease. Lancet 1984;2(8411):1055–8.

195. Newburger JW, Takahashi M, Burns JC, et al. The treatment of Kawasaki syndrome with intravenous gamma globulin. N Engl J Med 1986;315(6): 341–7.

196. Terai M, Shulman ST. Prevalence of coronary artery abnormalities in Kawasaki disease is highly dependent on gamma globulin dose but independent of salicylate dose. J Pediatr 1997;131(6):888–93.

197. Dajani AS, Taubert KA, Takahashi M, et al. Guidelines for long-term management of patients with Kawasaki disease. Report from the Committee on Rheumatic Fever, Endocarditis, and Kawasaki Disease, Council on Cardiovascular Disease in the Young, American Heart Association. Circulation 1994;89(2):916–22.

198. Durongpisitkul K, Soongswang J, Laohaprasitiporn D, et al. Immunoglobulin failure and retreatment in Kawasaki disease. Pediatr Cardiol 2003;24(2):145–8.

199. Wallace CA, French JW, Kahn SJ, et al. Initial intravenous gammaglobulin treatment failure in Kawasaki disease. Pediatrics 2000;105(6):E78.

200. Williams RV, Wilke VM, Tani LY, et al. Does Abciximab enhance regression of coronary aneurysms resulting from Kawasaki disease? Pediatrics 2002;109(1):E4.

201. Weiss JE, Eberhard BA, Chowdhury D, et al. Infliximab as a novel therapy for refractory Kawasaki disease. J Rheumatol 2004;31(4):808–10.

202. Myler RK, Schechtmann NS, Rosenblum J, et al. Multiple coronary artery aneurysms in an adult associated with extensive thrombus formation resulting in acute myocardial infarction: successful treatment with intracoronary urokinase, intravenous heparin, and oral anticoagulation. Cathet Cardiovasc Diagn 1991; 24(1):51–4.

203. Tsuda E, Kitamura S, Cooperative Study Group of Japan. National survey of coronary artery bypass grafting for coronary stenosis caused by Kawasaki disease in Japan. Circulation 2004;110(11 Suppl 1):II61–6.

204. Kitamura S, Tsuda E, Kobayashi J, et al. Twenty-five-year outcome of pediatric coronary artery bypass surgery for Kawasaki disease. Circulation 2009;120(1): 60–8.

205. Jennette JC, Falk RJ. Small-vessel vasculitis. N Engl J Med 1997;337(21): 1512–23.

206. Gibelin A, Maldini C, Mahr A. Epidemiology and etiology of Wegener granulomatosis, microscopic polyangiitis, Churg-Strauss syndrome and Goodpasture syndrome: vasculitides with frequent lung involvement. Semin Respir Crit Care Med 2011;32(3):264–73.

207. Davson J, Ball J, Platt R. The kidney in periarteritis nodosa. Q J Med 1948; 17(67):175–202.

208. Godman GC, Churg J. Wegener's granulomatosis: pathology and review of the literature. Arch Pathol 1954;58:533–53.

209. Zeek PM. Periarteritis nodosa; a critical review. Am J Clin Pathol 1952;22(8): 777–90.

210. Zeek PM, Smith CC, Weeter JC. Studies on periarteritis nodosa; the differentiation between the vascular lesions of periarteritis nodosa and of hypersensitivity. Am J Pathol 1948;24(4):889–917.

211. Klinger H. Grenzformen der Periarteriitis nodosa. Frankf Z Pathol 1931;42: 455–80 [in German].

212. Wegener F. Über eine eigenartige rhinogene Granulomatose mit besonderer Beteilgung des Arteriensystems und den Nieren. Beitr Pathol Anat Allg Pathol 1939;102:36–68 [in German].

213. Churg J, Strauss L. Allergic granulomatosis, allergic angiitis, and periarteritis nodosa. Am J Pathol 1951;27(2):277–301.

214. Kallenberg CG. Antineutrophil cytoplasmic autoantibody-associated small-vessel vasculitis. Curr Opin Rheumatol 2007;19(1):17–24.

215. Jennette JC, Falk RJ. Pathogenic potential of anti-neutrophil cytoplasmic auto-antibodies. Adv Exp Med Biol 1993;336:7–15.
216. Rarok AA, Limburg PC, Kallenberg CG. Neutrophil-activating potential of anti-neutrophil cytoplasm autoantibodies. J Leukoc Biol 2003;74(1):3–15.
217. Esnault VL, Testa A, Audrain M, et al. Alpha 1-antitrypsin genetic polymorphism in ANCA-positive systemic vasculitis. Kidney Int 1993;43(6):1329–32.
218. Mahr AD, Edberg JC, Stone JH, et al. Alpha(1)-antitrypsin deficiency-related alleles Z and S and the risk of Wegener's granulomatosis. Arthritis Rheum 2010; 62(12):3760–7.
219. Tsuchiya N, Kobayashi S, Hashimoto H, et al. Association of HLA-DRB1*0901-DQB1*0303 haplotype with microscopic polyangiitis in Japanese. Genes Immun 2006;7(1):81–4.
220. Vaglio A, Martorana D, Maggiore U, et al. HLA-DRB4 as a genetic risk factor for Churg-Strauss syndrome. Arthritis Rheum 2007;56(9):3159–66.
221. Wieczorek S, Hellmich B, Gross WL, et al. Associations of Churg-Strauss syndrome with the HLA-DRB1 locus, and relationship to the genetics of antineutrophil cytoplasmic antibody-associated vasculitides: comment on the article by Vaglio, et al. Arthritis Rheum 2008;58(1):329–30.
222. Gregorini G, Ferioli A, Donato F, et al. Association between silica exposure and necrotizing crescentic glomerulonephritis with p-ANCA and anti-MPO antibodies: a hospital-based case-control study. Adv Exp Med Biol 1993;336: 435–40.
223. Hogan SL, Cooper GS, Savitz DA, et al. Association of silica exposure with anti-neutrophil cytoplasmic autoantibody small-vessel vasculitis: a population-based, case-control study. Clin J Am Soc Nephrol 2007;2(2):290–9.
224. Nuyts GD, Van Vlem E, De Vos A, et al. Wegener granulomatosis is associated to exposure to silicon compounds: a case-control study. Nephrol Dial Transplant 1995;10(7):1162–5.
225. Gonzalez-Gay MA, Garcia-Porrua C, Guerrero J, et al. The epidemiology of the primary systemic vasculitides in northwest Spain: implications of the Chapel Hill Consensus Conference definitions. Arthritis Rheum 2003;49(3):388–93.
226. Koldingsnes W, Nossent H. Epidemiology of Wegener's granulomatosis in northern Norway. Arthritis Rheum 2000;43(11):2481–7.
227. Lane SE, Watts RA, Bentham G, et al. Are environmental factors important in primary systemic vasculitis? A case-control study. Arthritis Rheum 2003;48(3): 814–23.
228. Watts RA, Lane SE, Bentham G, et al. Epidemiology of systemic vasculitis: a ten-year study in the United Kingdom. Arthritis Rheum 2000;43(2):414–9.
229. Gaudin PB, Askin FB, Falk RJ, et al. The pathologic spectrum of pulmonary lesions in patients with anti-neutrophil cytoplasmic autoantibodies specific for anti-proteinase 3 and anti-myeloperoxidase. Am J Clin Pathol 1995;104(1):7–16.
230. Kallenberg CG. Churg-Strauss syndrome: just one disease entity? Arthritis Rheum 2005;52(9):2589–93.
231. Lanham JG, Elkon KB, Pusey CD, et al. Systemic vasculitis with asthma and eosinophilia: a clinical approach to the Churg-Strauss syndrome. Medicine (Baltimore) 1984;63(2):65–81.
232. Sinico RA, Di Toma L, Maggiore U, et al. Prevalence and clinical significance of antineutrophil cytoplasmic antibodies in Churg-Strauss syndrome. Arthritis Rheum 2005;52(9):2926–35.
233. Adu D, Howie AJ, Scott DG, et al. Polyarteritis and the kidney. QJM 1987;62: 221–37.

234. Guillevin L, Cohen P, Gayraud M, et al. Churg-Strauss syndrome. Clinical study and long-term follow-up of 96 patients. Medicine (Baltimore) 1999; 78(1):26–37.

235. Guillevin L, Durand-Gasselin B, Cevallos R, et al. Microscopic polyangiitis: clinical and laboratory findings in eighty-five patients. Arthritis Rheum 1999;42(3): 421–30.

236. Hogan SL, Nachman PH, Wilkman AS, et al. Prognostic markers in patients with antineutrophil cytoplasmic autoantibody-associated microscopic polyangiitis and glomerulonephritis. J Am Soc Nephrol 1996;7(1):23–32.

237. Lhote F, Guillevin L. Polyarteritis nodosa, microscopic polyangiitis, and Churg-Strauss syndrome. Clinical aspects and treatment. Rheum Dis Clin North Am 1995;21(4):911–47.

238. Savage CO, Winearls CG, Evans DJ, et al. Microscopic polyarteritis: presentation, pathology and prognosis. Q J Med 1985;56(220):467–83.

239. Specks U. Pulmonary vasculitis. In: Schwarz MI, King TE, editors. Interstitial lung disease. 3rd edition. Hamilton (Ontario): BC Decker; 1998. p. 507–34.

240. Agadi JB, Raghav G, Mahadevan A, et al. Usefulness of superficial peroneal nerve/peroneus brevis muscle biopsy in the diagnosis of vasculitic neuropathy. Clin Neurosci 2012;19(10):1392–6.

241. Alba MA, Flores-Suarez LF. Rituximab for the treatment of ANCA associated vasculitis: the future today? Reumatol Clin 2011;7(Suppl 3):S41–6 [in Spanish].

242. Roccatello D, Vangelista A, Pani A. The role of rituximab in the treatment of ANCA-associated systemic vasculitis. G Ital Nefrol 2011;28(5):474–88 [in Italian].

243. Gallagher H, Kwan JT, Jayne DR. Pulmonary renal syndrome: a 4-year, single-center experience. Am J Kidney Dis 2002;39(1):42–7.

244. Kaplan AA. Apheresis for renal disease. Ther Apher 2001;5(2):134–41.

245. Klemmer PJ, Chalermskulrat W, Reif MS, et al. Plasmapheresis therapy for diffuse alveolar hemorrhage in patients with small-vessel vasculitis. Am J Kidney Dis 2003;42(6):1149–53.

246. Gaskin G, Pusey CD. Plasmapheresis in antineutrophil cytoplasmic antibody-associated systemic vasculitis. Ther Apher 2001;5(3):176–81.

247. Aydin Z, Gursu M, Karadag S, et al. Role of plasmapheresis performed in hemodialysis units for the treatment of anti-neutrophilic cytoplasmic antibody-associated systemic vasculitides. Ther Apher Dial 2011;15(5):493–8.

248. Yamagata K, Hirayama K, Mase K, et al. Apheresis for MPO-ANCA-associated RPGN-indications and efficacy: lessons learned from Japan nationwide survey of RPGN. J Clin Apheresis 2005;20(4):244–51.

249. Hogan SL, Falk RJ, Chin H, et al. Predictors of relapse and treatment resistance in antineutrophil cytoplasmic antibody-associated small-vessel vasculitis. Ann Intern Med 2005;143(9):621–31.

250. Weinkauf J, Puttagunta L, Stewart K, et al. Lung transplantation for severe anti-neutrophilic cytoplasmic antibody-associated vasculitis. Transplant Proc 2010; 42(7):2707–10.

251. Frohnert PP, Sheps SG. Long-term follow-up study of periarteritis nodosa. Am J Med 1967;43(1):8–14.

252. Leib ES, Restivo C, Paulus HE. Immunosuppressive and corticosteroid therapy of polyarteritis nodosa. Am J Med 1979;67(6):941–7.

253. Nachman PH, Hogan SL, Jennette JC, et al. Treatment response and relapse in antineutrophil cytoplasmic autoantibody-associated microscopic polyangiitis and glomerulonephritis. J Am Soc Nephrol 1996;7(1):33–9.

254. Szpirt WM, Heaf JG, Petersen J. Plasma exchange for induction and cyclosporine A for maintenance of remission in Wegener's granulomatosis–a clinical randomized controlled trial. Nephrol Dial Transplant 2011;26(1):206–13.
255. Gassman A. Zur Histologie der Roentgenulcere. Fortschr Geb Röntgenstrahlen 1899;2:199 [in German].
256. Fonkalsrud EW, Sanchez M, Zerubavel R, et al. Serial changes in arterial structure following radiation therapy. Surg Gynecol Obstet 1977;145(3):395–400.
257. Butler MJ, Lane RH, Webster JH. Irradiation injury to large arteries. Br J Surg 1980;67:341–3.
258. Lindsay S, Entenman C, Ellis EE, et al. Aortic arteriosclerosis in the dog after localized aortic irradiation with electrons. Circ Res 1962;10:61–7.
259. Fajardo LF. The pathology of ionizing radiation as defined by morphologic patterns. Acta Oncol 2005;44(1):13–22.
260. Fokkema M, den Hartog AG, van Lammeren GW, et al. Radiation-induced carotid stenotic lesions have a more stable phenotype than de novo atherosclerotic plaques. Eur J Vasc Endovasc Surg 2012;43(6):643–8.
261. Modrall JG, Sadjadi J. Early and late presentations of radiation arteritis. Semin Vasc Surg 2003;16(3):209–14.
262. Chuang VP. Radiation-induced arteritis. Semin Roentgenol 1994;29(1):64–9.
263. Himmel PD, Hassett JM. Radiation-induced chronic arterial injury. Semin Surg Oncol 1986;2(4):225–47.
264. Carmody BJ, Arora S, Avena R, et al. Accelerated carotid artery disease after high-dose head and neck radiotherapy: is there a role for routine carotid duplex surveillance? J Vasc Surg 1999;30:1045–51.
265. Moritz MW, Higgins RF, Jacobs JR. Duplex imaging and incidence of carotid radiation injury after high-dose radiotherapy for tumors of the head and neck. Arch Surg 1900;125:1181–3.
266. Buden JA, Casarella WJ, Hariasiadis L. Subclavian artery occlusion following radiotherapy for carcinoma of the breast. Radiology 1976;118:169–73.
267. Kretschmer G, Niederle B, Polterauer P, et al. Irradiation-induced changes in the subclavian and axillary arteries after radiotherapy for carcinoma of the breast. Surgery 1986;99(6):658–63.
268. Lawson JA. Surgical treatment of radiation induced atherosclerotic disease of the iliac and femoral arteries. J Cardiovasc Surg 1985;26:151–6.
269. Bates MC, Almehmi A. Carotid stenting for symptomatic radiation-induced arteritis complicated by recurrent aneurysm formation. Catheter Cardiovasc Interv 2004;63(4):507–11.
270. Koenigsberg RA, Grandinetti LM, Freeman LP, et al. Endovascular repair of radiation-induced bilateral common carotid artery stenosis and pseudoaneurysms: a case report. Surg Neurol 2001;55(6):347–52.
271. Ross HB, Sales JE. Post-irradiation femoral aneurysm treated by iliopopliteal bypass via the obturator foramen. Br J Surg 1972;59(5):400–5.
272. Tallarita T, Oderich GS, Lanzino G, et al. Outcomes of carotid artery stenting versus historical surgical controls for radiation-induced carotid stenosis. J Vasc Surg 2011;53(3):629–636.e1–5.
273. Fokkema M, den Hartog AG, Bots ML, et al. Stenting versus surgery in patients with carotid stenosis after previous cervical radiation therapy: systematic review and meta-analysis. Stroke 2012;43(3):793–801.
274. Sadek M, Cayne NS, Shin HJ, et al. Safety and efficacy of carotid angioplasty and stenting for radiation-associated carotid artery stenosis. J Vasc Surg 2009;50(6):1308–13.

275. Protack CD, Bakken AM, Saad WE, et al. Radiation arteritis: a contraindication to carotid stenting? J Vasc Surg 2007;45(1):110–7.
276. Shin SH, Stout CL, Richardson AI, et al. Carotid angioplasty and stenting in anatomically high-risk patients: safe and durable except for radiation-induced stenosis. J Vasc Surg 2009;50(4):762–7 [discussion: 767–8].
277. Atkinson JL, Sundt TM Jr, Dale AJ, et al. Radiation-associated atheromatous disease of the cervical carotid artery: report of seven cases and review of the literature. Neurosurgery 1989;24(2):171–8.
278. Kashyap VS, Moore WS, Quinones-Baldrich WJ. Carotid artery repair for radiation-associated atherosclerosis is a safe and durable procedure. J Vasc Surg 1999;29(1):90–6 [discussion: 97–9].
279. Cormier F, Korso F, Fichelle JM, et al. Post-irradiation axillo-subclavian arteriopathy: surgical revascularization. J Mal Vasc 2001;26(1):45–9 [in French].
280. Goldstein LJ, Ayers JD, Hollenbeck S, et al. Successful revascularization for delayed presentation of radiation-induced distal upper extremity ischemia. Ann Vasc Surg 2010;24(2):257.e5–8.
281. Melliere D, Desgranges P, Berrahal D, et al. Radiation-induced aorto-ilio-femoral arterial arteritis. Mediocrity of the long-term results after conventional surgery. J Mal Vasc 2000;25(5):332–5.
282. Baerlocher MO, Rajan DK, Ing DJ, et al. Primary stenting of bilateral radiation-induced external iliac stenoses. J Vasc Surg 2004;40(5):1028–31.
283. Farrugia M, Gowda KM, Cheatle TR, et al. Radiotherapy-related axillary artery occlusive disease: percutaneous transluminal angioplasty and stenting. Two case reports and review of the literature. Cardiovasc Intervent Radiol 2006; 29(6):1144–7.
284. McBride KD, Beard JD, Gaines PA. Percutaneous intervention for radiation damage to axillary arteries. Clin Radiol 1994;49(9):630–3.
285. Goundry B, Bell L, Langtree M, et al. Diagnosis and management of Raynaud's phenomenon. BMJ 2012;344:e289.
286. Kaiser H. Maurice Raynaud (1834-1881) and the syndrome named after him. Z Rheumatol 2011;70(7):620–4 [in German].
287. Wigley FM, Flavahan NA. Raynaud's phenomenon. Rheum Dis Clin North Am 1996;22(4):765–81.
288. Cooke JP, Marshall JM. Mechanisms of Raynaud's disease. Vasc Med 2005; 10(4):293–307.
289. Herrick AL. Pathogenesis of Raynaud's phenomenon. Rheumatology (Oxford) 2005;44(5):587–96.
290. Herrick AL. Contemporary management of Raynaud's phenomenon and digital ischaemic complications. Curr Opin Rheumatol 2011;23(6):555–61.
291. Belch JJ. Raynaud's phenomenon. Curr Opin Rheumatol 1991;3(6):960–6.
292. Generini S, Kahaleh B, Matucci-Cerinic M, et al. Raynaud's phenomenon and systemic sclerosis. Ann Ital Med Int 1996;11(2):125–31.
293. Wigley FM, Wise RA, Mikdashi J, et al. The post-occlusive hyperemic response in patients with systemic sclerosis. Arthritis Rheum 1990;33(11):1620–5.
294. Agache I, Radoi M, Duca L. Platelet activation in patients with systemic scleroderma–pattern and significance. Rom J Intern Med 2007;45(2):183–91.
295. Polidoro L, Barnabei R, Giorgini P, et al. Platelet activation in patients with the Raynaud phenomenon. Intern Med J 2012;42(5):531–5.
296. Walmsley D, Goodfield MJ. Evidence for an abnormal peripherally mediated vascular response to temperature in Raynaud's phenomenon. Br J Rheumatol 1990;29(3):181–4.

297. Carter SA, Dean E, Kroeger EA. Apparent finger systolic pressures during cooling in patients with Raynaud's syndrome. Circulation 1988;77(5):988–96.
298. Maricq HR, Weinrich MC, Valter I, et al. Digital vascular responses to cooling in subjects with cold sensitivity, primary Raynaud's phenomenon, or scleroderma spectrum disorders. J Rheumatol 1996;23(12):2068–78.
299. Rosato E, Borghese F, Pisarri S, et al. Laser Doppler perfusion imaging is useful in the study of Raynaud's phenomenon and improves the capillaroscopic diagnosis. J Rheumatol 2009;36(10):2257–63.
300. Rosato E, Rossi C, Molinaro I, et al. Laser Doppler perfusion imaging in systemic sclerosis impaired response to cold stimulation involves digits and hand dorsum. Rheumatology (Oxford) 2011;50(9):1654–8.
301. Bilgi C, Pelmear PL. Hand-arm vibration syndrome: a guide to medical impairment assessment. J Occup Med 1993;35(9):936–42.
302. Pyykko I. Clinical aspects of the hand-arm vibration syndrome. A review. Scand J Work Environ Health 1986;12(5):439–47.
303. Hummers LK, Wigley FM. Management of Raynaud's phenomenon and digital ischemic lesions in scleroderma. Rheum Dis Clin North Am 2003;29(2):293–313.
304. Thompson AE, Pope JE. Calcium channel blockers for primary Raynaud's phenomenon: a meta-analysis. Rheumatology (Oxford) 2005;44(2):145–50.
305. Thompson AE, Shea B, Welch V, et al. Calcium-channel blockers for Raynaud's phenomenon in systemic sclerosis. Arthritis Rheum 2001;44(8):1841–7.
306. Dziadzio M, Denton CP, Smith R, et al. Losartan therapy for Raynaud's phenomenon and scleroderma: clinical and biochemical findings in a fifteen-week, randomized, parallel-group, controlled trial. Arthritis Rheum 1999;42(12):2646–55.
307. Wigley FM, Seibold JR, Wise RA, et al. Intravenous iloprost treatment of Raynaud's phenomenon and ischemic ulcers secondary to systemic sclerosis. J Rheumatol 1992;19(9):1407–14.
308. Brueckner CS, Becker MO, Kroencke T, et al. Effect of sildenafil on digital ulcers in systemic sclerosis: analysis from a single centre pilot study. Ann Rheum Dis 2010;69(8):1475–8.
309. Herrick AL, van den Hoogen F, Gabrielli A, et al. Modified-release sildenafil reduces Raynaud's phenomenon attack frequency in limited cutaneous systemic sclerosis. Arthritis Rheum 2011;63(3):775–82.
310. Shenoy PD, Kumar S, Jha LK, et al. Efficacy of tadalafil in secondary Raynaud's phenomenon resistant to vasodilator therapy: a double-blind randomized crossover trial. Rheumatology (Oxford) 2010;49(12):2420–8.
311. Chung L, Shapiro L, Fiorentino D, et al. MQX-503, a novel formulation of nitroglycerin, improves the severity of Raynaud's phenomenon: a randomized, controlled trial. Arthritis Rheum 2009;60(3):870–7.
312. Teh LS, Manning J, Moore T, et al. Sustained-release transdermal glyceryl trinitrate patches as a treatment for primary and secondary Raynaud's phenomenon. Br J Rheumatol 1995;34(7):636–41.
313. Gordon A, Zechmeister K, Collin J. The role of sympathectomy in current surgical practice. Eur J Vasc Surg 1994;8(2):129–37.
314. Coveliers HM, Hoexum F, Nederhoed JH, et al. Thoracic sympathectomy for digital ischemia: a summary of evidence. J Vasc Surg 2011;54(1):273–7.
315. Maga P, Kuzdzal J, Nizankowski R, et al. Long-term effects of thoracic sympathectomy on microcirculation in the hands of patients with primary Raynaud disease. J Thorac Cardiovasc Surg 2007;133(6):1428–33.

316. Tomaino MM, Goitz RJ, Medsger TA. Surgery for ischemic pain and Raynaud's' phenomenon in scleroderma: a description of treatment protocol and evaluation of results. Microsurgery 2001;21(3):75–9.
317. Tham S, Grossman JA. Limited microsurgical arteriolysis for complications of digital vasospasm. J Hand Surg 1997;22(3):359–61.

Aneurysmal Disease
The Abdominal Aorta

Toshio Takayama, MD, PhD, Dai Yamanouchi, MD, PhD*

KEYWORDS

- Abdominal aortic aneurysm • Asymptomatic • Ruptured • Open repair
- Endovascular aneurysm repair • Endoleak

KEY POINTS

- The mortality for ruptured abdominal aortic aneurysms (AAAs) is 80% to 90%. Ruptured AAA is the 15th leading cause of death in the United States.
- Approximately 80% of AAAs occur in the infrarenal portion of the abdominal aorta.
- Smoking is the risk factor most strongly associated with AAA. Smoking cessation is crucial to avoiding the condition.
- Contrast-enhanced computed tomography is the most reliable imaging modality, both for diagnosis and decision making.
- Open aneurysm repair is more invasive initially but more durable. Endovascular aneurysm repair is less invasive initially but less durable.
- Continuous follow-up after aneurysmal repair improves long-term outcome.

INTRODUCTION
Abdominal Aortic Aneurysm: Impact of Rupture

If diseases were action movie characters, abdominal aortic aneurysm (AAA) would be a *Ninja*: remaining quietly concealed for much of the plot, but reliably terminating the patient once out of hiding. Ruptured AAA is the 15th leading killer overall and the 10th leading killer for men older than 55 years in the United States.[1,2] More than 5000 people die from ruptured AAA every year, and 4% to 5% of sudden deaths are caused by ruptured AAA.[3–5] Roughly half of patients with ruptured AAA die before they reach the hospital, whereas half of those who do arrive do not survive despite treatment.[3,6] Under all circumstances, ruptured AAAs result in an overall mortality of 80% to 90%.

Division of Vascular Surgery, Department of Surgery, University of Wisconsin School of Medicine and Public Health, 600 Highland Avenue, CSC G5/325, Madison, WI 53792, USA
* Corresponding author.
E-mail address: yamano@surgery.wisc.edu

Surg Clin N Am 93 (2013) 877–891
http://dx.doi.org/10.1016/j.suc.2013.05.005
0039-6109/13/$ – see front matter © 2013 Elsevier Inc. All rights reserved.

Definition and Location of AAA

According to the Ad Hoc Committee on Reporting Standards of the Society for Vascular Surgery, an aneurysm is defined as a permanent, localized (ie, focal) dilation of an artery having at least a 50% increase in diameter compared with the expected normal diameter of the artery in question.[7] More than 80% of AAAs are located in the infrarenal portion of the aorta.[3,8] Thus, because the normal diameter of this portion in patients older than 50 years is estimated to be 10 to 20 mm, an infrarenal abdominal aorta larger than 30 mm is considered to be an AAA.[3,9–11]

CAUSE AND RISK FACTORS
Cause

Degeneration
A degenerative process in the aortic wall is the most common cause, and more than 90% of AAAs are degenerative.[12] Moreover, there is usually some degree of calcification and atherosclerotic disease present in such AAAs, meaning that atherosclerosis is also associated with degeneration of the aortic wall.[13] Metalloproteinases, a family of elastases, are abundant in AAA walls to degrade the extracellular matrix proteins such as elastin and collagen, making the aortic wall fragile and prone to forming aneurysms.[14,15] Smoking is strongly related to this process.

Inflammation
AAAs sometimes occur with a marked inflammatory change consisting of a thick, fibrotic process in the retroperitoneum. These inflammatory AAAs account for 5% to 10% of all AAAs.[16] Special attention should be paid, especially when performing open aneurysm repair, because inflammation often involves surrounding organs such as the duodenum and ureter. Although some specific diseases such as Takayasu arteritis and Behçet disease can cause aortic inflammation,[17,18] the underlying cause is unclear in most cases. Steroids are useful for remission of the inflammatory change.[19]

Infection
Infectious or mycotic AAAs are a rare condition, but the mortality for them is high. Oderich and colleagues[20] analyzed 6137 patients who had undergone an aortic reconstruction procedure and found that only 43 cases (0.7%) were related to infection; however, their operative mortality was 21% and 5-year mortality was 50%. Rapid destruction of the arterial wall resulting in rupture and persistent infection after the aneurysm repair accounts for the poor outcomes of infectious AAAs.

Connective tissue abnormalities
AAAs in patients with Marfan syndrome or Ehlers-Danlos syndrome often extend up to the thoracic region and persist as a chronic state after aortic dissection. Patients with such connective tissue abnormalities tend to develop larger AAAs at a younger age than patients with ordinary, degenerative AAAs.[21,22]

Risk Factors

The common risk factors of AAA are smoking, male gender, white race, older age, chronic obstructive pulmonary disease (COPD), hypertension, dyslipidemia, coronary artery disease (CAD), peripheral artery disease (PAD), and positive family history.[3,23–30]

Smoking
Smoking is the independent risk factor most strongly associated with AAA. Lederle and colleagues[28] reported that the odds ratio for AAAs larger than 40 mm is

5.57 compared with normal aortas, and the association between smoking and AAA increases significantly with the number of years of smoking and decreases significantly with the number of years after quitting smoking. The odds ratio is 12.13 for patients smoking 1 pack or more a day for more than 35 years, whereas the odds ratio is 0.42 for patients quitting smoking for more than 10 years.[30]

Gender, ethnicity, and age
The odds ratio for male gender is 5.71 and for white race the odds ratio is 1.45.[30] Age also affects AAA formation: approximately 1% of men between 55 and 64 years old have AAAs larger than 40 mm, and the prevalence increases by 2% to 4% per decade thereafter.[29,31]

COPD
COPD itself is an independent risk factor for AAA, although it is profoundly related to smoking. A case-control study of 308 patients revealed that the odds ratio for COPD is 3.0 (95% confidence interval, 1.6–5.5).[32]

Hypertension and dyslipidemia
The odds ratio for hypertension is 1.25.[30] In addition, hypertension is not only associated with AAA formation but also increases rupture risk in patients with established AAAs.[28,33] The odds ratio for high cholesterol is 1.34.[30] In particular, high serum total cholesterol has a positive association with AAA prevalence, whereas high-density lipoprotein cholesterol has an inverse association.[34] Patients with diabetes mellitus have a lower chance of developing AAAs (odds ratio, 0.75).[26,30,35]

CAD and PAD
Because most AAAs are caused by a degenerative process, CAD and PAD have a high affinity with AAA. The odds ratio of CAD is 1.72, and that of PAD is 1.59. The prevalence of AAA in patients with CAD is approximately 5%, and that of patients with CAD is approximately 10%.[25,26,30]

Family history
A positive family history is also a major risk factor (odds ratio, 3.30).[30] First-degree relatives of a patient with AAA have a 12-fold increased risk of aneurysm development; moreover, brothers of a patient with an AAA have an 18-fold increased risk.[36,37] Although almost 80% of AAAs occur in men, this familial clustering tendency is more common in women.[38,39]

ASYMPTOMATIC AAA
Screening

Screening with ultrasonography (US) on specific high-risk patients is established as the most effective way to filter asymptomatic AAAs, which are usually found accidentally by various imaging modalities performed for other purposes in clinical settings.[3] For patient cohort selection, 2 reliable guidelines were established based on the statement by Kent and colleagues,[40] the 2005 American College of Cardiology(ACC)/ American Heart Association (AHA) guidelines, and the United States Preventive Service Task Force (USPSTF) recommendation statement.

The 2005 ACC/AHA guidelines recommend: (1) men 60 years of age or older who are either siblings or offspring of patients with AAAs should undergo a physical examination and US screening, (2) men 65 to 75 years of age who have a smoking history should undergo a physical examination and a 1-time US screening.[11] USPSTF recommends US screening for men between 65 and 75 years of age who have a smoking history.[41]

History Taking, Physical Examination, and Laboratory Workups

The important information that should be taken from AAA patients' clinical histories are: (1) when and how the AAA was diagnosed; (2) the underlying medical conditions, especially hypertension, dyslipidemia, diabetes mellitus, renal dysfunction, cerebrovascular diseases, heart disease, pulmonary disease, peripheral vascular disease, and previous surgical history; (3) allergic history and current medications; (4) smoking history; (5) family history of any aortic aneurysms or dissections.

An AAA can be palpable as a pulsatile mass at or above the umbilicus, but the accuracy of manipulation highly depends on the patient's physique and the size of the AAA. Investigations for any other PAD or peripheral arterial aneurysms are also important. From 1% to 10% of AAAs complicate other peripheral arterial aneurysms, synchronously or metachronously, particularly in the femoral arteries and popliteal arteries.[42,43] The pulsation of the carotid artery, radial artery, ulnar artery, femoral artery, popliteal artery, posterior tibial artery, and dorsalis pedis artery should be checked. The auscultation at the neck, chest, abdomen, and groin should also be obtained; the presence of a bruit indicates possible stenotic lesions or arteriovenous fistula.[3]

A basic blood test, electrocardiography, echocardiography, spirometry, measurement of angle-brachial pressure index, and US for carotid and lower extremity arteries are all useful in estimating the patient's systemic baseline conditions.

Imaging Modalities and Diagnosis

Diagnosis of an AAA is confirmed by several imaging modalities, including abdominal US, computed tomography (CT), magnetic resonance imaging (MRI), or angiography. A combination of each finding provides accurate location, shape, and size of an AAA.

US

The merits of US are its noninvasiveness and low cost.[3,27] The sensitivity and specificity are more than 90% when it is performed by well-trained doctors or technicians,[27,41] suggesting that the quality of US is operator dependent. The patient's physique and the location of the aneurysm also affect quality; the findings around the suprarenal or pelvic regions are often poor because of intestinal gas. In clinical practice, US is most useful for periodic follow-up to measure AAA size after the initial diagnosis.

CT

Contrast-enhanced CT is the most reliable, indispensable modality, not only for diagnosis but also for decision making for AAAs, and is the current gold standard. CT can accurately and objectively detect AAA formation regardless of location or the patient's physique (**Fig. 1**). In addition, three-dimensional CT angiography composed of thin-slice (<3 mm) images obtained by multidetector row CT scanners clearly describes the details of the lesion, such as the location and length of the aneurysmal neck, the anatomic relationship to the visceral branches, the patency of the lumbar arteries, and the existence of concomitant iliac arterial aneurysms: all important observations for deciding how to treat the AAA, either by open repair or endovascular aneurysm repair (EVAR).

The disadvantages of CT are unavoidable exposure to radiation, the requirement for a contrast medium, and higher cost compared with US.[3] However, nonenhanced CT

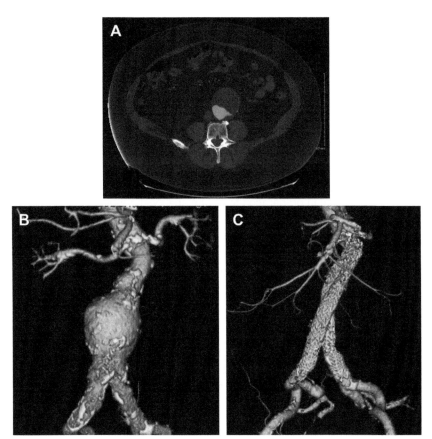

Fig. 1. (A) Contrast-enhanced CT scan image of infrarenal AAA with a maximum diameter of 6.5 cm. (B) Three-dimensional reconstruction image of infrarenal AAA. (C) Three-dimensional reconstruction image of AAA status after EVAR.

images still provide much valuable information. Therefore, all asymptomatic patients with AAA should be evaluated by CT with or without contrast medium.

MRI
Contrast-enhanced magnetic resonance (MR) angiography describes the detailed structure of an AAA as well as does contrast-enhanced CT angiography. Also, because nonenhanced MR angiography alone can describe the whole shape of an AAA, it is useful when planning an EVAR for patients with renal dysfunction. Avoidance of exposure to radiation is a big advantage. However, MR angiography is a time-consuming process, with contraindication for patients with claustrophobia or magnetic material implantation, and higher cost compared with CT might be the reason why MRI is not yet universally available.[44]

Angiography
Diagnostic angiography has been almost completely replaced by other modalities because of its invasiveness and the administration of contrast medium. However, the basic methods of angiography, such as the Seldinger technique, are still necessary for many endovascular treatments, which are called interventional radiology.

Management Before the Aneurysm Repair

The risk of rupture in AAAs smaller than 40 mm is very low. Brewster and colleagues[45] reported that the annual rupture risk of AAAs between 40 and 50 mm was less than 5%, whereas that of AAAs larger than 50 mm was more than 10%. Moreover, this risk increases as the size grows larger, and the estimated annual rupture risk of AAAs larger than 80 mm was 30% to 50% in the same report.[45] In addition, Conway and colleagues[46] reported that most AAAs larger than 55 mm resulted in rupture when they remained untreated. Taking account of these facts, the indication size of elective repair for infrarenal asymptomatic AAA without rapid expansion is generally 55 mm.[10,11]

Patients with small AAAs are managed conservatively. The purpose of such treatments is to reduce the expansion rate of AAAs and to optimize each patient's underlying medical condition in preparation for future aneurysm repair.

Smoking cessation

The priority in preventing AAA is to educate the patients into quitting smoking if they are current smokers. Continued smoking alone increases the rate of AAA growth by 20% to 25%.[29] Smoking cessation is also important for reducing pulmonary complications after aneurysm repair procedures. Moreover, patients should never smoke again even after a successful aneurysm repair, because smoking increases the risk of postoperative mortality and morbidity.[47,48]

β-blockers and statins

β-Blockers are reported to significantly reduce the expansion rate of AAAs, especially when they are larger than 50 mm.[49] Long-term statin use is reported to reduce all-cause and cardiovascular mortality after successful AAA repair.[50] The 2005 ACC/AHA guidelines recommend that patients with AAAs as well as patients with atherosclerotic disease should have their blood pressure and lipids controlled.[11]

Elective Aneurysm Repair: Open Repair or EVAR?

The best time for a patient with an asymptomatic AAA to have an aneurysm repair must be the moment when the benefit of the repair exceeds the risk of the repair. This decision-making strategy seems simple but is complicated in practice. The benefit of an AAA repair is to prevent aneurysm rupture. The risk of the repair is, on the other hand, different for the 2 major options: conventional open repair or EVAR, each of which has its own advantages and limitations (**Table 1**).

Open repair, the elimination of AAA

Since the first graft replacement was reported by Dubost in 1951,[51] open repair was the only option for preventing AAA ruptures until the first EVAR was reported by Parodi in 1991.[52] After EVAR was approved by the US Food and Drug Administration in 1999, 2 pivotal randomized trials comparing elective open repair and EVAR proved that the 30-day mortality was significantly lower for EVAR.[53,54] Now, more than 70% of AAAs are repaired by EVAR in the United States,[55,56] and the more limited invasiveness has been widely perceived as beneficial by both patients and surgeons.

Nevertheless, the conventional invasive option, open repair, which consists of directly opening the aneurysmal sac and implanting a synthetic graft with physical suture stitches, is still the only curative treatment of AAAs. Once an AAA is resected and replaced with a synthetic graft, the aneurysm has certainly disappeared, and the patient essentially needs no further follow-up radiologic studies.[10]

Table 1
Results of randomized control trials comparing open repair with EVAR

Series	Year	No. of Patients	Median Follow-Up (y)	30-d Mortality (%)			Long-term Mortality (%)			Graft-related Complication or Reintervention (%)		
				Open Repair	EVAR	P Value	Open Repair	EVAR	P Value	Open Repair	EVAR	P Value
The United Kingdom EVAR Trial[a]	2010	1252	6	4.3	1.8	.02	42	41	.72	12	45	<.001
DREAM Study[b]	2010	351	6.4	4.6	1.2	.1	30	31	.97	18	30	.03
ACE trial[c]	2011	316	3	0.6	2	NS	8	11.3	NS	2.7	16	<.0001

Abbreviation: NS, not significant.

[a] Endovascular versus open repair of abdominal aortic aneurysm.
[b] Long-term outcome of open or endovascular repair of abdominal aortic aneurysm.
[c] A randomized controlled trial of endovascular aneurysm repair versus open surgery for abdominal aortic aneurysms in low- to moderate-risk patients.
Data from Refs.[57–59]

Open repair is a more invasive treatment than EVAR, because patients need a large skin incision and aortic cross clamp, while experiencing a greater amount of blood loss, a longer operation time, and so on. However, the early benefit of the EVAR disappears in the long-term; moreover, EVAR is associated with increased rates of graft-related complications and reinterventions.[57–59]

One important factor that improves the outcome after open repair is case volume. Dimick and colleagues[60] reported that the mortality of the procedure was 3.0% when performed in a high-volume center that has more than 35 AAA repairs annually, whereas the mean mortality in low-volume centers is 5.5%.

EVAR, the decompression of AAA

Based on the concept that pressure reduction inside the aneurysm can prevent its future rupture, the initial purpose of EVAR is not to delete the aneurysm but to decompress it. Although some successful EVARs can eliminate AAAs by complete decompression leading to aneurysmal wall remodeling and shrinkage after several months, AAAs still remain after EVAR in most cases.

Therefore, the only way to judge whether an EVAR has been successful is to continue observing the aneurysm size after each procedure. Patients treated with EVAR are routinely examined for AAA size by CT or US at 1, 6, and 12 months after the procedure, and annually thereafter. If the size is decreasing, it means the EVAR has been successful; if the size remains the same, it means the intrasac pressure is still not high enough to expand; but if the size is increasing, it calls for action in response to endoleaks.

Endoleaks after EVAR

Endoleaks are a complication unique to endovascular repair for aortic aneurysms; they are defined as the remaining blood flow inside the aneurysmal sac after the endograft insertion (**Fig. 2**). Endoleaks are classified into 4 types: type I (perigraft blood flow caused by an inadequate seal at the proximal or distal end of the endograft); type II

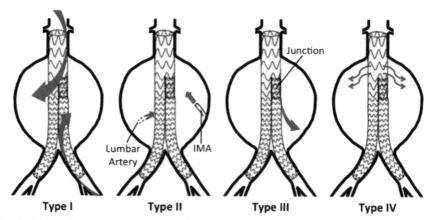

Type I   Type II   Type III   Type IV

Fig. 2. Endoleak types. Type I: perigraft blood flow caused by an inadequate seal at the proximal or distal end of the endograft. Type II: retrograde blood flow into the AAA from visceral vessels (such as the lumbar artery, inferior mesenteric artery, accessory renal artery, or hypogastric artery) without attachment site connection. Type III: perigraft blood flow from module disconnection or fabric disruption. Type IV: perigraft blood flow from porous fabric. (*Data from* Chaikof EL, Blankensteijn JD, Harris PL, et al. Reporting standards for endovascularaortic aneurysm repair. J Vasc Surg 2002;35(5):1048–60.)

(retrograde blood flow into the AAA from visceral vessels [such as the lumbar artery, inferior mesenteric artery, accessory renal artery, or hypogastric artery] without attachment site connection); type III (perigraft blood flow from module disconnection or fabric disruption); and type IV (perigraft blood flow from porous fabric).[61] The occurrence rate of endoleaks differs between endograft types.

Type I and type III endoleaks are usually detected at the time of the EVAR procedure by completion of an angiogram and are then treated properly; however, they sometimes appear at a later stage to cause chronic AAA size expansion. Type II endoleaks, especially from patent lumbar arteries or the inferior mesenteric artery, cause chronic expansion in many cases. Type IV endoleaks often disappear spontaneously within several weeks.

Management of endoleaks

Chronic endoleaks after EVAR can cause delayed AAA rupture; Mehta and colleagues[62] reported that 63% of delayed AAA ruptures after EVAR were caused by type I endoleaks with endograft migration, 11% by type I without migration, 19% by type II, and the rest of unknown type.

To distinguish the type of endoleak, time-resolved CT angiography and color duplex US are useful,[63,64] but sometimes diagnostic angiography is necessary. If a type I or type III endoleak is detected in an expanding AAA, it gives a yellow signal. A late type I/III endoleak is often caused by endograft migration or dilatation of the host artery (neck dilatation), and should be repaired immediately, because the existence of such foreflow endoleaks means the AAA is not decompressed and is still exposed to a high blood pressure environment (as high as the systemic blood pressure). Additional endograft insertion covering the endoleak site is usually effective in stopping the perigraft blood flow. Some extreme cases, like massive neck dilatation resulting in aneurysmal rupture, require open repair.

A type II endoleak also needs proper treatment when the AAA size increases. In contrast to the treatment of type I/III endoleaks, the treatment of type II endoleaks is not always urgent, because the intrasac pressure caused by such retrograde blood flow is low compared with the systemic blood pressure. But the treatment itself can be more complicated, because selecting the feeding artery is usually difficult after an endograft insertion; it is usually achieved retrogradely via various collateral networks with very fine microcatheters and microwires. Also, there are as yet no established criteria for when to treat a type II endoleak. The following conditions seem reasonable: AAAs increasing more than 5 mm over a 6-month period or increasing more than 10 mm when compared with the pre-EVAR diameter.[65]

Decision making

Simply stated, open repair is more invasive initially but more durable, whereas EVAR is less invasive initially but less durable. We expect that continuous improvements will provide us with a durable EVAR device in the future, but our patients cannot wait for that day. The 2005 ACC/AHA guideline is still valid for decision making: (1) open repair of infrarenal AAAs or common iliac aneurysms is indicated in patients who are good or average surgical candidates (class I, evidence level B), (2) endovascular repair of infrarenal aortic or common iliac aneurysms is reasonable in patients at high risk of complications from open operations because of cardiopulmonary or other associated diseases (class IIa, evidence level B).[11]

In some special situations, open repair may be suitable for AAAs in the upper abdominal aorta with highly tortuous necks, because reconstruction of blood flow into visceral arteries with an endovascular technique is complicated and not commonly available yet for AAAs in patients with a highly stenosed or occluded lesion at the iliac or femoral arteries that are unsuitable for device insertion (access to arteries should be wide enough for at least a 16-Fr sheath for commercially available EVAR devices). By contrast, EVAR may be suitable for AAAs in patients with hostile abdomen, for AAAs in patients with horseshoe kidneys, or for perianastomotic false aneurysms after open repair.

For surgeons treating AAAs, what matters most is not simply which option is better, but to have sufficient knowledge with regard to the characteristics of each option.

SYMPTOMATIC OR RUPTURED AAA
Clinical Presentation and Management

When a patient with an AAA presents with back, abdominal, or groin pain, it should be regarded as a red flag. Such symptoms often come from the rapid expansion of the AAA, and they are clear signs of rupture.[10] Outcomes for repair of symptomatic AAAs are significantly worse than for asymptomatic AAAs. Sullivan and colleagues[66] analyzed open repair cases to show that the mortality of emergency procedures for symptomatic AAA was 26% and for ruptured AAA was 35%, whereas the mortality for elective procedures was 5.1%. Symptomatic AAAs should be treated in essentially the same way as ruptured AAAs.

The classic triad of symptoms for ruptured AAA is: (1) hypotension, (2) abdominal or back pain, and (3) a pulsatile abdominal mass. When a patient with known infrarenal AAA that is larger than 55 mm presents with this triad and the general status is unstable, the patient should be brought to the operating room immediately to open the abdomen and clamp the AAA neck as quickly as possible. If the patient is clinically stable, an urgent CT with or without contrast medium and duplex US are useful for ruling out rupture. But the patient should at least be hospitalized for close observation even if rupture is ruled out, and a quick repair of the AAA is desirable. Also, a quick repair is necessary for some rapidly expanding AAAs even if they are asymptomatic, because they are considered to be at risk of rupture if the expansion rate is more than 5 mm per 6 months.

EVAR for Ruptured AAAs

In life-threatening situations like aneurysmal ruptures, initial lifesaving matters more than long-term durability. Hence, EVAR is preferable for ruptured AAAs. The lower invasiveness of EVAR has been proved beneficial by many studies since the first successful EVAR for ruptured AAA was reported by Marin and colleagues[67] in 1994. According to recent reports investigating treatment of ruptured AAAs, the 30-day mortality was 15.7% to 18.5% for EVAR and 49% to 54.2% for open repair.[68,69]

However, there are reasons why EVAR for ruptured AAA is not yet widespread. Essential for this procedure are high-performance CT scanners, rapid evaluation of aneurysm anatomy and selection of optimal devices, an ample stock of devices, a hybrid operating room suite, and well-trained endovascular staff,[68,70] but the availability of these essentials is limited in most emergency settings.

As EVAR expertise becomes more widespread, this technology has the potential to reduce the mortality from ruptured AAA.

SUMMARY

The impact of ruptured AAA is substantial. Its mortality is as high as 90% and it is the 15th leading cause of death in the United States. Approximately 80% of AAAs occurs in the surgically tractable infrarenal portion of the abdominal aorta. Most of these lesions are caused by degenerative processes in the aortic wall. Smoking, male gender, white race, advanced age, COPD, hypertension, dyslipidemia, and positive family history are major risk factors; among these, smoking is the risk factor most strongly associated with AAA. Hence, smoking cessation is crucial for prevention of this condition. Of the available imaging modalities, contrast-enhanced CT is most reliable, both for diagnosis and decision making.

Two options are available for aneurysm repair: open repair or EVAR. Open repair is more invasive initially but more durable, whereas EVAR is less invasive initially but less durable. However, as degradation of the aorta progresses with age, treatment of an AAA cannot be completed by a 1-time procedure. Continuous follow-up after aneurysmal repair improves the long-term outcome regardless of whether open repair or EVAR is used.

REFERENCES

1. Bobadilla JL, Kent KC. Screening for abdominal aortic aneurysms. Adv Surg 2012;46:101–9.
2. National Center for Injury Prevention and Control. WISQARS leading causes of death reports, 1999-2005. Atlanta: Centers for Disease Control and Prevention. Available at: http://webappa.cdc.gov/sasweb/ncipc/leadcaus10.html.
3. Aggarwal S, Qamar A, Sharma V, et al. Abdominal aortic aneurysm: a comprehensive review. Exp Clin Cardiol 2011;16(1):11–5.
4. Schermerhorn MA. 66-year-old man with an abdominal aortic aneurysm: review of screening and treatment. JAMA 2009;302(18):2015–22.
5. O'Sullivan JP. The coroner's necropsy in sudden death: an under-used source of epidemiological information. J Clin Pathol 1996;49(9):737–40.
6. Harris LM, Faggioli GL, Fiedler R, et al. Ruptured abdominal aortic aneurysms: factors affecting mortality rates. J Vasc Surg 1991;14(6):812–8 [discussion: 819–20].
7. Johnston KW, Rutherford RB, Tilson MD, et al. Suggested standards for reporting on arterial aneurysms. Subcommittee on Reporting Standards for Arterial Aneurysms, Ad Hoc Committee on Reporting Standards, Society for Vascular Surgery and North American Chapter, International Society for Cardiovascular Surgery. J Vasc Surg 1991;13(3):452–8.
8. Olsen PS, Schroeder T, Agerskov K, et al. Surgery for abdominal aortic aneurysms. A survey of 656 patients. J Cardiovasc Surg (Torino) 1991;32(5): 636–42.
9. Lederle FA, Johnson GR, Wilson SE, et al. Relationship of age, gender, race, and body size to infrarenal aortic diameter. The Aneurysm Detection and Management (ADAM) Veterans Affairs Cooperative Study Investigators. J Vasc Surg 1997;26(4):595–601.
10. Upchurch GR Jr, Schaub TA. Abdominal aortic aneurysm. Am Fam Physician 2006;73(7):1198–204.
11. Hirsch AT, Haskal ZJ, Hertzer NR, et al. ACC/AHA 2005 Practice Guidelines for the management of patients with peripheral arterial disease (lower extremity, renal, mesenteric, and abdominal aortic): a collaborative report from the American Association for Vascular Surgery/Society for Vascular Surgery, Society for Cardiovascular Angiography and Interventions, Society for Vascular Medicine and Biology, Society of Interventional Radiology, and the ACC/AHA Task Force on Practice Guidelines (Writing Committee to Develop Guidelines for

the Management of Patients With Peripheral Arterial Disease): endorsed by the American Association of Cardiovascular and Pulmonary Rehabilitation; National Heart, Lung, and Blood Institute; Society for Vascular Nursing; TransAtlantic Inter-Society Consensus; and Vascular Disease Foundation. Circulation 2006; 113(11):e463–654.

12. Nordon IM, Hinchliffe RJ, Holt PJ, et al. Review of current theories for abdominal aortic aneurysm pathogenesis. Vascular 2009;17(5):253–63.

13. Zarins CK, Glagov S, Vesselinovitch D, et al. Aneurysm formation in experimental atherosclerosis: relationship to plaque evolution. J Vasc Surg 1990; 12(3):246–56.

14. Wassef M, Baxter BT, Chisholm RL, et al. Pathogenesis of abdominal aortic aneurysms: a multidisciplinary research program supported by the National Heart, Lung, and Blood Institute. J Vasc Surg 2001;34(4):730–8.

15. Brophy CM, Marks WH, Reilly JM, et al. Decreased tissue inhibitor of metalloproteinases (TIMP) in abdominal aortic aneurysm tissue: a preliminary report. J Surg Res 1991;50(6):653–7.

16. Hellmann DB, Grand DJ, Freischlag JA. Inflammatory abdominal aortic aneurysm. JAMA 2007;297(4):395–400.

17. Matsumura K, Hirano T, Takeda K, et al. Incidence of aneurysms in Takayasu's arteritis. Angiology 1991;42(4):308–15.

18. Matsumoto T, Uekusa T, Fukuda Y. Vasculo-Behcet's disease: a pathologic study of eight cases. Hum Pathol 1991;22(1):45–51.

19. Yabe T, Hamada T, Kubo T, et al. Inflammatory abdominal aortic aneurysm successfully treated with steroid therapy. J Am Coll Cardiol 2010;55(25):2877.

20. Oderich GS, Panneton JM, Bower TC, et al. Infected aortic aneurysms: aggressive presentation, complicated early outcome, but durable results. J Vasc Surg 2001;34(5):900–8.

21. Takayama T, Miyata T, Nagawa H. True abdominal aortic aneurysm in Marfan syndrome. J Vasc Surg 2009;49(5):1162–5.

22. Kuivaniemi H, Elmore JR. Opportunities in abdominal aortic aneurysm research: epidemiology, genetics, and pathophysiology. Ann Vasc Surg 2012;26(6): 862–70.

23. Alcorn HG, Wolfson SK Jr, Sutton-Tyrrell K, et al. Risk factors for abdominal aortic aneurysms in older adults enrolled in The Cardiovascular Health Study. Arterioscler Thromb Vasc Biol 1996;16(8):963–70.

24. Lederle FA, Johnson GR, Wilson SE, et al. The aneurysm detection and management study screening program: validation cohort and final results. Aneurysm Detection and Management Veterans Affairs Cooperative Study Investigators. Arch Intern Med 2000;160(10):1425–30.

25. Bengtsson H, Ekberg O, Aspelin P, et al. Ultrasound screening of the abdominal aorta in patients with intermittent claudication. Eur J Vasc Surg 1989;3(6):497–502.

26. Cabellon S Jr, Moncrief CL, Pierre DR, et al. Incidence of abdominal aortic aneurysms in patients with atheromatous arterial disease. Am J Surg 1983;146(5): 575–6.

27. Fleming C, Whitlock EP, Beil TL, et al. Screening for abdominal aortic aneurysm: a best-evidence systematic review for the U.S. Preventive Services Task Force. Ann Intern Med 2005;142(3):203–11.

28. Lederle FA, Johnson GR, Wilson SE, et al. Prevalence and associations of abdominal aortic aneurysm detected through screening. Aneurysm Detection and Management (ADAM) Veterans Affairs Cooperative Study Group. Ann Intern Med 1997;126(6):441–9.

29. Powell JT, Greenhalgh RM. Clinical practice. Small abdominal aortic aneurysms. N Engl J Med 2003;348(19):1895–901.
30. Kent KC, Zwolak RM, Egorova NN, et al. Analysis of risk factors for abdominal aortic aneurysm in a cohort of more than 3 million individuals. J Vasc Surg 2010;52(3):539–48.
31. Singh K, Bonaa KH, Jacobsen BK, et al. Prevalence of and risk factors for abdominal aortic aneurysms in a population-based study: The Tromso Study. Am J Epidemiol 2001;154(3):236–44.
32. Meijer CA, Kokje VB, van Tongeren RB, et al. An association between chronic obstructive pulmonary disease and abdominal aortic aneurysm beyond smoking: results from a case-control study. Eur J Vasc Endovasc Surg 2012;44(2):153–7.
33. Anjum A, von Allmen R, Greenhalgh R, et al. Explaining the decrease in mortality from abdominal aortic aneurysm rupture. Br J Surg 2012;99(5): 637–45.
34. Tornwall ME, Virtamo J, Haukka JK, et al. Life-style factors and risk for abdominal aortic aneurysm in a cohort of Finnish male smokers. Epidemiology 2001; 12(1):94–100.
35. Shantikumar S, Ajjan R, Porter KE, et al. Diabetes and the abdominal aortic aneurysm. Eur J Vasc Endovasc Surg 2010;39(2):200–7.
36. Johansen K, Koepsell T. Familial tendency for abdominal aortic aneurysms. JAMA 1986;256(14):1934–6.
37. Verloes A, Sakalihasan N, Koulischer L, et al. Aneurysms of the abdominal aorta: familial and genetic aspects in three hundred thirteen pedigrees. J Vasc Surg 1995;21(4):646–55.
38. Darling RC 3rd, Brewster DC, Darling RC, et al. Are familial abdominal aortic aneurysms different? J Vasc Surg 1989;10(1):39–43.
39. Powell JT, Greenhalgh RM. Multifactorial inheritance of abdominal aortic aneurysm. Eur J Vasc Surg 1987;1(1):29–31.
40. Kent KC, Zwolak RM, Jaff MR, et al. Screening for abdominal aortic aneurysm: a consensus statement. J Vasc Surg 2004;39(1):267–9.
41. U.S. Preventive Services Task Force. Screening for abdominal aortic aneurysm: recommendation statement. Ann Intern Med 2005;142(3):198–202.
42. Whitehouse WM Jr, Wakefield TW, Graham LM, et al. Limb-threatening potential of arteriosclerotic popliteal artery aneurysms. Surgery 1983;93(5):694–9.
43. Harbuzariu C, Duncan AA, Bower TC, et al. Profunda femoris artery aneurysms: association with aneurysmal disease and limb ischemia. J Vasc Surg 2008; 47(1):31–4 [discussion: 34–5].
44. Petersen MJ, Cambria RP, Kaufman JA, et al. Magnetic resonance angiography in the preoperative evaluation of abdominal aortic aneurysms. J Vasc Surg 1995;21(6):891–8 [discussion: 899].
45. Brewster DC, Cronenwett JL, Hallett JW Jr, et al. Guidelines for the treatment of abdominal aortic aneurysms. Report of a subcommittee of the Joint Council of the American Association for Vascular Surgery and Society for Vascular Surgery. J Vasc Surg 2003;37(5):1106–17.
46. Conway KP, Byrne J, Townsend M, et al. Prognosis of patients turned down for conventional abdominal aortic aneurysm repair in the endovascular and sonographic era: Szilagyi revisited? J Vasc Surg 2001;33(4):752–7.
47. Kakafika AI, Mikhailidis DP. Smoking and aortic diseases. Circ J 2007;71(8): 1173–80.
48. Koole D, Moll FL, Buth J, et al. The influence of smoking on endovascular abdominal aortic aneurysm repair. J Vasc Surg 2012;55(6):1581–6.

49. Gadowski GR, Pilcher DB, Ricci MA. Abdominal aortic aneurysm expansion rate: effect of size and beta-adrenergic blockade. J Vasc Surg 1994;19(4): 727–31.

50. Kertai MD, Boersma E, Westerhout CM, et al. Association between long-term statin use and mortality after successful abdominal aortic aneurysm surgery. Am J Med 2004;116(2):96–103.

51. Dubost C, Allary M, Oeconomos N. Resection of an aneurysm of the abdominal aorta: reestablishment of the continuity by a preserved human arterial graft, with result after five months. AMA Arch Surg 1952;64(3):405–8.

52. Parodi JC, Palmaz JC, Barone HD. Transfemoral intraluminal graft implantation for abdominal aortic aneurysms. Ann Vasc Surg 1991;5(6):491–9.

53. EVAR trial participants. Endovascular aneurysm repair versus open repair in patients with abdominal aortic aneurysm (EVAR trial 1): randomised controlled trial. Lancet 2005;365(9478):2179–86.

54. Prinssen M, Verhoeven EL, Buth J, et al. A randomized trial comparing conventional and endovascular repair of abdominal aortic aneurysms. N Engl J Med 2004;351(16):1607–18.

55. Carpenter JP, Baum RA, Barker CF, et al. Impact of exclusion criteria on patient selection for endovascular abdominal aortic aneurysm repair. J Vasc Surg 2001; 34(6):1050–4.

56. Schwarze ML, Shen Y, Hemmerich J, et al. Age-related trends in utilization and outcome of open and endovascular repair for abdominal aortic aneurysm in the United States, 2001-2006. J Vasc Surg 2009;50(4):722–9.e2.

57. Greenhalgh RM, Brown LC, Powell JT, et al. Endovascular versus open repair of abdominal aortic aneurysm. N Engl J Med 2010;362(20):1863–71.

58. De Bruin JL, Baas AF, Buth J, et al. Long-term outcome of open or endovascular repair of abdominal aortic aneurysm. N Engl J Med 2010;362(20):1881–9.

59. Becquemin JP, Pillet JC, Lescalie F, et al. A randomized controlled trial of endovascular aneurysm repair versus open surgery for abdominal aortic aneurysms in low- to moderate-risk patients. J Vasc Surg 2011;53(5):1167–73.e1161.

60. Dimick JB, Cowan JA Jr, Stanley JC, et al. Surgeon specialty and provider volumes are related to outcome of intact abdominal aortic aneurysm repair in the United States. J Vasc Surg 2003;38(4):739–44.

61. Chaikof EL, Blankensteijn JD, Harris PL, et al. Reporting standards for endovascular aortic aneurysm repair. J Vasc Surg 2002;35(5):1048–60.

62. Mehta M, Paty PS, Roddy SP, et al. Treatment options for delayed AAA rupture following endovascular repair. J Vasc Surg 2011;53(1):14–20.

63. Sommer WH, Becker CR, Haack M, et al. Time-resolved CT angiography for the detection and classification of endoleaks. Radiology 2012;263(3):917–26.

64. Gray C, Goodman P, Herron CC, et al. Use of colour duplex ultrasound as a first line surveillance tool following EVAR is associated with a reduction in cost without compromising accuracy. Eur J Vasc Endovasc Surg 2012;44(2): 145–50.

65. Patatas K, Ling L, Dunning J, et al. Static sac size with a type II endoleak post-endovascular abdominal aortic aneurysm repair: surveillance or embolization? Interact Cardiovasc Thorac Surg 2012;15(3):462–6.

66. Sullivan CA, Rohrer MJ, Cutler BS. Clinical management of the symptomatic but unruptured abdominal aortic aneurysm. J Vasc Surg 1990;11(6):799–803.

67. Marin ML, Veith FJ, Cynamon J, et al. Initial experience with transluminally placed endovascular grafts for the treatment of complex vascular lesions. Ann Surg 1995;222(4):449–65 [discussion: 465–9].

68. Nedeau AE, Pomposelli FB, Hamdan AD, et al. Endovascular vs open repair for ruptured abdominal aortic aneurysm. J Vasc Surg 2012;56(1):15–20.
69. Starnes BW, Quiroga E, Hutter C, et al. Management of ruptured abdominal aortic aneurysm in the endovascular era. J Vasc Surg 2010;51(1):9–17 [discussion: 17–8].
70. Albuquerque FC Jr, Tonnessen BH, Noll RE Jr, et al. Paradigm shifts in the treatment of abdominal aortic aneurysm: trends in 721 patients between 1996 and 2008. J Vasc Surg 2010;51(6):1348–52 [discussion: 1352–3].

Aneurysmal Disease: Thoracic Aorta

Andrew W. Hoel, MD

KEYWORDS

- Thoracic aorta • Thoracoabdominal aorta • Aneurysm • Endovascular surgery

KEY POINTS

- Aneurysmal degeneration of the thoracic aorta is a condition requiring surgical repair to either prevent or treat aortic rupture, a condition with high morbidity and mortality.
- Maximum aortic diameter is currently the best indicator of risk of aneurysm rupture. Elective repair of a thoracic aortic aneurysm is typically undertaken when aortic diameter reaches 6 cm.
- Although medical therapy, including risk-factor modification, can slow aneurysmal degeneration and decrease rupture risk, the only definitive treatment is surgical repair.
- Open repair of thoracic and thoracoabdominal aneurysms is a highly invasive procedure with a measurable risk of major morbidity and mortality. Endovascular aneurysm repair has been developed as an alternative strategy for treatment of thoracic aortic aneurysms, and is currently being developed for the treatment of thoracoabdominal aortic aneurysms.
- Spinal cord ischemia is an important complication of thoracic aortic aneurysm repair, and multiple adjunctive strategies including cerebrospinal fluid drainage have been developed to minimize the risk of neurologic complications.

Although thoracic aortic aneurysms (TAAs) are uncommon relative to the full spectrum of cardiovascular disease, they are clinically important for the high potential acuity of symptomatic patients and the attendant risks of surgical intervention.

This article focuses on aneurysms of the descending thoracic aorta (DTAAs) and thoracoabdominal aorta (TAAAs). Aneurysms isolated to the abdominal aorta are discussed in detail in an article elsewhere in this issue. Although aneurysms of the ascending aorta are clinically important and can also be classified as TAAs, they have a pathophysiology distinct (though overlapping) to that of DTAAs. More importantly, however, aneurysms of the aortic root and ascending thoracic aorta require clinical evaluation and treatment that is quite distinct from that for DTAAs, and are therefore not discussed in this article.

Disclosures: No funding sources, no conflicts of interest (A.W. Hoel).
Division of Vascular Surgery, Feinberg School of Medicine, Northwestern University, 676 North Saint Clair Street, Suite #650, Chicago, IL 60611, USA
E-mail address: awhoel@nmh.org

In the discussion of TAAs the natural history and pathophysiology of thoracic aortic aneurysms is reviewed, the evaluation of these patients is discussed, and treatment options and their associated outcomes detailed.

TAA IN THE POPULATION

Although the precise incidence of TAAs is difficult to ascertain, 2 studies on a discrete population estimated the prevalence of aneurysms of the ascending, arch and descending aorta at between 6 and 10 per 100,000 person-years. These studies included all TAAs, of which the most common type was of the ascending aorta (40%), with the descending aorta accounting for 35% and the thoracoabdominal aorta 10%.[1,2] A population-based study of aortic disease in Sweden suggests that there is an increase in the prevalence of thoracic aortic aneurysms over time. While there is almost certainly increased detection of TAAs as a result of more widespread imaging, there also does appear to be a true increase in TAA incidence in the population.[3]

Risk Factors

Not surprisingly, there is an age-dependent increase in the incidence of TAA, with an average age of 65 years at diagnosis. Women tend to present, on average, more than 10 years later than men. Despite this, there is only a slight male predominance of TAA, in contrast to the strong male predominance of abdominal aortic aneurysms (AAAs).[2] The subset of patients with a genetic predisposition to aneurysm formation, including those with connective tissue disorders (see section on pathobiology), by contrast, tend to present at a much younger age and tend to have a more malignant course. Including this subset, it is estimated that approximately 20% of all patients with a TAA have at least 1 family member with a known aortic aneurysm.[4] In addition, there is a well-established relationship between the development of TAAs and aortic dissection. It is estimated that 20% of TAAs are preceded by aortic dissection.[5]

Natural History

Like the study of TAA incidence, the study of the natural history is challenging. Longitudinal study of patients undergoing surveillance demonstrates the clear tendency for the aorta to enlarge over time at an average rate of nearly 3 mm per year.[6] However, the rate of expansion tends to accelerate over time and is more rapid for larger-diameter aneurysms.[7] That said, the rate of expansion is clearly not uniform over time, and there appear to be periods of no growth interspersed with periods of expansion. In general, rates of expansion greater than 0.5 cm per 6-month period are considered rapidly expanding, and fall into the category of aneurysms warranting repair.

Although rapid expansion is an important element in the decision to intervene, the single most important component of surgical decision making is maximal aortic diameter. In most cases, a TAA with a diameter of 6 cm warrants repair. This size is based on our understanding of the diameter-dependent risk of aneurysm rupture. The longitudinal evaluation of rupture risk at 5 years was estimated in one study to be 16% from aneurysms from 4 to 5.9 cm and 31% for aneurysms greater than 6 cm.[2] Another series of 370 patients demonstrated a median diameter of 7.2 cm at the time of rupture.[8] This finding is not surprising given that, in the absence of rupture, the tendency of aneurysms is to expand over time.

The risk of aneurysm rupture is also increased with increasing age, the presence of chronic obstructive pulmonary disease (COPD), and the presence of chronic back pain. We can also reasonably extrapolate from our understanding of AAAs that continued tobacco abuse, in particular, may increase the likelihood of aneurysm rupture.[9,10]

PATHOBIOLOGY

The thoracic aorta collects a portion of the kinetic energy generated by ventricular contraction (systole). The elasticity of the thoracic aorta returns this stored kinetic energy during diastole, and is an important component of diastolic perfusion. Aneurysmal degeneration is a process characterized by chronic inflammation, smooth muscle cell death, and degradation of elastin in the aortic wall. This combination of events leads to stiffening of the aortic wall. Decreased compliance of the aortic wall combined with increased aortic diameter (that is not compensated by increased wall thickness) leads to increased wall stress on the aorta. This central sequence of events can lead to aneurysm rupture. The most predominant type of TAAs follows this degenerative pattern, although a small but important subset of aneurysmal disease is directly related to congenital etiology.

Connective Tissue Disorders

Congenital TAAs are grouped together broadly as connective tissue disorders, comprising 4 (primary) types:

- Marfan syndrome. A mutation of the fibrillin-1 gene confers a clinical syndrome characterized by cardiovascular, ocular, and musculoskeletal symptoms. These patients are at particular risk for aortic root dilation, ascending aortic aneurysms, and aortic dissection, which represent the greatest risk of premature death to these patients. However, descending aortic aneurysms, typically associated with aortic dissection, are also an important clinical component of this disease.[11]
- Ehlers-Danlos syndrome (EDS). One part of the spectrum of connective tissue disorders, type IV or "vascular" EDS is an autosomal dominant defect in type III procollagen. This syndrome can manifest in a broad spectrum of hemorrhagic complications, owing to arterial fragility. This spectrum includes aortic dissection with high risk of rupture that does not necessarily correlate with aortic diameter.[12]
- Loeys-Dietz syndrome (LDS). Recently described and a manifestation of a mutation of transforming growth factor β, LDS has a spectrum of craniofacial, skeletal, and cardiovascular abnormalities. There is a significant risk of aortic aneurysm rupture even at smaller diameters.[13]
- Nonsyndromic TAAs. There is an emerging spectrum of congenital TAAs with an autosomal dominant inheritance pattern and variable penetrance/expression. Patients tend to present at a younger age than those with degenerative TAAs, and tend to have a significant family history. In contrast to the disease pattern of degenerative aneurysms, there is an apparent predominance of descending aortic abnormality.[4]

EVALUATION OF PATIENTS
Asymptomatic TAA

The majority of TAAs are discovered incidentally on imaging studies conducted for other reasons. Such imaging includes plain chest radiographs on which a spectrum of findings in the mediastinum can suggest a TAA, such as a widened mediastinum, enlargement of the aortic knob, displacement of the trachea to the right, displacement of the aortopulmonary window, and occasional direct visualization of the calcified wall of a dilated aorta (**Fig. 1**).[14] Recognition of these findings typically warrants further evaluation with cross-sectional imaging. Unfortunately, there are scant clinical signs of an asymptomatic aneurysm on examination.

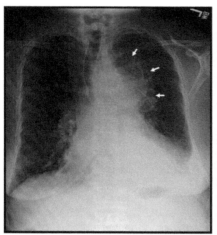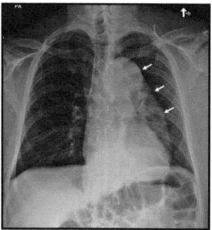

Fig. 1. Two representative chest radiographs of patients with an asymptomatic thoracic aortic aneurysm (TAA) demonstrating loss of the aortopulmonary window and a hilar mass (*white arrows*).

Imaging

As already discussed, the critical determinant of need for aneurysm repair is the maximal diameter of the aorta. Therefore, high-resolution imaging is the single most important step in evaluating a patient with a TAAs. High-resolution imaging also provides critical information about the aortic anatomy. This aspect is particularly important when considering endovascular repair of the aneurysm, although a great deal of operative planning can be made based on preoperative imaging even for open repair. Dilation of the aortic wall occurs in 3 dimensions, meaning that while diameter and circumference increase, so does length, leading to a marked increase in aortic tortuosity. Although this has some relevance for open repair, understanding the angulation and tortuosity of the thoracic aorta is critical in evaluation for endovascular repair. Multiple imaging modalities are available and are routinely used.

- Computed tomography (CT) angiography. The CT scan is the most common modality used for evaluation of the aorta. It provides high-resolution axial imaging and excellent quality reconstructions in coronal and sagittal planes, as well as 3-dimensional reconstructions. Advanced imaging software allows precise measurement of the aorta and its branches. In particular, measurements for endovascular repair are greatly aided by measurements in an orthogonal plane, at a right angle to the center line of the aorta. The disadvantages of CT are small, but there is a risk of renal injury with contrast administration, particularly in patients with baseline renal insufficiency. There is also emerging evidence of increased risk of radiation-induced malignancy in patients undergoing serial CT imaging. In planning an endovascular repair, it is extremely important to image the entire aorta and iliac system, as endograft delivery systems are large and there is a well-documented risk of access complications that can be minimized by an appreciation of iliofemoral pathology.
- Magnetic resonance (MR) angiography. The imaging resolution of MR angiography is generally of a lesser quality than CT. Further, MR angiography provides less information about aortic-wall calcification and atheroma, which has significant implications for surgical planning. The advantage is that there is no radiation exposure. Although there is a well-documented risk of nephrogenic systemic sclerosis in

patients with renal insufficiency who are exposed to the MR contrast agent gadolinium, there are methods that eliminate the need for contrast exposure.

- Angiography. Fluoroscopic, 2-dimensional angiography is an important secondary imaging technique that is largely required intraoperatively to accurately deploy an endograft. However, its utility is limited as a diagnostic modality for TAAs because it is only effective at imaging the flow lumen of the aorta. It does not adequately image mural thrombus or calcifications and, as such, the landing zones for an endograft and the sewing ring of an open repair may not be accurately interpreted. In addition, like CT, angiography uses iodinated contrast with its attendant renal risk. Finally, it is an invasive procedure that confers a limited procedural risk. These factors have made it largely obsolete as a diagnostic modality.
- Intravascular ultrasonography (IVUS). As an imaging modality, IVUS can be extremely helpful intraoperatively in understanding the aortic anatomy, particularly in the setting of aortic dissection. IVUS offers the additional benefit of potentially decreasing the need for intraoperative contrast angiography in the setting of renal insufficiency.
- Transesophageal echocardiography (TEE). TEE is a useful adjunct intraoperatively to assess the aortic arch and proximal descending aorta. It is useful in open repair for the anesthesia assessment of cardiac function around the time of proximal aortic clamping. It provides less direct benefit in thoracic endovascular aneurysm repair (TEVAR); however, it can be a useful adjunct if there is concern for retrograde aortic dissection at the time of endograft deployment.

Symptomatic TAAA

The key symptoms of thoracic aortic rupture or impending rupture are acute onset of back and/or chest pain. In addition, the presence of concurrent abdominal pain can be present in patients with symptomatic thoracoabdominal aneurysms. In patients with overt aortic rupture, there is typically rapid progression of hemodynamic instability with subsequent cardiovascular collapse. Rapid, concurrent respiratory failure is a feature of free rupture into the left hemithorax. Rarely, erosion into mediastinal structures can result in hemoptysis from aortobronchial fistula or hematemesis from an aortoesophageal fistula.

The ruptured TAA requires prompt evaluation for surgical repair, often including cross-sectional imaging as well as typical preoperative evaluation and surgical planning that would occur with any emergency surgery. This evaluation should be performed expeditiously and concurrently with resuscitation and stabilization. It is important that this does not necessarily require normalization of hemodynamics, as there is likely access to permissive hypotension in a contained rupture.

Less common is a TAAA causing subacute or chronic symptoms that do not indicate current or impending rupture. These signs and symptoms are generally related to compression or stretch of the aneurysmal aorta on adjacent structures including the esophagus (dysphagia, odynophagia, weight loss) (**Fig. 2**), the duodenum (early satiety), trachea (dyspnea), and recurrent laryngeal nerve (hoarseness, aspiration). Chronic, stable back pain can also be a feature of thoracic aneurysms, although this symptom is often difficult to separate from musculoskeletal pain because it is common for these patients to have concurrent degenerative disease of their spine. Occasionally, after repair and full recovery, chronic back pain can be attributed to a TAA by its absence after repair. Of course, change in severity or character of back pain in a patient with a known TAA warrants prompt evaluation with cross-sectional imaging and a low threshold for surgical intervention.

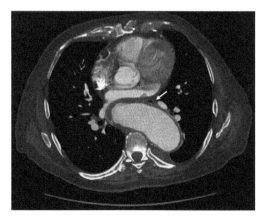

Fig. 2. Esophageal compression (*white arrow*) in a patient with a large, tortuous type II thoracoabdominal aortic aneurysm (TAAA). This patient required a gastrostomy tube before aneurysm repair for nutritional optimization.

Patients with chronic and stable symptoms that may be attributed to their aneurysm should undergo prompt risk stratification and risk-factor modification, as described later, in anticipation of repair.

THERAPEUTIC OPTIONS

There is an expanding spectrum of options for the surgical treatment of TAAs. Open repair remains the best studied and most inclusive repair, and technical improvements over time have improved outcomes. Closely following advancements in open repair, the treatment of TAA has been dramatically altered in the past 15 years with the advent of TEVAR. Medical therapy has incrementally improved the treatment of patients with TAAs.

Medical Therapy

Degenerative aneurysms, broadly speaking, are a chronic progressive condition. However, there are clear opportunities for medical optimization to mitigate the risks of aneurysm expansion and rupture. This factor is particularly relevant for patients with small aneurysms undergoing surveillance and patients who are not candidates for any repair. Even in patients undergoing repair, medical optimization is important and should not be overlooked. Furthermore, patients with connective tissue disorders are additionally susceptible to increased risk of adverse outcomes in the absence of risk modification.

- Smoking cessation. There is a clear relationship between smoking and cardiovascular disease. This relationship extends to aortic aneurysms, whereby smoking is a significant risk factor for both expansion[9] and rupture[10,15] of aneurysms. Because of this, there is no single more important modifiable risk factor than tobacco abuse in patients with TAAs.
- Statin medications. HMG-CoA reductase inhibitors have become a mainstay of treatment for a broad array of cardiovascular disease extending beyond their established lipid-lowering indications. Indeed, one can extrapolate a benefit to patients with TAAs from a meta-analysis with meta-regression of clinical studies that demonstrates benefit to statins in preventing the expansion of AAAs.[16] In a retrospective review, there was a demonstrated increase in survival for patients

with a TAA who were taking statins. This increased survival was attributed to decreased expansion of aneurysms and a decreased need for surgical repair.[17] This finding has been hypothesized to be related to an apparent pleiotropic effect that decreases inflammation and stabilizes the arterial wall.

- β-Blockade. Reduction in blood pressure, as well as cardiac ionotropy and chronotropy, seem to be intuitively beneficial for patients with TAA. Indeed, benefit for β-blockade was demonstrated for patients with Marfan syndrome, with a reduction in formation and enlargement of TAA with propranolol.[18] However, subsequent evaluation of β-blockade in patients with degenerative aortic aneurysms did not demonstrate clear benefit. That said, β-blockade remains generally accepted for perioperative risk reduction before cardiovascular surgery. There is therefore a strong basis for β-blockade in patients with TAA who are facing surgical intervention.
- Angiotensin-converting enzyme (ACE) inhibitors. Despite experimental evidence of a relationship between angiotensin II and the development of paravisceral aneurysms and their subsequent suppression by ACE inhibition,[19] there are conflicting data on the clinical benefit to suppression of angiotensin II. A large-scale population study in Canada demonstrated a decreased risk of aneurysm rupture in patients taking ACE inhibitors.[20] In stark contrast, results from the United Kingdom Small Aneurysm Trial demonstrated disproportionate aneurysm expansion with ACE inhibitors.[21] Clearly this area is open to further investigation.
- Doxycycline. Matrix metalloproteinases (MMPs) have been implicated in the degradation of elastin in the aortic wall and have been linked to the formation of AAAs. As a nonspecific inhibitor of MMPs, doxycycline is being investigated as a medical therapy for aortic aneurysms, based on experimental and preliminary clinical studies that suggest doxycycline decreases MMP expression in the aortic wall and inhibits the expansion of AAAs.[22] There is currently a phase III randomized trial evaluating doxycycline as medical therapy for small AAAs. Even if doxycycline is effective in the treatment of AAAs, it would not necessarily translate to equal benefit in the treatment of TAAs. However, doxycycline is an important example of a targeted medical therapy that may be included in the future scope of care for TAAs.

Although medical optimization is an important element of management of aneurysmal disease, there has been no demonstrated medical treatment for TAAs that eliminates the risk of future rupture. Therefore, surgery is the mainstay of therapy for patients meeting criteria for treatment. Determining optimal surgical therapy for a patient with a TAA requires an understanding of the aortic anatomy and the patient's medical fitness for a procedure.

Surgical Treatment

Open surgical repair of TAA is complex, care intensive, and carries significant risk of morbidity and mortality. For these reasons careful patient selection based on patient anatomy and medical comorbidities is mandatory.

Anatomic considerations

TAAs and TAAAs are commonly categorized by the extent of repair required. This classification, devised by Crawford and colleagues,[23] divides the anatomic type into 4 categories based on the extent of repair required:

- Type I aneurysm repair is performed distal to the left carotid extending below the diaphragm to above the renal arteries.

- Type II repair originates distal to the left carotid artery but above the sixth intercostal space, and extends to below the renal arteries.
- Type III repair originates in the mid-thoracic aorta below the sixth intercostal space but above the diaphragm, and extends below the renal arteries.
- Type IV aneurysm repair originates below the diaphragm but above the renal arteries, and terminates below the renal arteries.

In addition to providing a uniform description of the anatomic repair required, this classification also summarizes the potential for morbidity and mortality of repair. Type II aneurysms, in particular, have the greatest potential for morbidity and mortality owing to the extent of repair. By contrast, type IV aneurysms tend to have lower risk of morbidity and mortality, particularly if repair can be accomplished while remaining in the abdominal cavity.

Preoperative risk stratification

Patients who are anatomic candidates for open repair also require assessment of their medical fitness for surgery, in particular assessment with respect to cardiac, pulmonary, and renal impairment. As already noted, TAA patients tend to be older and are likely to have significant comorbidity that requires thorough consideration before surgery:

- Cardiac. In general, patients should undergo complete cardiac risk stratification. In the majority of patients with degenerative aneurysms this will involve a nuclear or echocardiographic stress test. Reversible ischemia is generally considered a contraindication to elective open TAAA repair without prior coronary revascularization. In addition, patients with baseline reduced ejection fraction and abnormal ventricular function are at particularly high risk for perioperative mortality.[24,25]
- Pulmonary. While preoperative pulmonary dysfunction is predictive of postoperative pulmonary complications, this is an even greater consideration in patients requiring thoracotomy for treatment of their TAA. Patients with a 1-second forced expiratory volume of less than 70% of predicted carry a diagnosis of COPD and are at particular risk for postoperative pulmonary complications and mortality.[25] Preoperative smoking cessation is critical in these patients.
- Renal. Renal insufficiency is a significant predictor of perioperative morbidity and mortality.[26] In particular, a baseline creatinine level of greater than 2.5 mg/dL is a relative contraindication to open repair. However, some would argue that patients with renal artery stenosis who are capable of undergoing revascularization during their procedure should be considered candidates for repair.

Patients at high risk for open repair can still be considered for repair by a hybrid or endovascular approach (see later discussion). However, of importance is that high-risk patients for open repair are still at increased risk of complications even with a less invasive procedure.

Open surgical treatment of TAA

Because open surgery for TAAs is so invasive, it is a procedure whereby treatment at centers with high volume and/or significant experience can lead to improved outcomes. Coselli and colleagues[27] reported an operative mortality of 6.6% and a rate of spinal cord ischemia of 4% in 2286 patients undergoing open TAAA repair. This result represents some of the best outcomes available in the literature, in contrast to perioperative mortality rates of 19% for elective TAAA repair in a review of claims data in California from 1991 to 2002.[28] This higher mortality rate points to the variation in outcome across centers, and suggests that outcomes from high-volume centers do not necessarily reflect "real-world" practice. Similarly, the risk of paraplegia is estimated to be as high as 14% in other series. Additional risks of open TAA are not trivial, and include an estimated 20% risk of cardiac events including myocardial infarction, a 20% to 50% risk of pulmonary complications, and a 13% to 20% risk of renal failure.[25,29,30]

There are many specific ways to gain adequate surgical exposure to a TAA. In general, efficient progress in aortic reconstruction is facilitated by wide exposure, and the author therefore does not compromise in the extent of dissection before beginning reconstruction. In open DTAA repair, the aneurysmal aorta is exposed through a posterior-lateral thoracotomy in the sixth intercostal space, with posterior division and shingling of the sixth rib for additional exposure. The left lung is reflected anteriorly after dividing the inferior pulmonary ligament. TAAAs require extension of the incision through the abdominal wall with retroperitoneal dissection and circumferential division of the diaphragm, to expose the entire involved aorta including the visceral segment.

Left heart bypass, sequentially moving the distal clamp further down the aorta as the reconstruction progresses, is an important adjunct that is used by many surgeons to maintain renal and spinal cord perfusion to a maximal extent during repair. This maneuver is typically accomplished by cannulation of the left atrial appendage or inferior pulmonary ligament proximally and the left femoral artery distally. Distal perfusion is facilitated with a Biomedicus pump, which can adjust perfusion pressure as necessary throughout the reconstruction and also allows selective perfusion of the visceral and renal arteries during reconstruction. Venoatrial bypass in the left groin and clamp-and-sew followed by antegrade perfusion via a side-arm graft just below the proximal anastomosis are other methods used successfully for end-organ protection.

Regardless of the precise method of end-organ protection, reconstruction typically proceeds with a Carrel patch of the celiac, superior mesenteric artery, and right renal artery, and a short branch to the left renal artery. A second patch to intercostal branches is often indicated as well. However, precise reconstruction is tailored to the specific anatomy of the patient, and careful review of preoperative axial imaging greatly facilitates procedure planning. The important exception to the use of a Carrel patch is in the setting of connective tissue disorders, whereby a multiple-branched Dacron graft and reinforcement of anastomoses is warranted to prevent late degeneration (**Fig. 3**).

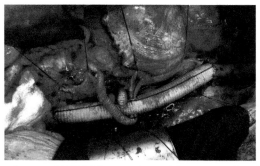

Fig. 3. Open repair of a type III TAAA in a patient with a connective tissue disorder. Note that each renal and visceral artery has a separate branch to prevent future aortic degeneration.

Perioperative adjuncts As already noted, in addition to cardiac, pulmonary, and renal morbidity associated with TAA repair, there is significant risk of spinal cord ischemia associated with aortic cross-clamping. Multiple adjuncts have been developed to minimize the risk of paraplegia associated with TAA repair. These methods are generally centered on maintaining spinal perfusion pressure intraoperatively and in the immediate postoperative period. The most widely studied, used, and accepted of these adjuncts is spinal fluid drainage, whereby a catheter is inserted into the intrathecal space at the L3-L4 interspace. Maintenance of low intracranial cerebrospinal fluid pressure (ICP) augments spinal cord perfusion pressure (SCPP) and has been demonstrated to be effective in multiple studies.[31] Maintenance of mean arterial pressure (MAP) greater than 90 is also an effective adjunct in maintaining perfusion pressure (SCPP = MAP − ICP). Passive hypothermia, distal aortic perfusion, and intravenous naloxone infusion have also been demonstrated to contribute to the prevention of spinal cord ischemia.[32] The real-time, intraoperative monitoring of spinal cord function with somatosensory and/or motor evoked potentials have been demonstrated to be a useful adjunct to tailoring therapy to the patient's physiology and anatomy.[33]

Endovascular treatment of DTAA

As previously noted, endovascular repair has dramatically altered the management of TAAs. The first report detailing this treatment strategy is commonly attributed to Dake and colleagues[34] at Stanford. Since that time the technology has advanced significantly, and TEVAR currently markedly outpaces open aneurysm repair. There are clear theoretical advantages to an endovascular repair that eliminates the need for thoracotomy and single lung ventilation as well as avoiding cross-clamping of the thoracic aorta. The periprocedural superiority of TEVAR was demonstrated in a 2.1% perioperative mortality in comparison with 11.7% for an open surgical cohort.[29] As might be expected, perioperative complications and length of stay were significantly reduced in patients undergoing TEVAR. Indeed, a systematic review of available studies demonstrated a significant reduction in mortality and major neurologic complications.[35] The risk of neurologic complications including spinal cord ischemia remains present in TEVAR, just as in open repair.[36] Therefore, the adjuncts for spinal cord protection as described herein are also likely to be beneficial in the endovascular repair of TAAs and TAAAs.

However, the long-term benefit of TEVAR has not yet been clearly established. In fact, although an analysis of Medicare patients demonstrated early benefit for TEVAR, that benefit did not persist. By 5 years, open repair of DTAAs had better survival (72%, vs 62% for TEVAR; $P = .001$), an effect that persisted with risk adjustment and propensity matching.[37] There are many potential explanations for this finding, but what is clear is that patient selection remains extremely important for any thoracic aortic procedure.

As discussed earlier, preoperative axial imaging with CT angiography supplemented with advanced imaging software is critical to the accurate assessment of patient suitability for TEVAR. There are 3 crucial elements to appropriately selecting an endograft for implantation:

1. Assurance of adequate proximal and distal seal zones. Current commercially available devices require at least 2 cm of nondiseased parallel aortic wall for proximal and distal landing zones (**Fig. 4**).
2. Accurate sizing of devices. In general, measurements of aortic diameter are obtained at multiple points along the length of the seal zone. Selection of appropriately sized devices involves oversizing by approximately 20% to achieve appropriate radial force on the aortic wall.

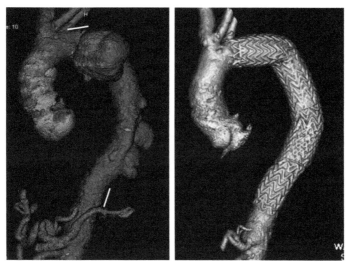

Fig. 4. Thoracic endovascular aneurysm repair requires 2 cm of proximal and distal landing zone for adequate seal of the endograft (*white bars on left panel*). Completion imaging demonstrates good position of devices and exclusion of the aneurysm.

3. Assessment of access vessels. It is critical and often overlooked that device deployment requires delivery of a large (20F to 24F) sheath to the aorta. It is not uncommon that the iliac arteries are of inadequate size to deliver the device, and therefore require additional procedures for access, such as a graft to the iliac artery as a conduit.

Although there is evidence for efficacy of TEVAR in the treatment of degenerative aneurysms, the treatment of connective tissue disorders with TEVAR is not widely accepted, largely because of concerns that more fragile aortic tissue in connective tissue disease would not be suitable as a seal zone for a stable and durable endograft seal.

Hybrid procedures: aortic debranching
Aortic arch debranching In patients with inadequate proximal seal zones for standard TEVAR, aortic arch debranching may be a reasonable alternative to cardiopulmonary bypass with hypothermic circulatory arrest. The aortic arch is divided into zones for the purposes of accurately describing the necessary proximal landing zone of the aortic arch (**Fig. 5**). Endovascular repair is appropriate for aneurysms originating in zone 4, with aneurysms in zone 0 to 3 frequently requiring debranching procedures.

The most common and least invasive debranching procedure is a left carotid to subclavian transposition or bypass. The procedure is generally well tolerated and is achieved through a small left supraclavicular incision. A single-center series demonstrated a 63% risk of stroke or vertebrobasilar insufficiency without revascularization, and a 9% rate of left vocal cord paresis with revascularization,[38] suggesting efficacy for revascularization. A systemic review and meta-analysis of related literature resulted in a Society for Vascular Surgery practice guideline recommending left subclavian revascularization in most circumstances.[39] This procedure allows endograft placement into zone 2 of the aortic arch, and can provide a suitable proximal seal zone for TEVAR.

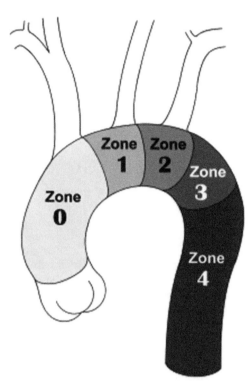

Fig. 5. The zones of the aortic arch relative to proximal endograft attachment sites. (*From* Adams JD, Garcia LM, Kern JA. Endovascular repair of the thoracic aorta. Surg Clin North Am 2009;89:895–912.)

A carotid-carotid bypass allows coverage of the left carotid artery origin by an endograft and extends the proximal seal into zone 1 of the arch. However, the anatomy of the left carotid origin is variable, and if the distance between the innominate artery and left carotid is short there is potentially little benefit to this procedure. The procedure is performed by end-to-side anastomosis on each carotid artery with a prosthetic conduit in either a retropharyngeal or retroesophageal tunnel, followed by proximal ligation of the left common carotid artery. Additional left carotid to left sub-clavian bypass, as already described, is also recommended in this circumstance. Patency of the carotid-carotid bypass is excellent[40] and avoids the median sternotomy required for total arch debranching.

To extend the proximal seal of an endograft into zone zero, arch debranching via median sternotomy is necessary. This procedure entails proximalization of great vessel perfusion using a bifurcated or trifurcated synthetic conduit, with proximal anastomosis to the proximal ascending aorta using a side-biting clamp. Distal anastomoses are then performed with proximal ligation of each of the supra-aortic trunk vessels (**Fig. 6**).

Visceral debranching Debranching of the celiac, superior mesenteric, and renal arteries to a more distal origin allows the use of thoracic endografts in the treatment of thoracoabdominal aneurysms. In this procedure, a multibranch bypass is taken from either the distal aorta or iliac arteries with separate distal anastomoses to the visceral and renal arteries. The procedure is typically performed via a midline

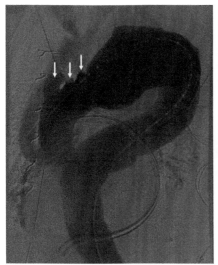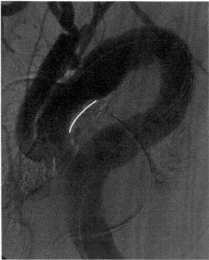

Fig. 6. Aortic arch debranching with a common trunk from the ascending aorta. Arrows in the image on the left demonstrate the origins of the innominate, left carotid, and left subclavian arteries. At the time of stent-graft deployment in the image on the right, an additional 4 cm of proximal seal was obtained with the debranching (*curved white line*).

laparotomy, which allows ready access to all vessels. Less common is a retroperitoneal approach, which allows extraperitoneal dissection but limits exposure of the right renal artery. The precise configuration of graft origin and orientation is highly dependent on patient anatomy and requires careful review of a preoperative CT angiogram. In planning the debranching, the CT is important in ensuring that the aneurysm will be adequately covered by the endograft without compromising the debranching bypasses. In addition, the CT should be reviewed to ensure that there is no occlusive disease in either the inflow or outflow that could interfere with durability of the debranching procedure. Iliac access for the subsequent endograft is preferred on the contralateral side of the debranching inflow site to minimize the risk of anastomotic injury, but this is not always possible in the setting of small or diseased iliac arteries. For patients with small iliac access, aortic debranching can be done in conjunction with an iliofemoral conduit (**Fig. 7**).

Completion of the aneurysm repair with endograft coverage of the aneurysm can be completed at the time of debranching, or as a staged procedure with endograft deployment as a separate procedure. A single-stage procedure may be more convenient from a vascular exposure standpoint. However, because these patients tend to be more medically fragile, it is common to stage the procedure to limit morbidity.

There are clear theoretical advantages to aortic debranching and endograft placement when compared with open repair. Advantages include eliminating the need for a thoracotomy and its attendant pulmonary morbidity, avoiding aortic clamping in most cases, and minimizing the ischemic time to kidneys and viscera. Indeed, there have been single-center series with excellent results of 0% to 4% mortality and spinal cord ischemia of 1% to 6%.[41–43] However, these results represent the very best of outcomes, and a systematic review of published series between 2000 and 2010 analyzed results from 507 patients with a pooled 12.8% 30-day/in-hospital mortality and a 7.5% rate of spinal cord ischemia.[44] The variability in these results highlights

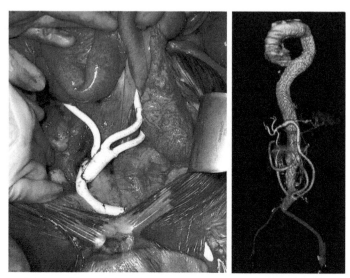

Fig. 7. Visceral debranching of the celiac, superior mesenteric, and bilateral renal arteries with polytetrafluoroethylene from a left iliac artery conduit origin (*left*). After endograft repair, CT demonstrates good position of all grafts and patency of bypass grafts (*right*).

the importance of both patient selection and surgical expertise. As the technology of branched and fenestrated endografts expands to treat the full spectrum of complex aneurysms, aortic debranching will become more rarely used.

Branched endografts

When TEVAR (and EVAR in the case of type IV and juxtarenal aneurysms) is not appropriate because of aneurysmal involvement of the visceral segment, total endovascular TAAA exclusion, particularly the branched endograft, is becoming the best remaining alternative in patients who are not candidates for open repair.

Branched endovascular aneurysm repair (BEVAR) is an emerging technology that builds on and customizes existing endograft technology. Fenestrations are placed in the endograft, which allow cannulation and stenting of the visceral and renal arteries to maintain branch patency in a segment of treated aorta. The initial iteration of this technology was a custom device for the treatment of juxtarenal and type IV thoracoabdominal aneurysms. Studies by Verhoeven and colleagues[45] and Amiot and colleagues[46] demonstrated very good outcomes in the perioperative period, with 99% technical success and 30-day mortality of less than 2%. Using the same technology, Greenberg and colleagues[47] compared 372 open and 352 endovascularly treated DTAAs and TAAAs in a single-institution study. Although the endovascular patients had more significant medical comorbidities, they had an equal 30-day and 1-year survival as well as equivalent rates of spinal cord ischemia.

The development of an endograft using a caudally directed branch technique is also undergoing evaluation in a multicenter clinical trial. The current iteration of this device is an off-the-shelf graft designed to treat approximately 80% of TAAA anatomy (**Fig. 8**).[48] A single-center evaluation of this technique demonstrated excellent outcomes in treatment of 81 high-risk patients, with a 6.2% 30-day mortality and a 3.7% rate of paraplegia. A total of 306 branches were placed in the 81 study subjects, with a primary patency rate of 95% at a mean 21-month follow-up.[49] In general,

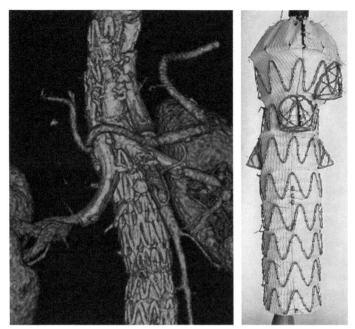

Fig. 8. Postoperative CT of the Cook T-branch device (*left*) using the caudally directed cuff technique and designed for the endovascular treatment of TAAAs. The device is shown on the right.

effective use of these devices requires sophisticated imaging evaluation, precise multidimensional measurement of anatomy, and a higher-order operative skill set than that required for TEVAR. Although this technology is some time away from widespread clinical use, it has the potential to effectively treat high-risk patients in the near term and, potentially, standard-risk patients in the future.

SUMMARY

TAAs and TAAAs are uncommon vascular abnormalities. However, the high mortality associated with aneurysm rupture and the indolent course of aneurysm formation captures the attention of patients and providers when an aneurysm is discovered. The treatment of TAAs has advanced markedly over the last 20 years, with improvements in adjuncts for open aneurysm repair and the development and refinement of endovascular therapy. The technology will continue to advance, and the prospect of broadly available branched and fenestrated endografts for the treatment of TAAAs has the potential to provide improved outcomes to patients with this severe disease.

REFERENCES

1. Bickerstaff LK, Pairolero PC, Hollier LH, et al. Thoracic aortic aneurysms: a population-based study. Surgery 1982;92(6):1103–8.
2. Clouse WD, Hallett JW Jr, Schaff HV, et al. Improved prognosis of thoracic aortic aneurysms: a population-based study. JAMA 1998;280(22):1926–9.
3. Olsson C, Thelin S, Stahle E, et al. Thoracic aortic aneurysm and dissection: increasing prevalence and improved outcomes reported in a nationwide

population-based study of more than 14,000 cases from 1987 to 2002. Circulation 2006;114(24):2611–8.

4. Albornoz G, Coady MA, Roberts M, et al. Familial thoracic aortic aneurysms and dissections—incidence, modes of inheritance, and phenotypic patterns. Ann Thorac Surg 2006;82(4):1400–5.

5. Cambria RA, Gloviczki P, Stanson AW, et al. Outcome and expansion rate of 57 thoracoabdominal aortic aneurysms managed nonoperatively. Am J Surg 1995; 170(2):213–7.

6. Coady MA, Rizzo JA, Hammond GL, et al. What is the appropriate size criterion for resection of thoracic aortic aneurysms? J Thorac Cardiovasc Surg 1997; 113(3):476–91 [discussion: 489–91].

7. Dapunt OE, Galla JD, Sadeghi AM, et al. The natural history of thoracic aortic aneurysms. J Thorac Cardiovasc Surg 1994;107(5):1323–32 [discussion: 1332–3].

8. Coady MA, Rizzo JA, Hammond GL, et al. Surgical intervention criteria for thoracic aortic aneurysms: a study of growth rates and complications. Ann Thorac Surg 1999;67(6):1922–6 [discussion: 1953–8].

9. Lederle FA, Johnson GR, Wilson SE, et al. The aneurysm detection and management study screening program: validation cohort and final results. Aneurysm Detection and Management Veterans Affairs Cooperative Study Investigators. Arch Intern Med 2000;160(10):1425–30.

10. Fillinger MF, Racusin J, Baker RK, et al. Anatomic characteristics of ruptured abdominal aortic aneurysm on conventional CT scans: implications for rupture risk. J Vasc Surg 2004;39(6):1243–52.

11. Adams JN, Trent RJ. Aortic complications of Marfan's syndrome. Lancet 1998; 352(9142):1722–3.

12. Pepin M, Schwarze U, Superti-Furga A, et al. Clinical and genetic features of Ehlers-Danlos syndrome type IV, the vascular type. N Engl J Med 2000; 342(10):673–80.

13. Loeys BL, Schwarze U, Holm T, et al. Aneurysm syndromes caused by mutations in the TGF-beta receptor. N Engl J Med 2006;355(8):788–98.

14. von Kodolitsch Y, Nienaber CA, Dieckmann C, et al. Chest radiography for the diagnosis of acute aortic syndrome. Am J Med 2004;116(2):73–7.

15. Brown LC, Powell JT. Risk factors for aneurysm rupture in patients kept under ultrasound surveillance. UK Small Aneurysm Trial Participants. Ann Surg 1999; 230(3):289–96 [discussion: 296–7].

16. Takagi H, Yamamoto H, Iwata K, et al. Effects of statin therapy on abdominal aortic aneurysm growth: a meta-analysis and meta-regression of observational comparative studies. Eur J Vasc Endovasc Surg 2012;44(3):287–92.

17. Jovin IS, Duggal M, Ebisu K, et al. Comparison of the effect on long-term outcomes in patients with thoracic aortic aneurysms of taking versus not taking a statin drug. Am J Cardiol 2012;109(7):1050–4.

18. Shores J, Berger KR, Murphy EA, et al. Progression of aortic dilatation and the benefit of long-term beta-adrenergic blockade in Marfan's syndrome. N Engl J Med 1994;330(19):1335–41.

19. Daugherty A, Manning MW, Cassis LA. Angiotensin II promotes atherosclerotic lesions and aneurysms in apolipoprotein E-deficient mice. J Clin Invest 2000; 105(11):1605–12.

20. Hackam DG, Thiruchelvam D, Redelmeier DA. Angiotensin-converting enzyme inhibitors and aortic rupture: a population-based case-control study. Lancet 2006;368(9536):659–65.

21. Sweeting MJ, Thompson SG, Brown LC, et al. Use of angiotensin converting enzyme inhibitors is associated with increased growth rate of abdominal aortic aneurysms. J Vasc Surg 2010;52(1):1–4.

22. Curci JA, Mao D, Bohner DG, et al. Preoperative treatment with doxycycline reduces aortic wall expression and activation of matrix metalloproteinases in patients with abdominal aortic aneurysms. J Vasc Surg 2000;31(2):325–42.

23. Crawford ES, Crawford JL, Safi HJ, et al. Thoracoabdominal aortic aneurysms: preoperative and intraoperative factors determining immediate and long-term results of operations in 605 patients. J Vasc Surg 1986;3:389–404.

24. Suzuki S, Davis CA 3rd, Miller CC 3rd, et al. Cardiac function predicts mortality following thoracoabdominal and descending thoracic aortic aneurysm repair. Eur J Cardiothorac Surg 2003;24(1):119–24 [discussion: 124].

25. Svensson LG, Crawford ES, Hess KR, et al. Experience with 1509 patients undergoing thoracoabdominal aortic operations. J Vasc Surg 1993;17(2): 357–68 [discussion: 368–70].

26. LeMaire SA, Miller CC 3rd, Conklin LD, et al. A new predictive model for adverse outcomes after elective thoracoabdominal aortic aneurysm repair. Ann Thorac Surg 2001;71(4):1233–8.

27. Coselli JS, Bozinovski J, LeMaire SA. Open surgical repair of 2286 thoracoabdominal aortic aneurysms. Ann Thorac Surg 2007;83(2):S862–4 [discussion: S890–2].

28. Rigberg DA, Zingmond DS, McGory ML, et al. Age stratified, perioperative, and one-year mortality after abdominal aortic aneurysm repair: a statewide experience. J Vasc Surg 2006;43(2):224–9.

29. Bavaria JE, Appoo JJ, Makaroun MS, et al. Endovascular stent grafting versus open surgical repair of descending thoracic aortic aneurysms in low-risk patients: a multicenter comparative trial. J Thorac Cardiovasc Surg 2007;133(2): 369–77.

30. Kieffer E, Chiche L, Cluzel P, et al. Open surgical repair of descending thoracic aortic aneurysms in the endovascular era: a 9-year single-center study. Ann Vasc Surg 2009;23(1):60–6.

31. Khan SN, Stansby G. Cerebrospinal fluid drainage for thoracic and thoracoabdominal aortic aneurysm surgery. Cochrane Database Syst Rev 2012;(10):CD003635.

32. Acher CW, Wynn M. A modern theory of paraplegia in the treatment of aneurysms of the thoracoabdominal aorta: an analysis of technique specific observed/expected ratios for paralysis. J Vasc Surg 2009;49(5):1117–24 [discussion: 1124].

33. Estrera AL, Sheinbaum R, Miller CC 3rd, et al. Neuromonitor-guided repair of thoracoabdominal aortic aneurysms. J Thorac Cardiovasc Surg 2010;140(Suppl 6): S131–5 [discussion: S142–6].

34. Dake MD, Miller DC, Semba CP, et al. Transluminal placement of endovascular stent-grafts for the treatment of descending thoracic aortic aneurysms. N Engl J Med 1994;331(26):1729–34.

35. Walsh SR, Tang TY, Sadat U, et al. Endovascular stenting versus open surgery for thoracic aortic disease: systematic review and meta-analysis of perioperative results. J Vasc Surg 2008;47(5):1094–8.

36. Gravereaux EC, Faries PL, Burks JA, et al. Risk of spinal cord ischemia after endograft repair of thoracic aortic aneurysms. J Vasc Surg 2001;34(6):997–1003.

37. Goodney PP, Travis L, Lucas FL, et al. Survival after open versus endovascular thoracic aortic aneurysm repair in an observational study of the Medicare population. Circulation 2011;124(24):2661–9.

38. Peterson BG, Eskandari MK, Gleason TG, et al. Utility of left subclavian artery revascularization in association with endoluminal repair of acute and chronic thoracic aortic pathology. J Vasc Surg 2006;43(3):433–9.

39. Matsumura JS, Lee WA, Mitchell RS, et al. The Society for Vascular Surgery Practice Guidelines: management of the left subclavian artery with thoracic endovascular aortic repair. J Vasc Surg 2009;50(5):1155–8.

40. Byrne J, Darling RC 3rd, Roddy SP, et al. Long term outcome for extra-anatomic arch reconstruction. An analysis of 143 procedures. Eur J Vasc Endovasc Surg 2007;34(4):444–50.

41. Quinones-Baldrich W, Jimenez JC, DeRubertis B, et al. Combined endovascular and surgical approach (CESA) to thoracoabdominal aortic pathology: a 10-year experience. J Vasc Surg 2009;49(5):1125–34.

42. Patel HJ, Upchurch GR Jr, Eliason JL, et al. Hybrid debranching with endovascular repair for thoracoabdominal aneurysms: a comparison with open repair. Ann Thorac Surg 2010;89(5):1475–81.

43. Kuratani T, Kato M, Shirakawa Y, et al. Long-term results of hybrid endovascular repair for thoraco-abdominal aortic aneurysms. Eur J Cardiothorac Surg 2010; 38(3):299–304.

44. Moulakakis KG, Mylonas SN, Avgerinos ED, et al. Hybrid open endovascular technique for aortic thoracoabdominal pathologies. Circulation 2011;124(24): 2670–80.

45. Verhoeven EL, Vourliotakis G, Bos WT, et al. Fenestrated stent grafting for short-necked and juxtarenal abdominal aortic aneurysm: an 8-year single-centre experience. Eur J Vasc Endovasc Surg 2010;39(5):529–36.

46. Amiot S, Haulon S, Becquemin JP, et al. Fenestrated endovascular grafting: the French multicentre experience. Eur J Vasc Endovasc Surg 2010;39(5):537–44.

47. Greenberg RK, Lu Q, Roselli EE, et al. Contemporary analysis of descending thoracic and thoracoabdominal aneurysm repair: a comparison of endovascular and open techniques. Circulation 2008;118(8):808–17.

48. Sweet MP, Hiramoto JS, Park KH, et al. A standardized multi-branched thoracoabdominal stent-graft for endovascular aneurysm repair. J Endovasc Ther 2009;16(3):359–64.

49. Reilly LM, Rapp JH, Grenon SM, et al. Efficacy and durability of endovascular thoracoabdominal aortic aneurysm repair using the caudally directed cuff technique. J Vasc Surg 2012;56(1):53–63 [discussion: 63–4].

Peripheral Artery Aneurysm

Heather A. Hall, MD*, Samantha Minc, MD, Trissa Babrowski, MD

KEYWORDS

- Peripheral aneurysm • Femoral pseudoaneurysm • Axillary aneurysm
- Brachial aneurysm

KEY POINTS

- Peripheral aneurysms discovered in one location warrant screening for aneurysms in the contralateral limb as well as in other locations because of the high incidence of concurrent disease.
- Peripheral aneurysms typically present as asymptomatic findings in tests done for other reasons, or may present with symptoms when there is local compression of other structures, such as nerves or veins, with ischemia, or rarely with rupture.
- Larger aneurysms and those causing symptoms should be repaired.
- Ultrasonography, computed tomography angiography, and magnetic resonance angiography can be used to define inflow and outflow and better characterize the aneurysm, particularly its size and thrombus.
- Repair of peripheral aneurysms typically involves resection with interposition grafting, although certain anatomic sites may be amenable to endovascular approaches.
- Femoral pseudoaneurysms can be managed with observation, surgical repair, ultrasound-guided compression, or ultrasound-guided thrombin injection.

COMMON FEMORAL ARTERY ANEURYSMS

Common femoral artery (CFA) aneurysms are defined as a focal dilatation of the CFA to 1.5 times the size of an adjacent segment of artery of normal diameter. In men, the normal diameter of the CFA is 0.78 to 1.12 cm and in women, the normal diameter is 0.78 to 0.85 cm.[1] Cutler and Darling[2] classified CFA aneurysms into 2 categories: type 1, involving the CFA and ending proximal to the bifurcation; and type 2, involving the CFA and extending into the profunda femoris artery (PFA). Type 1 aneurysms account for 44% to 85% of all CFA aneurysms.

Epidemiology

CFA aneurysms are the second most common peripheral arterial aneurysm after popliteal aneurysms. The major risk factors for CFA aneurysms are male sex,

The authors have nothing to disclose.

Section of Vascular Surgery and Endovascular Therapy, The University of Chicago Medical Center, 5841 South Maryland Avenue, MC 5028, Chicago, IL 60636, USA

* Corresponding author.

E-mail address: hhall1@surgery.bsd.uchicago.edu

advanced age, hypertension, and tobacco use. The mean age at diagnosis is 65 years and the male to female predominance is significant at approximately 30:1. Most CFA aneurysms are degenerative in nature and caused by atherosclerotic disease. Other causes of CFA aneurysms include Behçet syndrome, acromegaly, and arteriomegaly. Patients with CFA aneurysms have a high risk for aneurysms elsewhere; 50% of patients present with bilateral CFA aneurysms, 27% to 44% of patients present with concurrent popliteal artery aneurysms, and 50% to 90% of patients present with aortic aneurysms. Patients presenting with CFA aneurysms must be thoroughly screened for concurrent aneurysmal disease and undergo lifelong surveillance for the development of future aneurysms.

Patient Presentation, Natural History, and Indications for Treatment

Approximately 30% to 40% of patients with CFA aneurysms are asymptomatic at the time of initial presentation and 30% to 40% of patients present with local symptoms such as pain or tenderness caused by mass effect, neuralgia caused by femoral nerve compression, or edema caused by vein compression. In reported series, 10% to 65% of patients present with an ischemic complication caused by the aneurysm, such as chronic thrombosis with claudication, acute thrombosis leading to critical limb ischemia (occurring in 15% of patients), and less commonly, distal embolization or rupture.[3]

Because of the rare nature of CFA aneurysms, the natural history is not well defined. Complications with aneurysms less than 2.5 cm are rare and have been reported at 1% to 2% annually. Multiple studies have confirmed that small aneurysms can be managed conservatively.[3] Treatment is indicated for the following:

- All symptomatic aneurysms
- Aneurysms greater than 2.5 cm
- Aneurysms being followed conservatively with expansion of aneurysm
- Aneurysms being followed conservatively with a change in baseline pulse examination (indicating an occult embolic event)

Diagnosis and Imaging

Diagnosis may be made on physical examination and patient history. However, often due to patient body habitus, physical examination alone is insufficient as a diagnostic tool. Duplex ultrasonography can be used for screening and surveillance, and can determine the size of femoral artery aneurysms, delineate the presence of thrombus in the sac, and show the extent of artery involved. Once the decision to treat has been made, magnetic resonance angiography (MRA) or computed tomography angiography (CTA) can be used for more precise measurements and detailed anatomic views, and to determine the patency of the proximal and distal vessels, which are useful for operative planning.

Surgical Treatment

Surgical management of CFA aneurysms depends on the type of aneurysm, patency of proximal and distal vessels, and the presence of other aneurysms. The open operative approach to a CFA aneurysm is through a vertical groin incision over the CFA. If access to the external iliac artery is necessary for proximal control, the vessel may be accessed by dividing the inguinal ligament or by making a retroperitoneal incision. Another option for achieving proximal control is using a percutaneous endovascular approach via the contralateral groin and occluding the external iliac artery with a balloon.

Type 1 aneurysms can be treated with a short interposition graft using Dacron or polytetrafluoroethylene (PTFE). Prosthetic graft works well in this location and autologous vein is reserved for cases of infection. Small aneurysms may be completely excised; larger aneurysms may be treated from within the sac using the graft inclusion technique used in abdominal aortic aneurysm repair. Type 2 aneurysms require either reimplantation of the profunda onto the CFA–femoral artery interposition graft, bypass to the profunda from the CFA–femoral artery graft, or an end-to-end CFA to profunda bypass with femoral artery ligation and division in the case of chronic femoral artery occlusion.

With regard to endovascular therapy, the anatomic location of the CFA in relation to the inguinal ligament and hip flexor as well as its proximity to the profunda make open repair the procedure of choice over stent grafting. Although technically possible, high rates of early and late stent thrombosis have been observed, and the potential for stent fracture or migration in this location is particularly troublesome.[4]

Results

Results of open CFA aneurysm repair are generally good, with 5-year patency rates of approximately 85% and mortality rates ranging from 2% to 5% in most series.[4]

FEMORAL ARTERY PSEUDOANEURYSMS

Femoral artery pseudoaneurysms (also known as false aneurysms) are caused by an arterial defect that becomes contained in the surrounding structures. The outer wall is composed of compressed thrombus and surrounding soft tissue rather than the 3 layers of the arterial wall (found in true aneurysms). The pseudoaneurysm has arterial flow with a defined neck that traces back to the site of the arterial defect. Causes of pseudoaneurysms include arterial access for interventional procedures, anastamotic leakage, infection, and noniatrogenic trauma.

Postcatheterization Femoral Pseudoaneurysms

Iatrogenic pseudoaneurysm formation is one of the most common complications of femoral artery catheterization, occurring in 0.6% to 6% of femoral interventions.[4] Risk factors for postcatheterization pseudoaneurysms include periprocedural anticoagulation/coagulopathy, obesity, large sheath size (7 Fr or greater), faulty puncture technique, inadequate manual compression, simultaneous catheterization of the artery and vein, puncture of the femoral artery or PFA, hypertension, heavily calcified vessels, female gender, and chronic renal failure requiring hemodialysis.

Patient Presentation, Natural History, and Indications for Treatment

Patients may present with a pulsatile mass, femoral thrill or bruit, pain caused by local compression, neuralgia from nerve compression, or edema from vein compression. Patients may also present with skin ischemia and necrosis from progressive enlargement, as well as distal embolization or rupture.

The main issue to be faced when managing a patient with a femoral pseudoaneurysm is whether or not the pseudoaneurysm will thrombose spontaneously. The main predictors of pseudoaneurysm thrombosis are size and anticoagulation status. In 1 study, spontaneous thrombosis occurred in 72 of 82 patients with pseudoaneurysms less than 3 cm at a mean of 23 days.[5] However, in another prospective study only 9 of 16 patients had spontaneous thrombosis at a mean of 22 days and failure to thrombose was associated with size greater than 1.8 cm and concomitant use of anticoagulation or antiplatelet agents.[6]

Because of the discrepancy in the data and because many of the studies were performed before the widespread use of antiplatelet agents and warfarin, it is generally agreed that pseudoaneurysms less than 2 cm can be safely observed[7] and that more aggressive surveillance and intervention should be considered for pseudoaneurysms measuring 2 to 3 cm. Symptomatic pseudoaneurysms and those greater than 3 cm should be treated. Absolute indications for repair include rapid expansion, infection, skin or soft tissue necrosis, neuropathy, distal ischemia, pain, or artery rupture.

Diagnosis and Imaging

Duplex ultrasonography is the imaging modality of choice for femoral pseudoaneurysms, with sensitivity and specificity of 94% and 97%, respectively, for symptomatic patients.[8] Duplex ultrasonography provides information on size, morphology, flow, neck anatomy, and feeding vessels. On B-mode imaging, the pseudoaneurysm appears as an echolucent mass connected to the artery that may expand and contract with the cardiac cycle. Color Doppler reveals a swirling flow pattern (sometimes referred to as a yin-yang sign) and when a pulsed wave Doppler is placed in the pseudoaneurysm tract, a classic to-and-fro signal is obtained, indicating flow in and out of the pseudoaneurysm space.

Treatment

The most common approaches to treat femoral pseudoaneurysms are surgery, ultrasound-guided compression, and ultrasound-guided thrombin injection. Endovascular approaches using coils, fibrin glue, and stent graft exclusion have been attempted with variable success.

Surgical Management

Surgical repair is indicated in patients presenting with pseudoaneurysms due to previous vascular surgical interventions (ie, suture line disruption), infection, or noniatrogenic trauma. Other indications for surgical repair include skin or soft tissue ischemia, associated arteriovenous fistula, injury to the vessel above the inguinal ligament, and in patients undergoing general anesthesia for another procedure (most often cardiac). Urgent surgical repair should be performed in any patient with rupture, an expanding pulsatile mass, or compression of surrounding structures causing neuropathy, claudication, or critical limb ischemia.

The open operative approach to femoral pseudoaneurysm repair is through a vertical groin incision, with the goal of obtaining proximal and distal control around the site of arterial injury. Proximal control may require a retroperitoneal incision or division of the inguinal ligament to access the external iliac artery, or contralateral femoral artery access for endovascular placement of an occlusion balloon. The pseudoaneurysm sac is then entered, the hematoma evacuated, and the arterial injury repaired with interrupted, transverse sutures. If debridement of the artery is required or there is extensive injury to the vessel, saphenous vein from the contralateral thigh may be used for either patch angioplasty or interposition graft. If the pseudoaneurysm is infected, the artery must be debrided to noninfected tissue. If the affected area is limited, a saphenous vein patch may be performed with sartorius flap for coverage, otherwise all infected tissue should be debrided with ligation of the artery. Once the wound is closed and covered, an obturator bypass may then be performed.

In cases of rupture with hemodynamic instability, the pseudoaneurysm may be entered without first obtaining proximal or distal control with the goal of evacuating the hematoma and applying digital pressure on the site of injury until the patient is stabilized. The procedure can then proceed in the standard fashion.

Ultrasound-Guided Compression

Duplex ultrasonography was introduced in 1991 and is used to locate the pseudoaneurysm tract; pressure is applied to the tract and sac to the point of flow cessation, as seen on Doppler imaging. Pressure is held in cycles of 10 to 20 minutes and the pseudoaneurysm is then reassessed. If flow persists, compression is held for another cycle, typically stopping after 1 or 2 attempts. Patients are then put on bed rest for 6 hours and duplex ultrasonography is performed 24 to 48 hours later to confirm thrombosis.

Success rates for ultrasound-guided compression are 66% to 86%, with average compression times of 30 to 44 minutes. Recurrence is 4% and the likelihood of success decreases to less than 40% in the setting of anticoagulation.[9] Other limitations are aneurysm size (larger aneurysms are more difficult to thrombose), patient body habitus, and pain. Complications occur in 2% to 4% of cases and include pseudoaneurysm rupture, femoral vein thrombosis, femoral artery thrombosis with resultant limb ischemia, and hypotension from vasovagal events or sedation during the procedure.

Ultrasound-Guided Thrombin Injection

Thrombin directly converts fibrinogen to fibrin and maintains its efficacy in patients on heparin or warfarin as it bypasses their effects on the clotting cascade. In ultrasound-guided thrombin injection (UGTI), duplex ultrasonography is used to identify the pseudoaneurysm cavity. The cavity is then punctured under direct visualization, and the needle tip position confirmed; 0.1 to 0.2 mL of 1000 units/mL of thrombin is then injected over 10 to 15 seconds until flow in the cavity ceases. A second injection may be performed; however, it is important to stop injecting as soon as thrombosis occurs to avoid thrombin entering the rest of the circulation. The patient is placed on bed rest for 1 hour and duplex ultrasonography is performed 24 hours later to confirm thrombosis.

Success rates for UGTI are 93% to 100% and recurrence rates are 3%. Complication rates have been reported at 0% to 4% and include distal embolization of thrombin, groin abscess, femoral artery and/or vein thrombosis, and anaphylaxis in patients previously exposed to bovine thrombin.[4] Distal embolization has been reported in up to 2% of patients, however the risk can be minimized by slow injection and avoiding aneurysms with short wide necks. In cases of embolization, the patient should be placed on intravenous heparin and if symptoms do not resolve rapidly, catheter-directed thrombolysis with tissue plasminogen activator should be instituted. Contraindications to UGTI include aneurysms with short wide necks, patients with infection or overlying skin necrosis, allergy to bovine thrombin (a skin test may be helpful to assess for hypersensitivity in patients with a history of bovine thrombin exposure), presence of arteriovenous fistula, ischemic extremity, and pregnancy.

PFA ANEURYSMS

Aneurysms involving the PFA are rare and account for 0.5% of all peripheral aneurysms.[2] Because of their rarity, data are limited. According to the current literature, 58% of cases present with a complication at initial presentation[10] and synchronous aneurysms are present in up to 81% of patients. In a series from Mayo, 11/15 patients (73%) had aneurysms in other locations and rupture occurred in 13%.[11] Again, because of the paucity of data, it is difficult to determine whether these aneurysms are more likely to rupture than others.

Surgical Treatment

The profunda is approached via a vertical groin incision, proximal control is obtained via the CFA or external iliac artery as needed, and the course of the artery is followed from the CFA, laterally and inferiorly to the site of the profunda aneurysm. The sartorius and rectus femoris muscles should be reflected laterally and distal control of the profunda branches may be obtained using vessel loops or balloons. Care should be taken to preserve branches of the femoral nerve and the crossing branch of the deep femoral vein should be ligated when it is encountered. An interposition graft using saphenous vein or prosthetic material should be performed once the aneurysm is excised. Ligation of the profunda femoris is highly discouraged unless absolutely necessary, and should not be performed in the setting of an occluded superficial femoral artery.

SUPERFICIAL FEMORAL ARTERY ANEURYSMS

Superficial femoral artery (SFA) aneurysms are typically found in the setting of arteriomegaly or as an extension of an existing popliteal artery aneurysm. There is a high male preponderance, with 75% to 85% of cases presenting in men. There is some discrepancy in the literature regarding the rate of rupture as the initial presenting symptom, however most reviews report a rupture prevalence of 30% to 50% among patients presenting with SFA aneurysms.[12] Other presenting symptoms include thrombosis, distal embolism, and asymptomatic thigh mass. In a series by Rigdon and colleagues,[13] 65% of patients presented with a complication. Thirty-five percent presented with rupture, 18% with thrombosis, and 18% with distal embolization. Despite the high rate of initial complications, this series demonstrated a 94% limb salvage rate.

Surgical Treatment

If possible, preoperative arteriography is valuable to assess for inflow and outflow vessels when assessing these aneurysms. Exposure is obtained via incision at the mid thigh, although groin exposure can be obtained for proximal control if needed. Otherwise, the surgical approach is nearly identical to popliteal aneurysm repair, with end-to-end interposition grafts for small aneurysms and proximal and distal ligation and bypass for larger aneurysms. Saphenous vein is the preferred conduit if the knee joint is crossed, otherwise prosthetic can be used.

POPLITEAL ARTERY ANEURYSMS

Popliteal artery aneurysms are relatively rare but potentially morbid aneurysms that can occur in isolation or in conjunction with other large-vessel aneurysms. They are the most common peripheral artery aneurysm, accounting for 85% of all peripheral aneurysms and are reported to occur in 1% of men aged 65 to 80 years.[14] They are bilateral 53% of the time and are associated with abdominal aortic aneurysms 40% to 50% of the time.[15] Up to 40% of patients have a concomitant femoral aneurysm.[16] With modern screening techniques, the incidence of popliteal artery aneurysms found in patients with abdominal aortic aneurysms is 14%.[17] Often atherosclerotic in origin, they can also be associated with conditions such as Behçet disease, Marfan syndrome, and mycotic degeneration. Up to 75% of all popliteal artery aneurysms are discovered in symptomatic patients, manifested as claudication, chronic distal ischemia caused by chronic embolization, or acute limb-threatening ischemia caused by either aneurysm thrombosis or acute thromboembolism. Patients may also present with swelling or pain. When diagnosed in asymptomatic patients, they are commonly detected during screening examinations in individuals diagnosed with some form of vascular disease. Rupture of popliteal artery aneurysms is an uncommon occurrence, however when rupture occurs, it is often limb threatening and associated with an amputation rate of 50% to 70%.[18]

Anatomy

The popliteal artery is the distal extension of the femoral artery, which courses through the popliteal fossa. It extends from the opening in the adductor magnus downward and lateral to the intercondyloid fossa of the femur then vertically to the lower border of the popliteus where it divides into the tibial arteries. Popliteal artery aneurysms are true aneurysms, meaning all 3 layers of the wall are involved (intima, media, and adventitia). The artery is considered to be aneurysmal when its diameter is greater than 2 cm or 1.5 times the normal caliber.

Pathogenesis

The popliteal artery is more typical of a central elastic artery than most peripheral muscular arteries. Thus, aneurysmal changes likely follow a similar mechanism to those seen in abdominal aortic aneurysms.[19] Aneurysm formation is caused by a disruption between the production and degradation of vascular wall constituents such as collagen and elastin. The process is likely complex and multifactorial. Inflammation is often found in the wall of aneurysmal popliteal arteries.[20] The release of reactive oxygen species and matrix metalloproteinases leads to elastin and collagen degradation, and the degradation of the smooth muscle of the media via apoptosis impairs arterial wall repair. Although deranged autoimmune responses have been identified in the setting of abdominal aortic aneurysms, the role of immunity in the development of popliteal aneurysms has not been investigated.[21] Mechanical factors are also believed to play an important role in the formation of these aneurysms. Shear stress forces as a result of hypertension and disturbed flow beyond a relative stenosis causes dilation in the distal segment. The arcuate popliteal ligament may represent an area of relative stenosis; popliteal entrapment caused by abnormal insertion of the thigh muscle tendons can also contribute to aneurysm formation.[22]

Clinical Presentation

Approximately half of all patients are asymptomatic on presentation and are diagnosed by imaging studies performed for other reasons such as knee pain or in the course of screening related to aneurysmal disease elsewhere. If the patient does not have adequate blood flow around a thrombosed aneurysm, chronic limb ischemia develops, which may be indistinguishable from occlusive atherosclerotic disease. Individuals with chronic ischemia often present with claudication, which may improve as collateral blood flow develops or may progress to critical limb ischemia. Some individuals initially present with thromboemboli manifested as blue toe syndrome. Patients with acute limb ischemia from thrombosis present with the abrupt onset of foot or leg pain, numbness, or coolness. A small number of individuals present with compressive symptoms such as pain, or sensory or motor deficits from compression of the sciatic, tibial, or peroneal nerves.[23] Deep venous thrombosis, varicose veins, or phlebitis are other rare occurrences.

Diagnosis

Routine vascular examination should include an examination of the popliteal fossa. Popliteal artery aneurysm is often suggested on physical examination by the presence of an exaggerated popliteal pulse; 60% of patients with popliteal aneurysms have a pulsatile mass. If the popliteal pulse is not appreciated secondary to thrombosis, the presence of a contralateral prominent popliteal pulse or bounding aortic pulsation should raise suspicion.[24] Examination should also involve looking for clinical signs of distal embolization. Popliteal aneurysms are confirmed with a noninvasive imaging technique such as duplex ultrasonography, CTA, or MRA. The choice of modality depends on resources as well as presentation.

Duplex ultrasonography is the first-line examination in cases of suspected popliteal aneurysm. It provides information about patency of the popliteal and outflow vessels, identifies thrombus, and allows screening for coexisting aneurysmal disease. When elective repair is planned, it is essential to have good imaging of both inflow and outflow vessels. CTA allows for measurement of true arterial lumen size, which is important if endovascular therapy is being considered.[24] Conventional arteriography is a reasonable approach in a patient with acute symptoms if thrombolytic therapy is an option. Patients with limb-threatening ischemia should always be evaluated in the operating room.

Natural History of Asymptomatic Popliteal Artery Aneurysms

Popliteal artery aneurysms become symptomatic at a rate of 5% to 24% per year.[25] Left untreated, asymptomatic popliteal artery aneurysms cause complications in 60% to 75% of patients at 5 years. Approximately one-third of patients go on to develop acute ischemia either from thrombosis of the aneurysm or distal embolization. About one-quarter of patients develop intermittent claudication. Pain and discomfort is a common complaint due to local compression from large aneurysms. Compression of the popliteal vein occurs in about 5% of cases leading to deep vein thrombosis. Rupture is a potential, yet rare, complication of these aneurysms. Even after repair, approximately 1% of patients have residual symptoms.[25] The natural history of popliteal aneurysm growth is not well defined; expansion rates are variable and difficult to predict. Published rates for small (1.5–2.0 cm) popliteal aneurysms range from 0.7 to 1.5 mm per year, whereas larger aneurysms (>2 cm) grow from 1.5 to 3.7 mm per year with a significant number of aneurysms not showing any expansion at all.[26]

Risk Factors for Thrombosis

Multiple characteristics of popliteal artery aneurysms have been studied to determine when repair should be considered.

Size
Most practitioners recommend repairing popliteal artery aneurysms once they have reached 2 cm in size as size relates to development of symptoms.[27] One recent study of a large population found that the median diameter of asymptomatic popliteal aneurysms was 2.0 cm (range 1.5–4.8 cm), the median diameter of aneurysms producing symptoms of acute ischemia was 3 cm (range 1.4–4.6 cm), and 3.45 cm (range 3.0–5.6 cm) for those producing compression.[28]

Distortion
The popliteal artery is relatively fixed at its upper and lower extents so as the diameter of the artery increases, so does its degree of distortion. Increasing distortion correlates to increased symptoms; the median distortion of asymptomatic popliteal aneurysms is reported to be 0°, median distortion of aneurysms producing compression is 45° and for those producing acute ischemic symptoms, it is 60°.[29]

Thrombus within popliteal aneurysm
Larger aneurysms are more likely to contain thrombus. Chronic embolization from aneurysms containing thrombus may eventually lead to occluded run-off. Some

investigators have demonstrated greater risk of complications in patients with popliteal aneurysms associated with absent distal pulses.[30] Thus, many surgeons consider the presence of thrombus within an aneurysm combined with poor run-off to be an indication for repair.

Management

Popliteal artery aneurysms may be repaired surgically, with an endovascular approach, or managed conservatively depending on the clinical presentation, size, and patient factors. Any individual who is symptomatic or presents with acute limb ischemia should undergo repair. Patients with patent popliteal aneurysms greater than 2.0 cm in diameter should consider undergoing repair as results are superior in the setting of elective repair in these individuals with 5-year graft patency rates greater than 85%.[24]

Popliteal aneurysms smaller than 2.0 cm in diameter are typically managed conservatively. Between 18% and 35% of these individuals risk becoming symptomatic. If nonoperative management is pursued, individuals should undergo serial ultrasonography examinations with the consideration of anticoagulation.

Patients who are incidentally noted to have thrombosed popliteal artery aneurysms are managed similar to patients with occlusive atherosclerotic disease and claudication. An effort is made to mitigate cardiovascular risk factors and these patients may also benefit from an exercise program as well as a trial of cilostazol. Patients with from chronic limb ischemia as a result of chronic embolization may benefit from lower extremity revascularization.

Thrombolytic therapy for acutely thrombosed popliteal artery aneurysms is useful when it succeeds in clearing thrombus from run-off vessels. Multiple small series have demonstrated some value in this technique in patients with Rutherford Class I or IIa ischemia. Excellent graft patency rates of 68% to 100% and limb salvage rates of 73% to 100% have been reported.[31,32] Any patient who has progression of symptoms while undergoing thrombolytic therapy should have therapy terminated and be immediately taken to the operating room.

Surgical management of popliteal artery aneurysms is most commonly approached by a medial incision with proximal and distal ligation of the aneurysm, followed by bypass grafting. The preferred conduit is autologous vein.[33] Some investigators have suggested that up to 30% of aneurysms treated this way either retain or redevelop flow after ligation[34] as this approach does not allow side branches to be ligated. These lesions may be repaired via an open posterior approach with opening of the aneurysm and insertion of an interposition graft.

With the increase in endovascular techniques, a less invasive approach than open surgical repair of these aneurysms has been investigated. A recent meta-analysis of endovascular versus open approaches to nonthrombosed popliteal aneurysm repair demonstrated a significantly greater 30-day graft thrombosis and reintervention rate compared with open repair. There were 13 early and late stent-related complications in 9 patients in a group of 67 popliteal artery aneurysms. Complications included stent migration with or without endoleak, stenosis, and stent disruption.[35] Endoleak has been reported in 20% of endovascular popliteal artery aneurysm repairs in other studies.[36]

Any patient with multiple large-vessel aneurysms must have intervention tailored to their specific needs. In general, an abdominal aortic aneurysm is treated first unless in the setting of acute limb ischemia. When concomitant ipsilateral femoral artery aneurysms are present, popliteal artery aneurysms are repaired at the same time; contralateral peripheral aneurysms are typically approached in a staged fashion.

AXIAL ARTERY ANEURYSMS

Causes

Axillary artery aneurysms are rare and almost always occur as a result of penetrating or blunt trauma.[37] Posttraumatic aneurysms have been described in athletes who repeatedly perform forceful extension of the upper extremity such as baseball pitchers. In pitching, repetitive mechanical trauma is caused by the throwing motion, which involves abduction and external rotation of the arm and compression of the axillary artery by the humeral head.[38] Other sources of axillary aneurysm formation include repetitive use injury from crutches, and pseudoaneurysm formation from anterior shoulder dislocation, humeral fractures, and penetrating trauma.

Presentation and Diagnosis

Symptoms of axillary artery aneurysms include mass effect from brachial plexus compression and thromboembolic events with hand and finger ischemia. Diagnosis is made with arteriography or CTA depending on the acuity of symptoms.

Surgical Treatment

Surgical treatment of axillary artery aneurysms involves resection of the aneurysm and interposition vein grafting. Care should be taken to protect the axillary vein and brachial plexus during dissection. Saphenous vein is the conduit of choice due to higher patency rates than prosthetic.[39] Brachial and axillary vein should be avoided as conduits as they are thin walled and may have aneurysmal degeneration over time. Long-term results for surgical repair are excellent, with 1 report showing a 100% graft patency rate over a follow up period of 3.2 ± 0.41 years. In this report, symptom resolution occurred in all patients except for 1, who had presented with nerve impingement caused by compression from the aneurysmal mass and hemorrhage.[37]

Endovascular repair using endograft placement to exclude the aneurysm has been described. There are limited data in the literature to recommend this approach and endovascular repair should be limited to high-risk patients with major comorbidities.

BRACHIAL ARTERY ANEURYSMS

Causes

Brachial artery aneurysms are rare upper extremity aneurysms that typically occur as a result of trauma or infection. Many of these patients have a history of intravenous drug use.[40] Injuries sustained during deliberate puncture for angiography or cardiac catheterization lead to pseudoaneurysm formation 0.3% of the time.[41] Brachial artery aneurysms are also associated with various congenital connective tissue disorders including Kawasaki syndrome, Burger disease, Ehlers-Danlos syndrome, Kaposi sarcoma, and cystic adventitial disease.[42] However, in a significant number of patients, no clear cause can be identified. In this situation aneurysms are considered idiopathic.[43]

Presentation

Brachial artery aneurysms often present as a mass in the upper extremity. Pain and rapid expansion are also common findings. They may be associated with a thrill or bruit. Distally, there may be a loss of pulse and paresthesias from median nerve compression or compartment syndrome. In rare circumstances, initial presentation can be from embolic or thrombotic complications, including ischemia or gangrene necessitating amputation.[44] These aneurysms have a low risk of rupture and rarely present in this setting.

Diagnosis

Duplex ultrasonography is the initial diagnostic test of choice. CTA is also a reasonable approach for operative planning. Conventional angiography may be used in select cases.

Management

As with most aneurysmal disease, surgical repair is recommended for a brachial artery aneurysm between 1.5 and 2 times the normal arterial diameter.[45] Nonoperative management may be considered when brachial artery aneurysms are small, asymptomatic, and likely to spontaneously thrombose. However, the morbidity of surgical repair is so low that careful consideration should be made to repair these aneurysms promptly. Both open and endovascular techniques have been used, although open surgical repair remains the gold standard. Typically, the aneurysmal segment of artery is resected and the artery is reconstructed with either vein or prosthetic graft material. Careful consideration must be made when putting prosthetic material in patients who develop aneurysms related to intravenous drug abuse. If the aneurysm is small, suture repair may be adequate. A small body of literature exists reviewing the use of stent graft placement in brachial artery pseudoaneurysms from dialysis access with favorable early results.[46]

REFERENCES

1. Johnston KW, Rutherford RB, Tilson MD, et al. Suggested standards for reporting on arterial aneurysms. Subcommittee on Reporting Standards for Arterial Aneurysms, Ad Hoc Committee on Reporting Standards, Society for Vascular Surgery and North American Chapter, International Society for Cardiovascular Surgery. J Vasc Surg 1991;13:452–8.
2. Cutler BS, Darling RC. Surgical management of arteriosclerotic femoral aneurysms. Surgery 1973;74:764–73.
3. Savolainen H, Widmer MK, Heller G, et al. Common femoral artery—uncommon aneurysms. Scand J Surg 2003;92:203–5.
4. Corriere MA, Guzman RJ. True and false aneurysms of the femoral artery. Semin Vasc Surg 2005;18:216–23.
5. Toursarkissian B, Allen BT, Petrinec D, et al. Spontaneous closure of selected iatrogenic pseudoaneurysms and arteriovenous fistulae. J Vasc Surg 1997;25:803–8.
6. Kent KC, McArdle CR, Kennedy B, et al. A prospective study of the clinical outcome of femoral pseudoaneurysms and arteriovenous fistulas induced by arterial puncture. J Vasc Surg 1993;17:125–31.
7. Webber GW, Jang J, Gustavson S, et al. Contemporary management of postcatheterization pseudoaneurysms. Circulation 2007;115:2666–74.
8. Coughlin BF, Paushter DM. Peripheral pseudoaneurysms: evaluation with duplex US. Radiology 1988;168:339–42.
9. Coley BD, Roberts AC, Fellmeth BD, et al. Postangiographic femoral artery pseudoaneurysms: further experience with US-guided compression repair. Radiology 1995;194:307–11.
10. Van Bockel JH, Hamming JF. Lower extremity aneurysms. In: Rutherford RB, editor. Vascular surgery. 5th edition. Philadelphia: Elsevier Saunders; 2005. p. 1534–51.
11. Harbuzariu C, Duncan AA, Bower TC, et al. Profunda femoris artery aneurysms: association with aneurysmal disease and limb ischemia. J Vasc Surg 2008;47: 31–4.

12. Leon LR Jr, Taylor Z, Psalms SB, et al. Degenerative aneurysms of the superficial femoral artery. Eur J Vasc Endovasc Surg 2008;35:332–40.
13. Rigdon EE, Monajjem N. Aneurysms of the superficial femoral artery: a report of two cases and review of the literature. J Vasc Surg 1992;16:790–3.
14. Trickett JP, Scott RA, Tilney HS. Screening and management of asymptomatic popliteal aneurysms. J Med Screen 2002;9:92–3.
15. Wychulis AR, Spittel JA Jr, Wallace RB. Popliteal aneurysms. Surgery 1970;68: 942–52.
16. Vermillion BD, Kimmins SA, Pace WG, et al. A review of one hundred forty-seven popliteal aneurysms with long-term follow-up. Surgery 1981;90:1009–14.
17. Diwan A, Sarkar R, Stanly JC, et al. Incidence of femoral and popliteal artery aneurysms in patients with abdominal aortic aneurysms. J Vasc Surg 2000;31: 863–9.
18. Mitchell ME, Carpenter JP. Popliteal artery aneurysms. In: Ernst CB, Stanley JC, editors. Current Therapy in Vascular Surgery. Saunders; 2001. p. 1017–29.
19. Debasso R, Astrand H, Bjarnegard N, et al. The popliteal artery, an unusual muscular artery with wall properties similar to the aorta: implications for susceptibility to aneurysm formation? J Vasc Surg 2004;39:836–42.
20. Jacob T, Hingorani A, Ascher E. Examination of the apoptotic pathway and proteolysis in the pathogenesis of popliteal artery aneurysms. Eur J Vasc Endovasc Surg 2001;22:77–85.
21. Jagadesham VP, Scott DJ, Carding SR. Abdominal aortic aneurysms: an autoimmune disease? Trends Mol Med 2008;14:522–9.
22. Lopez Garcia D, Arranz MA, Tagarro S, et al. Bilateral popliteal aneurysm as a result of vascular type IV entrapment in a young patient: a report of an exceptional case. J Vasc Surg 2007;46:1047–50.
23. Selvam A, Shetty K, James NV, et al. Giant popliteal aneurysm presenting with foot drop. J Vasc Surg 2006;44:882–3.
24. Robinson WP, Belkin M. Acute limb ischemia due to popliteal artery aneurysm: a continuing surgical challenge. Semin Vasc Surg 2009;22:17–24.
25. Michaels JA, Galland RB. Management of asymptomatic popliteal aneurysms: the use of a Markov decision tree to determine the criteria for a conservative approach. Eur J Vasc Surg 1993;7:136–43.
26. Magee R, Quigley F, McCann M, et al. Growth and risk factors for expansion of dilated popliteal arteries. Eur J Vasc Endovasc Surg 2010;39:606–11.
27. Varga ZA, Locke-Edmunds JC, Baird RN. A multicenter study of popliteal aneurysms. J Vasc Surg 1994;20:171–7.
28. Galland RB, Magee TR. Popliteal aneurysms: distortion and size related to symptoms. Eur J Vasc Endovasc Surg 2005;30:534–8.
29. Galland RB. Popliteal aneurysms: from John Hunter to the 21st century. Ann R Coll Surg Engl 2007;89:466–71.
30. Dawson I, Sie R, van Baalen JM, et al. Asymptomatic popliteal aneurysm: elective operation versus conservative follow-up. Br J Surg 1994;81:1504–7.
31. Mahmood A, Salaman R, Sintler M, et al. Surgery of popliteal artery aneurysms: a 12 year experience. J Vasc Surg 2003;37:586–93.
32. Aulivola B, Hamdan AD, Hile CN, et al. Popliteal artery aneurysms: a comparison of outcomes in elective versus emergent repair. J Vasc Surg 2004;39:1171–7.
33. Ravn H, Bergqvist D, Bjorck M. Nationwide study of the outcome of popliteal artery aneurysms treated surgically. Br J Surg 2007;94:970–7.
34. Kirkpatrick UJ, McWilliams RG, Martin J, et al. Late complications after ligation and bypass for popliteal aneurysm. Br J Surg 2004;91:174–7.

35. Lovegrove RE, Javid M, Magee TR, et al. Endovascular and open approaches to non-thrombosed popliteal artery aneurysm repair; a meta-analysis. Eur J Vasc Endovasc Surg 2008;36:96–100.
36. Curi MA, Geraghty PJ, Merino OA, et al. Mid-term outcomes of endovascular popliteal artery aneurysm repair. J Vasc Surg 2007;45:505–10.
37. Tetik O, Yilik L, Besir Y, et al. Surgical treatment of axillary artery aneurysm. Tex Heart Inst J 2005;32:186.
38. Rohrer MJ, Cardullo PA, Pappas AM, et al. Axillary artery compression and thrombosis in throwing athletes. J Vasc Surg 1990;11(6):761–8.
39. McCarthy WJ, Flinn WR, Yao JS, et al. Result of bypass grafting for upper limb ischemia. J Vasc Surg 1986;3:741.
40. Wahlgren CM, Lohman R, Pearce BJ, et al. Metachronous giant brachial artery pseudoaneurysms: a case report and review of the literature. Vasc Endovascular Surg 2007;41:467–72.
41. Babu SC, Piccorelli GO, Shah PM, et al. Incidence and results of arterial complications among 16,350 patients undergoing cardiac catheterization. J Vasc Surg 1989;10:113.
42. Wong SS, Roche-Nagle G. Giant true brachial artery aneurysm. Vasc Endovascular Surg 2012;46:492–4.
43. Gray RJ, Stone WM, Fowl RJ, et al. Management of true aneurysms distal to the axillary artery. J Vasc Surg 1998;28:606.
44. Wilson RM, McClellan WT. Management of bilateral brachial artery pseudoaneurysms in an intravenous drug user. Plast Reconstr Surg 2012;129:200–2.
45. Schunn CD, Sullivan TM. Brachial arteriomegaly and true aneurysmal degeneration: case report and literature review. Vasc Med 2002;7:25–7.
46. Vesely TM. Use of stent grafts to repair hemodialyssi graft-related pseudoaneurysms. J Vasc Interv Radiol 2005;16:1301–7.

Mesenteric Ischemia

Joseph L. Bobadilla, MD

KEYWORDS

- Mesenteric ischemia • Chronic mesenteric ischemia • Acute mesenteric ischemia
- Nonocclusive mesenteric ischemia • Median arcuate ligament syndrome

KEY POINTS

- For all forms of mesenteric ischemia, catheter-based angiography remains the diagnostic gold standard, but when not available high-quality, thin-slice computed tomographic angiography (CTA) is an acceptable alternative.
- Acute mesenteric ischemia must be diagnosed and intervened upon rapidly to prevent catastrophic outcomes. A high index of suspicion based on history and physical examination findings is essential for the proper diagnosis and expeditious treatment of this disease process.
- Endovascular treatment options, including catheter-directed thrombolysis and visceral vessel stenting, are emerging techniques in the treatment of acute mesenteric ischemia. These methods are best used when the diagnosis is made early and bowel integrity has not yet been compromised.
- Discovery of mesenteric venous thrombosis on delayed venous-phase CTA should prompt a thorough evaluation for underlying hypercoagulable states, including occult malignancy.
- Chronic mesenteric ischemia often demonstrates a significant delay in diagnosis. The triad of postprandial pain, weight loss, and food fear are most often present. Surgical bypass remains the therapy of choice, but endovascular techniques are increasingly used.
- Median arcuate ligament syndrome can be treated by open or laparoscopic release of the compressive bands followed by endovascular techniques if residual symptoms and stenosis are present after decompression.

INTRODUCTION

The recognition of mesenteric vascular insufficiency and subsequent intestinal compromise dates back to 1895, with the first description of 2 cases of bowel resection for compromised arterial inflow.[1] With these initial descriptions, the fundamental finding of "pain out of proportion to physical examination" was established. In

Disclosures: None.
Vascular & Endovascular Surgery, Department of Surgery, University of Kentucky, 800 Rose Street, Room C219, Lexington, KY 40536-0293, USA
E-mail address: jbo244@uky.edu

Surg Clin N Am 93 (2013) 925–940
http://dx.doi.org/10.1016/j.suc.2013.04.002
0039-6109/13/$ – see front matter © 2013 Elsevier Inc. All rights reserved.

surgical.theclinics.com

addition, the recognition of the rapidity with which acute mesenteric ischemia can progress, and the gravity of missed or delayed diagnosis, was also firmly established. It was not until later that the entity of chronic visceral ischemia was borne out in the literature, initially referred to as angina abdominis.[2,3] Nearly 40 years after these initial observations, the first successful surgical intervention was reported.[4] Shaw and Maynard described the first use of thromboendarterectomy for what is now termed acute-on-chronic mesenteric ischemia. Our understanding of mesenteric ischemia continues to evolve with new recognition of compressive syndromes, including median arcuate ligament syndrome.[5]

Although visceral ischemia remains rare (2 to 3 cases per 100,000 population), the dire consequences of missed or delayed diagnosis continue to make it a focus of great attention. The need for prompt and accurate diagnosis is essential in avoiding catastrophic complications, especially in acute and acute-on-chronic mesenteric ischemia. This article focuses on each of these entities with regard to relevant history, diagnosis, and treatment options.

MESENTERIC ANATOMY

The mesenteric circulation comprises 3 main branches of the abdominal aorta: the celiac axis (CA), the superior mesenteric artery (SMA), and the inferior mesenteric artery (IMA) (**Fig. 1**).[6] Each of these is richly collateralized, such that significant disease of 2 branches is often required to result in symptoms of chronic ischemia.

The CA gives rise to branches that perfuse the liver, stomach, spleen, and pancreas. It collateralizes via the superior anterior and posterior pancreaticoduodenal branches to the SMA. The origin of the CA often arises from the ventral surface of the abdominal

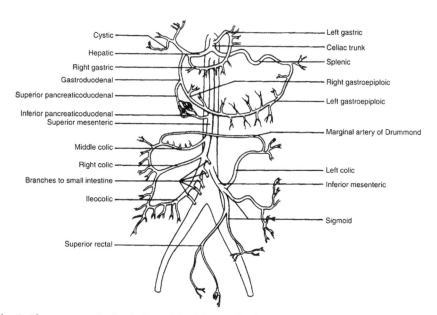

Fig. 1. The mesenteric circulation with abdominal collateral networks. (*From* Schwartz LB, Davis RD, Heinle JS, et al. The vascular system. In: Lyerly HK, Gaynor JW, editors. The handbook of surgical intensive care. 3rd edition. St Louis (MO): Mosby Year Book; 1992. p. 287; with permission.)

aorta between the T12 and L1 vertebral bodies. The median arcuate ligament runs across this origin, the implications of which are discussed later in this article. The most notable anatomic variant related to the CA is the replaced right hepatic. In approximately 12% of patients, the right hepatic artery arises from the SMA and not the proper hepatic branch of the CA.

The SMA is the next abdominal branch, arising from the ventral surface of the abdominal aorta between the L1 and L2 vertebral bodies. It collateralizes via the inferior anterior and posterior pancreaticoduodenal branches to the CA. In addition, it forms a collateral network via the marginal artery of Drummond to the IMA. The distribution of perfusion of the SMA includes partial pancreas and duodenum, the entire jejunum and ileum, and the ascending and transverse colon. Because of its relative size, long common segment, and proximal and distal collateral connection, the SMA is often a target for revascularization procedures.

The IMA arises from a slightly left anterolateral location on the abdominal aorta, usually a few centimeters above the aortic bifurcation. It collateralizes via the marginal artery of Drummond to the SMA and through the superior rectal branches to the hypogastric (internal iliac) artery. The IMA is most commonly compromised in patients with aneurysmal disease whereby mural thrombus occludes flow, or in those patients with significant tobacco abuse and subsequent severe aortoiliac occlusive disease.

ACUTE MESENTERIC ISCHEMIA

Acute mesenteric ischemia (AMI) has historically been associated with poor outcomes, with hospital mortalities rates ranging anywhere from 50% to 100%.[7–13] The essence of treatment has focused on a high clinical index of suspicion, early diagnosis, visceral revascularization, bowel resection, second-look laparotomy, and supportive care. There are 4 distinct pathophysiologies associated with acute mesenteric ischemia[9,14,15]:

- Arterial embolism (50%)
- Arterial thrombosis (20%)
- Nonocclusive pathologies (20%)
- Mesenteric venous thrombosis (10%)

Arterial Embolism

Ischemia caused by embolism is the most common form of AMI, accounting for roughly half of all patients. This condition results from embolism, usually from a cardiac source, to one of the visceral branches. The most common source of central embolism is atrial fibrillation with subsequent formation of atrial appendage thrombus.[16] Additional sources include left ventricular mural thrombus owing to hypokinesis in regions of prior myocardial infarction.[16,17] In addition, emboli may arise from cardiac valvular origins.

The branch most often affected is the SMA, because of its high basal flow rate and the anatomic angle of take-off.[18] The minority of emboli remain at the origin of the SMA (<15%), with most emboli resulting in more distal lodging, often just past the take-off of the middle colic vessel. Proximal SMA branch vessels may be preserved, as seen in **Fig. 2**.[19] Reactive vasospasm of the more distal mesenteric circulation can often compound the injury, and simultaneous embolism to other vascular beds is seen up to 15% of the time.

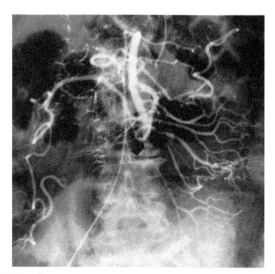

Fig. 2. Typical angiographic appearance of a superior mesenteric artery (SMA) embolism, with proximal branch sparing and mid-segment occlusion of the SMA; this is in contrast to an athro-occlusive lesion that most often results in flush occlusion at the aortic interface. (*Reproduced from* McKinsey JF, Gewertz BL. Acute mesenteric ischemia. Surg Clin North Am 1997;77:307–18.)

Arterial Thrombosis (Acute-on-Chronic)

Acute-on-chronic mesenteric ischemia implies an abrupt change overlaid on a preexisting picture of chronic mesenteric atherosclerosis. Because of the typical delay in diagnosis of chronic mesenteric ischemia, this form of acute ischemia accounts for nearly one-quarter of all AMI presentations. Careful questioning of the patient or family will most often reveal a history of weight loss, food fear, bloating, or other symptoms of chronic mesenteric ischemia, leading to acute clinical decline. Typically this form of ischemia results from slow progression of mesenteric atherosclerosis until a point of critical stenosis has developed; then, during a period of low flow, thrombosis of this critical lesion occurs. Contrary to embolic presentations, these lesions are most commonly flush to the origin of the vessel, and are often heavily calcified on computed tomography (CT) imaging. This pathophysiology has been described after myocardial infarction, acute viral illness, and even after other surgical interventions, including cardiac surgery.[20] Any clinical scenario leading to low flow and/or hypotension can result in acute-on-chronic arterial thrombosis.

Nonocclusive Mesenteric Ischemia

Nonocclusive causes of mesenteric ischemia are manyfold, but each results in a common final pathway, prolonged intestinal vasoconstriction and reduced intestinal blood flow. Typically these patients present with either shock/multisystem organ failure or after toxic pharmacologic ingestion. Common inciting pathology includes:

- Myocardial failure/cardiogenic shock[21]
- Septic shock[21]
- High-dose/prolonged vasopressor (α-agonist) infusions[21]
- Cocaine ingestion[22,23]
- Ergot poisoning[24]
- Digoxin toxicity[25,26]

This population historically has the worst in-hospital mortality rates among the various presentations of mesenteric ischemia. Presumably, this is due to the resulting mesenteric ischemia being a symptom of a more profound physiologic derangement, and not the primary disease process. This particular population is prone to significant delay in diagnosis, as they are often sedated or obtunded, which may further confound subjective reporting of symptoms. The gold standard for diagnosis is catheter-directed contrast angiography. Angiographic findings in nonocclusive mesenteric ischemia include[27]:

- SMA branch vessel origin narrowing
- Alternating dilation and narrowing "chain of lakes" or "string of sausages" sign
- Spasm of mesenteric arcades
- Impaired intramural vessel filling, "blush"

Mesenteric Venous Thrombosis

A less common form of AMI, caused by venous thrombosis, was first described in 1895 and later expounded by Warren and Eberhard.[1,28] Mesenteric vein thrombosis leads to impaired venous return, bowel-wall edema, impaired microvascular perfusion, bowel distention, and ultimately infarction of the involved segments of intestine. Mesenteric venous thrombosis is often secondary to a more global disease state. Possible predisposing pathology includes:

- Neoplastic disease processes
- Hypercoagulable syndromes
- Abdominal trauma
- Pancreatitis
- Severe dehydration
- Polycythemia vera

At present, neoplastic and hypercoagulable syndromes represent the most common inciting conditions. A thorough search for age-specific and gender-specific neoplasias as well as heritable hypercoagulable conditions (Leiden V, protein C and S deficiencies, antithrombin III deficiencies, prothrombin gene mutations, and antiphospholipid antibodies) should be undertaken as a secondary goal in the treatment of patients with mesenteric vein thrombosis. The most common vessels involved include the superior mesenteric vein (70%), the portal vein, and the inferior mesenteric vein.[29]

Presentation and Evaluation

Patients with acute and acute-on-chronic mesenteric ischemia will classically present with acute abdominal pain out of proportion to physical examination findings. A careful history may be all that is needed to diagnose each of these entities. A history of recent myocardial infarction or untreated atrial fibrillation combined with the acute onset of abdominal symptoms may be all that is needed to raise suspicion for central embolic sources. Furthermore, a prodrome of food fear, weight loss, and colicky abdominal pain that has acutely worsened may suggest acute-on-chronic arterial thrombosis.

It should be noted that the presence of bowel sounds does not exclude mesenteric ischemia. In fact, patients often experience increased expulsion of bowel contents with these processes. Presence of bowel sounds is a marker of early disease status, and if present should prompt aggressive movement toward therapeutic intervention in an attempt to maximize survival and reduce further complications. If diagnosis is delayed patients will precipitously decline, soon developing guarding, rebound, and other peritoneal signs. As the bowel becomes frankly necrotic, perforation ensues.

At this point, the "quiet abdomen" may be encountered, and this should be taken as an ominous sign. Beyond this, hemodynamic instability and multisystem organ dysfunction soon develop as acidosis worsens. Coagulopathy may also ensue. At this point, salvage becomes exceedingly more unrealistic, and mortality markedly increases.

Laboratory evaluation often shows evidence of hemoconcentration with marked leukocytosis. The leukocytosis often demonstrates a leftward shift with increased immature white cells. Increased base deficits along with elevated anion gap, lactate dehydrogenase, and amylase levels may also be seen.[30] These signs are all markers of late disease status, and, if present, should portend a guarded prognosis. Plain abdominal radiographs are helpful in ruling out alternative diagnoses, but have little utility in confirming the diagnosis of AMI.

Duplex ultrasonography of the mesenteric vessels is highly sensitive and specific; however, it is often technically limited by accompanying abdominal distention and overlying bowel gas.[31] The historical gold standard for the diagnosis of mesenteric ischemia was selective catheterization and mesenteric angiography. Although this continues to be a gold standard, CT, with its better image quality, expansion of availability, and ease of noninvasive image acquisition, has come to challenge catheter-based angiography.

Patients with nonocclusive mesenteric ischemia typically will show multiple areas of narrowing, consistent with a "string of beads" appearance. There will also be evidence of "pruning" of the more distal medium and small branch vessels, and loss of the submucosal blush normally seen with selective visceral angiography.

Patients with mesenteric venous thrombosis tend to present with a more protracted time course when compared with those patients with arterial-based ischemia syndromes. Often, symptoms will be present for 2 to 3 days before the diagnosis is made.[29] However, pain out of proportion to physical examination findings is still a hallmark of these patients' presentations. Rhee and colleagues[29] reviewed their 20-year experience with mesenteric venous thrombosis, and found that 75% of patients were symptomatic for more than 48 hours before diagnosis. In addition, abdominal pain (83%), anorexia (53%), and diarrhea (43%) were the most common presenting symptoms. Contrast-enhanced axial imaging with delayed venous phase is a key tool in the diagnosis of this abnormality. Failure to acquire delayed venous-phase images can hamper the diagnosis of this uncommon clinical entity. Duplex ultrasonography and magnetic resonance (MR) venography are alternative techniques for diagnosis, although they are less commonly used and not so readily available.

Treatment Options

Initial treatments should be aimed at stabilization and resuscitation of the patient, but these interventions should not delay or prolong the time to revascularization. Volume resuscitation, initiation of broad-spectrum antibiotics, and initiation of a heparin infusion are essential first steps. Secondary steps include insertion of nasogastric tubes, arterial lines, and Foley catheters, and central venous access. These interventions can be accomplished while the patient is prepared for anesthesia in the operating room, so as not to further delay revascularization.

The treatment of choice for arterial embolization is open surgical embolectomy and evaluation of bowel viability.[21] This procedure is performed via a generous midline laparotomy, and allows for rapid clearing of clot, both antegrade and retrograde, using transverse arteriotomy and embolectomy catheters. The transverse colon is retracted cephalad, and the duodenum mobilized to the ligament of Treitz. From here, the SMA can be palpated in the root of the mesentery. A transverse arteriotomy is made, and balloon-tipped embolectomy catheters are advanced proximally and distally. Clearance of clot should be confirmed with multiple clot-free passes of the catheter, after which heparin flushing and primary repair of the arteriotomy is completed. At this point the bowel can be assessed, clearly nonviable portions resected, and the abdomen packed for second-look laparotomy in 24 to 48 hours.

Others have advocated for a primary percutaneous approach, especially in the setting of early intervention where peritoneal signs have not yet ensued.[32–36] This approach remains somewhat controversial, as direct visualization of the bowel is not an option during percutaneous interventions. If endoluminally directed transcatheter therapy is selected there should be a low threshold for surgical exploration and bowel evaluation, based on patient data and clinical examination.

For the management of acute-on-chronic mesenteric ischemia, open thrombectomy with either endarterectomy or distal bypass are the treatments of choice. Visceral bypass can be performed either antegrade, using the supraceliac aorta for inflow, or retrograde, using the common iliac artery for inflow.[37] Choice of conduit is important, as bowel viability and bacterial translocation may very readily occur. Native venous conduit is ideal and if not available, cryopreserved alternatives may be used. Prosthetic reconstructions are discouraged because of the high risk of graft infection if bowel failure occurs. Others have advocated the use of classic open abdominal embolectomy with retrograde stenting of the primary lesion.[38] This approach is particularly useful in the setting of compromised bowel when native conduit for bypass is not available, or when inflow vessels are severely diseased, precluding safe antegrade or retrograde bypass techniques.

Nonocclusive intestinal ischemia remains a difficult entity to treat. The mainstay of therapy involves correcting the primary issue, leading to compromised intestinal perfusion. Observation and resuscitation in an intensive care environment are essential.[21] Transcatheter infusion of vasodilators has been described, especially in the setting of illicit drug overdose or accidental therapeutic drug overdoses.[39,40] Despite these interventions, this population has one of the poorest survival rates, primarily because of the severity of comorbid conditions leading to this condition.

The essential treatment of mesenteric venous thrombosis is systemic anticoagulation. Initiation of an unfractionated heparin bolus, followed by continuous infusion, is critical. Secondary therapies include bowel rest, nasogastric decompression, and the intravenous administration of broad-spectrum antibiotics to guard against sequelae of bacterial translocation. Patients who develop peritoneal signs will require exploration and bowel resection. There have been conflicting reports about the utility of percutaneous, transhepatic catheter-directed thrombolysis in these patients. Some groups have advocated for its use,[41–43] whereas others have found a significantly increased mortality rate when used.[44] Most patients can be treated conservatively with anticoagulation, bowel rest, and observation. Those patients requiring more aggressive intervention after failure to respond to conservative measures have been shown to have a worse prognosis.[44]

CHRONIC MESENTERIC ISCHEMIA
Presentation

Contrary to most cardiovascular conditions, chronic mesenteric ischemia is represented by a preponderance of female patients, up to 60% in most reported series. The average age at presentation is 50 to 60 years. More than 75% of patients have current or former tobacco exposure, and most have concurrent hypertension, coronary artery disease, prior cerebrovascular accident, and renal insufficiency. Despite the relatively common finding of significant celiac and SMA stenosis rates

(50% and 30%, respectively) during autopsy series, true chronic mesenteric ischemia remains relatively rare,[45,46] owing in part to the rich collateral networks described earlier. It has long been thought that significant disease of at least 2 of the 3 major visceral branches is needed to compromise overall mesenteric flow.

First described by Councilman nearly 120 years ago, the cardinal symptom of chronic mesenteric ischemia remains postprandial abdominal pain. This pain usually sets in 1 to 2 hours after a meal and results in dull, crampy, or spasmodic waves of pain in the epigastrium or periumbilical abdomen. The pain is often in disproportion to other clinical examination findings. Over time, patients will learn to equate food consumption with pain elicitation, and the classic "food fear" or avoidance will develop. Along with this, a history of unintentional weight loss is often present. Alternatively, patients may report a history of continual low-volume grazing habits, another strategy to avoid bolus feeding, which increases visceral blood flow in response to digestive needs and precipitates abdominal angina. Patients may also present with increasing complaints of nausea, vomiting, diarrhea, and/or bloating after meals.

Diagnosis

Visceral duplex scanning plays a significant role in the evaluation of chronic mesenteric ischemia, contrary to its modest role in AMI. Evaluation of mesenteric vessel waveforms and peak systolic velocity (PSV) calculation has been shown to be highly sensitive and specific (**Table 1**).[47] Others have added preprandial and postprandial scanning techniques, which slightly improve specificity.[48] PSVs greater than 275 cm/s in the SMA and greater than 200 cm/s in the celiac artery have been demonstrated to correlate to stenoses of greater than 70% in each vessel.[47] As with arterial stenosis in general, poststenotic dilation and the presence of a turbulent jet are also supportive findings on duplex evaluation. In addition, retrograde flow in the common hepatic artery can be seen if severe celiac stenosis is present.

Because of the high negative predictive value and sensitivity of duplex ultrasonography, it makes an excellent screening examination for chronic mesenteric ischemia. Confirmatory evaluation with thin-slice CT angiography (CTA) or MR angiography is recommended if surgical or transcatheter interventions are being entertained. In addition, selective catheter-based angiography remains the gold-standard diagnostic modality.

Treatment Options

Both endovascular and open revascularization options exist for the treatment of chronic mesenteric ischemia. However, open surgical revascularization remains the treatment of choice when the patient's condition allows, either by bypass or endarterectomy. Visceral bypass can be performed either antegrade, using the supraceliac aorta for inflow, or retrograde, using the common iliac artery for inflow.[37] Native venous conduit is ideal when suitable segments can be obtained. If native vein is not available, prosthetic or cryopreserved alternatives may be used.

Antegrade bypass is completed via a midline incision with exposure of the distal thoracic aorta.[49] The triangular ligaments of the liver are divided, and the left lobe of the liver protected and retracted laterally out of the operative field. The gastrohepatic ligaments are divided carefully with electrocautery to gain entry into the lesser sac and periesophageal space. The esophagus is then retracted to the left lateral position, and the diaphragmatic crus and median arcuate ligament are divided. Care must be taken to protect the esophagus from injury during these steps. Once the crus is divided, the distal thoracic aorta can be identified and cleared to allow clamping and anastomosis. The CA is often immediately visible during this dissection; it can be traced to the right,

Table 1
Moneta visceral duplex criterion

Specific Mesenteric Artery	Peak Systolic Velocity (cm/s)	Corresponding Percent Stenosis	Sensitivity (%)	Specificity (%)	PPV (%)	NPV (%)	Overall Accuracy (%)
SMA	>275	≥70	92	96	80	99	96
Celiac	>200	≥70	87	80	63	94	82

Abbreviations: NPV, negative predictive value; PPV, positive predictive value.
Data from Moneta GL, Lee RW, Yeager RA, et al. Mesenteric duplex scanning: a blinded prospective study. J Vasc Surg 1993;17:79–84 [discussion: 85–6].

allowing anastomosis to the hepatic or directly onto the bifurcation of the splenic and hepatic branches. If SMA revascularization is needed, blunt tunneling retrograde to the pancreas can be achieved to the left of the aorta (**Fig. 3**).[50]

Retrograde bypass can use the distal aorta or either iliac system as inflow. This region tends to be more prone to atherosclerotic change, but in many patients can be a suitable donor vessel. Care must be taken to avoid acute angulation or kinking of the bypass graft when this approach is used. Some have advocated the use of this approach only when:

- Emergency revascularization is needed
- Patient comorbidities preclude supraceliac clamping
- Prior foregut surgery prevents supraceliac dissection

The abdominal contents are packed to the right side of the abdomen, and the retroperitoneum overlying the distal aorta is incised in the usual fashion. A suitable portion of the distal aorta or iliac vessel is dissected free and prepared for anastomosis. The SMA is exposed as discussed previously, and if celiac revascularization is needed, exposure of the common hepatic artery can be accomplished with the same dissection described earlier for antegrade bypass. Blunt tunneling underneath the pancreas can again be used to bring the graft up to this region for anastomosis to the common hepatic artery, thus allowing for less anastomotic angulation and kinking associated

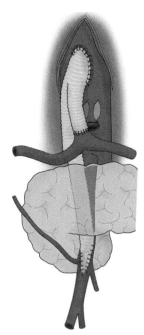

Fig. 3. Antegrade aortoceliac–superior mesenteric artery bypass. The proximal anastomosis originates from the supraceliac aorta, and the limbs of the graft are oriented on top of each other. The body of the graft should be left as short as possible. The celiac anastomosis can be performed in an end-to-end fashion. The inferior limb to the superior mesenteric artery is tunneled deep to the pancreas. The superior mesenteric anastomosis is performed end to side. (*From* Huber TS, Lee WA. Mesenteric vascular disease: chronic ischemia. In: Cronenwett JL, Johnston W, editors. Rutherford's vascular surgery. 7th edition. Philadelphia: Saunders/Elsevier; 2010; with permission.)

with the celiac revascularization. The bypass limb to the SMA should follow a "lazy reverse C" in the retroperitoneum to minimize the risk of kinking when the abdominal contents are returned to their native position (**Fig. 4**).[50]

Open surgical endarterectomy also remains a viable and durable option for chronic mesenteric ischemia. Endarterectomy offers definitive clearance of the obstructing lesions, and can be performed safely with excellent long-term results.[51] This procedure is best performed via a left thoracoabdominal incision. The diaphragm can be partially or completely divided radially; the retroperitoneal space is entered behind the left kidney, and the abdominal content rotated medially, along with the left kidney and spleen. The distal thoracic aorta is dissected free, and the crura overlying the CA divided only after the left renal vessel is clearly identified. The dissection is then carried distally to identify the SMA at its origin. Once proximal and distal control is obtained an aortic arteriotomy can be made, allowing eversion endarterectomy of the renal and visceral vessels. On completion, the arteriotomy can be closed primarily, or with a patch.

More recently, some have investigated the role of endovascular techniques for chronic mesenteric ischemia. Many groups have noted a reduced early mortality when endovascular techniques are used.[36,52] As with many endovascular techniques, the reduced early complication rate and mortality reduction comes with reduced long-term durability and increased need for reintervention.[53] When compared with open surgical revascularization, Kasirajan and colleagues[54] found an increased recurrence of symptoms in patients treated endovascularly. The Mayo group found that nearly

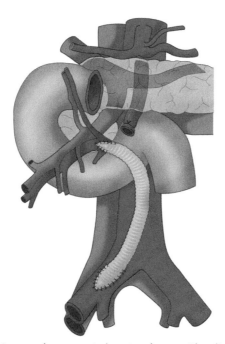

Fig. 4. Retrograde aorta–superior mesenteric artery bypass. The distal anastomosis is performed in an end-to-end or end-to-side fashion to the superior mesenteric artery after mobilization of the ligament of Treitz and the other duodenal peritoneal attachments. The bypass graft takes a gentle "reverse-C loop" as it transitions. (*From* Huber TS, Lee WA. Mesenteric vascular disease: chronic ischemia. In: Cronenwett JL, Johnston W, editors. Rutherford's vascular surgery. 7th edition. Philadelphia: Saunders/Elsevier; 2010; with permission.)

40% of endovascularly treated patients required reintervention within the first 2 years, but that this could be completed with low mortality, although complications related to the secondary procedure were as high as 27%.[53] The group at Dartmouth also confirmed the increased risk of restenosis and the need for reintervention with endovascular treatment.[55] However, these investigators did note that endovascular treatments served well to temporize some poor open surgical candidates, allowing for medical optimization, nutritional recovery, and subsequent open revascularization.[55]

COMPRESSIVE SYNDROMES
Median Arcuate Ligament Syndrome

Median arcuate ligament syndrome (MALS) shares many of the same presenting symptoms as the other forms of mesenteric ischemia. Episodic, crampy, upper abdominal pain associated with meal intake is a hallmark. Often an associated recent weight loss is also present, and many patients will also have symptoms of delayed gastric emptying. This process results from dynamic compression of the CA.[56] The hallmark diagnostic finding is dynamic compression of the celiac artery on expiration. On inspiration, the compression lessens or is absent. This disorder can be diagnosed with duplex ultrasonography, MR angiography, and conventional catheter-based angiography.[57] There has been much debate over the extent to which MALS contributes to potentially symptomatic mesenteric ischemia states, and MALS remains a diagnosis of exclusion.[58] Surgical treatment for MALS has been somewhat limited, and at present only case reports and small case series exist in the literature. There have been multiple reports of open or laparoscopic division of the ligament and crus with or without celiac ganglionectomy resulting in symptomatic relief.[59–62] The specific aim of treatment should encompass division of the restrictive fibroligamentous bands, with endovascular attempts at angioplasty and stenting as a secondary measure for persistent celiac stenosis.[61,63] Angioplasty alone, with or without stenting, is ineffective, if not contraindicated without proper decompression first and foremost.

SUMMARY

Mesenteric ischemia remains a rare clinical entity, but because of the grave consequences of missed or significantly delayed diagnosis, clinical suspicion must remain high. Abdominal pain, bloating, nausea, vomiting, and pain out of proportion to physical examination findings remain the hallmark of presentation. Catheter-based angiography is still the gold standard of diagnosis, but high-quality CTA is an acceptable alternative.

With regard to AMI, treatment options include open embolectomy, catheter-directed thrombolysis, visceral bypass, and/or mesenteric angioplasty and stenting. If percutaneous therapies are selected it is essential that the abdominal examination can be followed closely, and any concern over bowel integrity should prompt an exploratory intervention. Treatment of nonocclusive mesenteric ischemia includes therapy for the primary disease process, and some promising results have been seen with catheter-directed vasodilator infusions. Mesenteric venous thrombosis most often is a marker for systemic hypercoagulable states or occult malignancy. This disease can be treated most often with anticoagulation and a careful search for the inciting hypercoagulable-inducing condition.

Chronic mesenteric ischemia remains a disease of women in their fifth and sixth decade. Prolonged symptomatology and delayed diagnosis is often seen. Classic food fear, meal avoidance, and postprandial epigastric or periumbilical pain are hallmarks of this disease state. Open surgical revascularization is the mainstay of therapy, but in nonideal surgical candidates endovascular techniques are an acceptable alternative. These endovascular interventions are associated with lower early mortality rates but seem to be less durable in the long term, often requiring repeat intervention to maintain patency.

Finally, MALS results in dynamic compression of the celiac access, and can be confirmed as a diagnosis of exclusion. Laparoscopic or open division of the compressive bands is the treatment of choice. After complete operative lysis, persistent symptoms with residual angiographic findings of stenosis can be treated with endovascular approaches, including angioplasty and stenting. Endovascular therapy alone should not be attempted until external compression has been completely removed by other techniques.

REFERENCES

1. Elliot JW. II. The operative relief of gangrene of intestine due to occlusion of the mesenteric vessels. Ann Surg 1895;21:9–23.
2. Goodman G. Angina abdominus. Am J Med Sci 1918;155:524–8.
3. Dunphy J. Abdominal pain of vascular origin. Am J Med Sci 1936;192:109–13.
4. Shaw RS, Maynard EP 3rd. Acute and chronic thrombosis of the mesenteric arteries associated with malabsorption; a report of two cases successfully treated by thromboendarterectomy. N Engl J Med 1958;258:874–8.
5. Curl JH, Thopson NW, Stanley JC. Median arcuate ligament compression of the celiac and superior mesenteric arteries. Ann Surg 1971;173:314–20.
6. Schwartz LB, Davis RD, Heinle JS, et al. The vascular system. In: Lyerly HK, Gaynor JW, editors. The handbook of surgical intensive care. 3rd edition. St Louis (MO): Mosby Year Book; 1992. p. 287.
7. Ottinger LW, Austen WG. A study of 136 patients with mesenteric infarction. Surg Gynecol Obstet 1967;124:251–61.
8. Smith JS Jr, Patterson LT. Acute mesenteric infarction. Am Surg 1976;42:562–7.
9. Kairaluoma MI, Karkola P, Heikkinen D, et al. Mesenteric infarction. Am J Surg 1977;133:188–93.
10. Hertzer NR, Beven EG, Humphries AW. Acute intestinal ischemia. Am Surg 1978;44:744–9.
11. Sachs SM, Morton JH, Schwartz SI. Acute mesenteric ischemia. Surgery 1982; 92:646–53.
12. Bergan JJ, McCarthy WJ 3rd, Flinn WR, et al. Nontraumatic mesenteric vascular emergencies. J Vasc Surg 1987;5:903–9.
13. Klempnauer J, Grothues F, Bektas H, et al. Long-term results after surgery for acute mesenteric ischemia. Surgery 1997;121:239–43.
14. Stoney RJ, Cunningham CG. Acute mesenteric ischemia. Surgery 1993;114: 489–90.
15. Chang RW, Chang JB, Longo WE. Update in management of mesenteric ischemia. World J Gastroenterol 2006;12:3243–7.
16. Vokurka J, Olejnik J, Jedlicka V, et al. Acute mesenteric ischemia. Hepatogastroenterology 2008;55:1349–52.
17. Visser CA, Kan G, Meltzer RS, et al. Embolic potential of left ventricular thrombus after myocardial infarction: a two-dimensional echocardiographic study of 119 patients. J Am Coll Cardiol 1985;5:1276–80.
18. Cappell MS. Intestinal (mesenteric) vasculopathy. I. Acute superior mesenteric arteriopathy and venopathy. Gastroenterol Clin North Am 1998;27: 783–825, vi.

19. McKinsey JF, Gewertz BL. Acute mesenteric ischemia. Surg Clin North Am 1997;77:307–18.
20. Schutz A, Eichinger W, Breuer M, et al. Acute mesenteric ischemia after open heart surgery. Angiology 1998;49:267–73.
21. Hirsch AT, Haskal ZJ, Hertzer NR, et al. ACC/AHA 2005 Practice Guidelines for the management of patients with peripheral arterial disease (lower extremity, renal, mesenteric, and abdominal aortic): a collaborative report from the American Association for Vascular Surgery/Society for Vascular Surgery, Society for Cardiovascular Angiography and Interventions, Society for Vascular Medicine and Biology, Society of Interventional Radiology, and the ACC/AHA Task Force on Practice Guidelines (Writing Committee to Develop Guidelines for the Management of Patients With Peripheral Arterial Disease): endorsed by the American Association of Cardiovascular and Pulmonary Rehabilitation; National Heart, Lung, and Blood Institute; Society for Vascular Nursing; Trans-Atlantic Inter-Society Consensus; and Vascular Disease Foundation. Circulation 2006;113:e463–654.
22. Endress C, Gray DG, Wollschlaeger G. Bowel ischemia and perforation after cocaine use. AJR Am J Roentgenol 1992;159:73–5.
23. Sudhakar CB, Al-Hakeem M, MacArthur JD, et al. Mesenteric ischemia secondary to cocaine abuse: case reports and literature review. Am J Gastroenterol 1997;92:1053–4.
24. Liu JJ, Ardolf JC. Sumatriptan-associated mesenteric ischemia. Ann Intern Med 2000;132:597.
25. Weil J, Sen Gupta R, Herfarth H. Nonocclusive mesenteric ischemia induced by digitalis. Int J Colorectal Dis 2004;19:277–80.
26. Guglielminotti J, Tremey B, Maury E, et al. Fatal non-occlusive mesenteric infarction following digoxin intoxication. Intensive Care Med 2000;26:829.
27. Siegelman SS, Sprayregen S, Boley SJ. Angiographic diagnosis of mesenteric arterial vasoconstriction. Radiology 1974;112:533–42.
28. Warren S, Eberhard T. Mesenteric venous thrombosis. Surg Gynecol Obstet 1935;141:102–21.
29. Rhee RY, Gloviczki P, Mendonca CT, et al. Mesenteric venous thrombosis: still a lethal disease in the 1990s. J Vasc Surg 1994;20:688–97.
30. Graeber GM, Cafferty PJ, Reardon MJ, et al. Changes in serum total creatine phosphokinase (CPK) and its isoenzymes caused by experimental ligation of the superior mesenteric artery. Ann Surg 1981;193:499–505.
31. Harward TR, Smith S, Seeger JM. Detection of celiac axis and superior mesenteric artery occlusive disease with use of abdominal duplex scanning. J Vasc Surg 1993;17:738–45.
32. McBride KD, Gaines PA. Thrombolysis of a partially occluding superior mesenteric artery thromboembolus by infusion of streptokinase. Cardiovasc Intervent Radiol 1994;17:164–6.
33. Rivitz SM, Geller SC, Hahn C, et al. Treatment of acute mesenteric venous thrombosis with transjugular intramesenteric urokinase infusion. J Vasc Interv Radiol 1995;6:219–23 [discussion: 224–8].
34. Arthurs ZM, Titus J, Bannazadeh M, et al. A comparison of endovascular revascularization with traditional therapy for the treatment of acute mesenteric ischemia. J Vasc Surg 2011;53:698–704 [discussion:704–5].
35. Cortese B, Limbruno U. Acute mesenteric ischemia: primary percutaneous therapy. Catheter Cardiovasc Interv 2010;75:283–5.

36. Schermerhorn ML, Giles KA, Hamdan AD, et al. Mesenteric revascularization: management and outcomes in the United States, 1988-2006. J Vasc Surg 2009;50:341–348.e1.
37. Holdsworth RJ, Raza Z, Naidu S, et al. Mesenteric revascularisation for acute-on-chronic intestinal ischaemia. Postgrad Med J 1997;73:642–4.
38. Pisimisis GT, Oderich GS. Technique of hybrid retrograde superior mesenteric artery stent placement for acute-on-chronic mesenteric ischemia. Ann Vasc Surg 2011;25:132.e7–11.
39. Mitsuyoshi A, Obama K, Shinkura N, et al. Survival in nonocclusive mesenteric ischemia: early diagnosis by multidetector row computed tomography and early treatment with continuous intravenous high-dose prostaglandin E(1). Ann Surg 2007;246:229–35.
40. Habboushe F, Wallace HW, Nusbaum M, et al. Nonocclusive mesenteric vascular insufficiency. Ann Surg 1974;180:819–22.
41. Lopera JE, Correa G, Brazzini A, et al. Percutaneous transhepatic treatment of symptomatic mesenteric venous thrombosis. J Vasc Surg 2002;36:1058–61.
42. Kim HS, Patra A, Khan J, et al. Transhepatic catheter-directed thrombectomy and thrombolysis of acute superior mesenteric venous thrombosis. J Vasc Interv Radiol 2005;16:1685–91.
43. Zhou W, Choi L, Lin PH, et al. Percutaneous transhepatic thrombectomy and pharmacologic thrombolysis of mesenteric venous thrombosis. Vascular 2007; 15:41–5.
44. Grisham A, Lohr J, Guenther JM, et al. Deciphering mesenteric venous thrombosis: imaging and treatment. Vasc Endovascular Surg 2005;39:473–9.
45. Derrick JR, Pollard HS, Moore RM. The pattern of arteriosclerotic narrowing of the celiac and superior mesenteric arteries. Ann Surg 1959;149:684–9.
46. Reiner L, Jimenez FA, Rodriguez FL. Atherosclerosis in the mesenteric circulation. Observations and correlations with aortic and coronary atherosclerosis. Am Heart J 1963;66:200–9.
47. Moneta GL, Lee RW, Yeager RA, et al. Mesenteric duplex scanning: a blinded prospective study. J Vasc Surg 1993;17:79–84 [discussion: 85–6].
48. Gentile AT, Moneta GL, Lee RW, et al. Usefulness of fasting and postprandial duplex ultrasound examinations for predicting high-grade superior mesenteric artery stenosis. Am J Surg 1995;169:476–9.
49. Farber MA, Carlin RE, Marston WA, et al. Distal thoracic aorta as inflow for the treatment of chronic mesenteric ischemia. J Vasc Surg 2001;33:281–7 [discussion: 287–8].
50. Huber TS, Lee WA. Mesenteric vascular disease: chronic ischemia. In: Cronenwett JL, Johnston W, editors. Rutherford's vascular surgery. 7th edition. Philadelphia: Saunders/Elsevier; 2010. p. 2273–88.
51. Mell MW, Acher CW, Hoch JR, et al. Outcomes after endarterectomy for chronic mesenteric ischemia. J Vasc Surg 2008;48:1132–8.
52. Matsumoto AH, Angle JF, Spinosa DJ, et al. Percutaneous transluminal angioplasty and stenting in the treatment of chronic mesenteric ischemia: results and longterm followup. J Am Coll Surg 2002;194:S22–31.
53. Tallarita T, Oderich GS, Macedo TA, et al. Reinterventions for stent restenosis in patients treated for atherosclerotic mesenteric artery disease. J Vasc Surg 2011; 54:1422–1429.e1.
54. Kasirajan K, O'Hara PJ, Gray BH, et al. Chronic mesenteric ischemia: open surgery versus percutaneous angioplasty and stenting. J Vasc Surg 2001;33:63–71.

55. Brown DJ, Schermerhorn ML, Powell RJ, et al. Mesenteric stenting for chronic mesenteric ischemia. J Vasc Surg 2005;42:268–74.

56. Lindner HH, Kemprud E. A clinicoanatomical study of the arcuate ligament of the diaphragm. Arch Surg 1971;103:600–5.

57. Aschenbach R, Basche S, Vogl TJ. Compression of the celiac trunk caused by median arcuate ligament in children and adolescent subjects: evaluation with contrast-enhanced MR angiography and comparison with Doppler US evaluation. J Vasc Interv Radiol 2011;22:556–61.

58. Gloviczki P, Duncan AA. Treatment of celiac artery compression syndrome: does it really exist? Perspect Vasc Surg Endovasc Ther 2007;19:259–63.

59. Kohn GP, Bitar RS, Farber MA, et al. Treatment options and outcomes for celiac artery compression syndrome. Surg Innov 2011;18:338–43.

60. Tulloch AW, Jimenez JC, Lawrence PF, et al. Laparoscopic versus open celiac ganglionectomy in patients with median arcuate ligament syndrome. J Vasc Surg 2010;52:1283–9.

61. Baccari P, Civilini E, Dordoni L, et al. Celiac artery compression syndrome managed by laparoscopy. J Vasc Surg 2009;50:134–9.

62. Roseborough GS. Laparoscopic management of celiac artery compression syndrome. J Vasc Surg 2009;50:124–33.

63. van Petersen AS, Vriens BH, Huisman AB, et al. Retroperitoneal endoscopic release in the management of celiac artery compression syndrome. J Vasc Surg 2009;50:140–7.

Modern Advances in Vascular Trauma

Rachael A. Callcut, MD, MSPH[a], Matthew W. Mell, MD, MS[b],*

KEYWORDS

- Blunt thoracic aortic injury • Blunt cerebrovascular injury • Peripheral vascular injury
- Shunts • Tourniquets

KEY POINTS

- Early diagnosis and intervention are paramount for improving the likelihood of a favorable outcome for traumatic vascular injuries.
- As technology has rapidly diversified, the diagnostic and therapeutic approaches available for vascular injuries have evolved.
- Mortality and morbidity from vascular injury have declined over the last decade.
- The use of vascular shunts and tourniquets has become standard of care in military medicine.

INTRODUCTION

Vascular trauma is a major cause of significant morbidity and mortality with the highest rates of death from thoracic aortic transections and major abdominal venous injuries. Risk factors, diagnosis, and management considerations vary depending on the vessel injured. However, in general, early diagnosis and intervention are paramount for improving the likelihood of a favorable outcome.

Types of injuries range from subtle intimal arterial dissections to complete vascular disruption (**Box 1, Fig. 1**).[1,2] Isolated vascular injury is more common with penetrating mechanisms and prognosis is generally more favorable in these cases. In contrast, vascular trauma from blunt mechanisms is often found in patients with complex multisystem injuries, which can result in both delays in diagnosis and competing management principles (ie, blunt cerebrovascular injury and traumatic brain injury [TBI]).

Disclosures: Neither author has any relevant disclosures.
[a] Department of Surgery, San Francisco General Hospital, University of California-San Francisco (UCSF), San Francisco, CA, USA; [b] Division of Vascular Surgery, Department of Surgery, Stanford University School of Medicine, 300 Pasteur Drive, Suite H3600, Stanford, CA 94305-5642, USA
* Corresponding author.
E-mail address: mwmell@stanford.edu

Surg Clin N Am 93 (2013) 941–961
http://dx.doi.org/10.1016/j.suc.2013.04.010
0039-6109/13/$ – see front matter © 2013 Elsevier Inc. All rights reserved.

surgical.theclinics.com

| **Box 1** |
| **Types of vascular injury** |
| Intimal disruption or flap |
| Subintimal or intramural hematomas |
| Lacerations |
| Contusions (with or without thrombosis) |
| Focal wall defects with pseudoaneurysms or hemorrhage |
| Transections (complete or partial) |
| External compression (from a large hematoma) |
| Vasospasm |

As technology has rapidly diversified, the diagnostic and therapeutic approaches available for vascular injuries have evolved. The state of the art in blunt cerebrovascular trauma, blunt aortic injury, peripheral vascular trauma, and damage control techniques for vascular surgery are detailed in this article.

BLUNT CEREBROVASCULAR INJURY

The reported incidence of blunt cerebrovascular injury (BCVI) is variable between 0.1% and 2% of all traumas with most centers reporting rates around 1%.[3–6] The frequency of diagnosis seems proportional to the aggressiveness of screening.[3,4,7–10] Injury to the carotid and vertebral arteries is uncommon; however, when an injury occurs, poor outcomes are prevalent.[11,12] Overall, mortality is generally reported to be

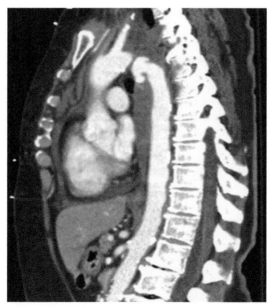

Fig. 1. Example of aortic injury. This computed tomography (CT) angiogram shows an aortic transection in a 50-year-old woman following a high-speed motor vehicle collision. Aortic transections are an example of significant arterial trauma.

20% to 30% and, for survivors, permanent neurologic impairment typically results from BCVI-related strokes.[4–6] A minority of BCVIs have overt signs or symptoms (**Box 2**) of injury. For those presenting with obvious worrisome signs or symptoms, a rapid assessment including angiography should be undertaken.[3,11,13]

Most (80%) injuries are asymptomatic at the time of initial trauma evaluation.[5] In the past, this has led to frequent delays in diagnosis, and stroke rates approach 40% to 60% without treatment.[4,5,8,9,14] The timing of strokes in initially asymptomatic patients ranges from a few hours to a week, with most BCVI strokes occurring at 12 to 72 hours.[5,12] In an effort to mitigate stroke risk, prediction algorithms have been developed to allow early identification of which asymptomatic patients have the highest risk for BCVI.[9,13,15]

In those who are asymptomatic, a high index of suspicion based on mechanism, associated injuries, and clinical presentation guides decision for screening. The Western Trauma Association (WTA) and the Eastern Association for the Surgery of Trauma (EAST) have adopted uniform criteria for screening for adults and children.[9,13,16] Screening with a minimal 16-slice computed tomography (CT) angiogram[9,17,18] is recommended in asymptomatic patients with the following risk factors[8,9,13]:

- Significant cervical hyperextension, rotation, or hyperflexion
- Le Fort II or III midface fractures
- Basilar skull fracture through the carotid canal
- Severe TBI (Glasgow Coma Scale <6) or associated with diffuse axonal injury
- Any C1 to C3 vertebral fracture
- C4 to C7 transverse foramen or vertebral body fracture
- Near hanging with associated anoxic injury
- Cervical seat belt sign associated with significant pain, swelling, or altered mental status
- High-risk mechanism with normal initial head CT and altered mental status not explained by other factors (eg, intoxication)

Recent work by Burlew and colleagues[15] advocated for expansion of these criteria to include additional associated injuries given that, in a 14-year database study, up to 20% of patients were not captured by the traditional screening criteria. Most of these missed patients were asymptomatic at the time of initial presentation. The expanded criteria include screening for patients with mandible fractures, complex skull fractures, TBI with associated thoracic injury, scalp degloving injury, and associated thoracic vascular injury.[15]

Box 2
Overt signs or symptoms of BCVI

Arterial hemorrhage from oropharynx, nasopharynx, or neck

Expanding cervical hematoma

New cervical bruit in patients less than 50 years old

Focal neurologic deficit (transient ischemic attack, hemiparesis, Horner syndrome, vertebral-basilar symptoms)

Asymmetric pupillary defect (small nonreactive pupil)

Neurologic deficit unexplained by initial imaging

Stroke on initial radiographic imaging

Despite general acceptance of the less inclusive EAST and WTA recommendations, screening remains controversial.[19] The incidence of BCVI has increased, but outcome has not universally improved, likely because of limitations in the ability to treat injury once it is discovered.[4,12] For example, even in patients aggressively screened for injury, approximately 25% to 40% have a concomitant hemorrhagic injury that has traditionally been considered a contraindication to therapy.[4,12,20] These competing injuries typically include TBIs and spinal cord injury (SCI) or traumatic neurologic injuries (TNI).

There is a general reluctance of neurosurgeons and spine surgeons to risk progression of TNI, especially cervical SCI or major intracranial bleeds. Thus, timing to initiation of treatment of the BCVI with concomitant TNI is largely variable and reflects individual practitioner preferences.[4] It is important to recognize that the perceived risk of worsening of TNI with pharmacologic therapy for BCVI is based largely on anecdotal cases and not on formal clinical studies. Most of the reported literature lacks a comparison group and this has contributed to a culture in which the presumption is that treatment of BCVI carries a higher risk of conversion of a hemorrhagic TNI to a worsening injury than the stroke risk of leaving patients unprotected from the BCVI.[4]

The first study to provide significant insight into whether treatment is safe and effective in concomitant TNI and BCVI was recently reported. An observational study followed cohort of 77 consecutive patients with concomitant TNI and at least 1 BCVI (115 BCVIs total) to determine timing of treatment, risk of TNI progression, and outcome.[4] This study represents the first direct comparison between equivalent patient populations with both BCVI and TNI and suggests that early initiation of therapy following the first 24 hours after injury is safe. Treatment was initiated on a case-by-case basis after a stable head CT was obtained in the first 24 hours of care for patients with TBI and a stable clinical examination for patients with SCI. Overall, 74% of the patients in the cohort were treated with either aspirin or therapeutic heparin.[4] The treated and untreated groups were equivalent with regard to important characteristics factoring into the decision to treat, including need for craniotomy or spine surgery and severity of injury.

In this patient cohort, the risk of worsening hemorrhagic injury in patients with TBI was equivalent in those treated and untreated for the BCVI, and no patients with SCI experienced any clinical deterioration from treatment.[4] The risk of progression was also independent of the type of pharmacologic therapy exposure (therapeutic heparin or aspirin). Benefit exceeded risk with 44% of patient deaths directly attributed to a potentially preventable BCVI-related stroke and all of the potential preventable stroke-related deaths were in the untreated group.[4] In contrast, no patients died as a result of worsening TBI caused by the initiation of BCVI pharmacologic treatment. Treatment was also effective, with failure to initiate treatment the most significant stroke predictor (adjusted odds ratio 4.4, 95% confidence interval 3.0–6.5, $P<.0001$).[4]

These findings, coupled with the increasing nontrauma literature in neurosurgery, suggest that earlier treatment of BCVI in this patient population is likely safe.[4,21–23] For example, the safety and early reinitiation of therapeutic anticoagulant therapy in patients with spontaneous intracranial hemorrhage in high-risk conditions (ie, mechanical heart valves) has also recently been investigated. The rebleed rate with therapeutic anticoagulation was small even when initiated within 2 days of the initial hemorrhage.[4,23]

However, it is likely that, despite the impressive results in the recent work, without a prospective, randomized trial of aspirin versus therapeutic heparin (which would be difficult to perform), the selection of agents and timing of BCVI treatment in concomitant TNI will remain provider dependent. Individual practitioner comfort with the choice of either agent is likely to remain variable despite theoretic arguments that could be made for one agent rather than the other.[4] Some might prefer intravenous heparin because it can be titrated and rapidly reversed if brain injury worsens,[13,24] whereas others may prefer aspirin because they fear the risk of overanticoagulation that can occur with the use of heparin.[4,5,12]

In patients without concomitant TNI, the decision to treat is less controversial, but debate continues regarding optimal treatment agent and duration of therapy. In general, BCVI treatment is guided by the grade of injury (**Box 3**).[13,25,26] In 2010, EAST published a systematic review of treatment recommendations for treatment by grade.[9] No level 1 recommendation could be made from the available data and the only level 2 recommendations (defined as reasonably justifiable by available scientific evidence and strongly supported by expert opinion) was that grade I or II injuries should be treated with pharmacotherapy.[9]

No clear data exist to recommend one therapy rather than another, and no prospective, randomized studies have examined the equipoise between aspirin and heparin.[9] Some experts continue to advocate using therapeutic heparin as the initial treatment of BCVI with no contraindication for heparinization because of an early study by Biffl and colleagues[27] suggesting improved outcome.[9] However, heparinization has not clearly been more beneficial in follow-up studies.[9] Some also prefer treating with heparin in those with the highest risk of bleeding from associated intra-abdominal or intrathoracic injury because of heparin's reversibility.[4–6] If heparin is used, EAST recommends (level 3 recommendation) starting heparin with no bolus and targeting a partial thromboplastin time (PTT) that is 1.5 to 2.0 times normal.[9] Some, but not all, advocate for no pharmacologic therapy in grade IV injuries because risk of stroke is theoretically fixed at the time of injury. No data exist to recommend duration of therapy for BCVI.

Operative and endovascular repair are generally reserved for symptomatic injury (transient ischemic attacks without frank stroke), asymptomatic high-risk injuries for stroke (ie, large intimal flap), worsening injury despite pharmacologic therapy, and rapidly expanding neck hematomas. If lesions are amenable to open repair, it is preferred to stent therapy. Although initially promising, routine stent therapy for grade III injuries (pseudoaneurysms) has fallen out of favor because of worse outcomes compared with pharmacologic therapy alone.[28] Angiography performed 7 days after injury is generally recommended to assess healing or progression for grade I to III injuries.[13,29]

BLUNT THORACIC AORTIC INJURY

Blunt thoracic aortic injury (TAI) is an uncommon, but extremely serious, injury. Historical studies using autopsy data have estimated that TAI is associated with less than

---

Box 3
Denver Grading Scale of BCVI

- Grade I: intimal irregularity with less than 25% narrowing

- Grade II: dissection or intramural hematoma with greater than 25% narrowing

- Grade III: pseudoaneurysm

- Grade IV: occlusion

- Grade V: transection with extravasation

From Biffl WL, Moore EE, Offner PJ, et al. Blunt carotid arterial injuries: implications of a new grading scale. J Trauma 1999;47(5):845–53.

1% of all major traumas, but it has an exceedingly high mortality (75%–90%).[30–33] Most the deaths from TAI occur at the time of initial injury.[33–36] For those who reach the hospital alive, timely diagnosis is imperative to improve likelihood of a favorable outcome.[37] The major risk factor for injury is a rapid deceleration mechanism that leads to a tear of the aortic isthmus just distal to the left subclavian artery.[33] As with BCVI, isolated injuries of the thoracic aorta are rare and most patients are severely injured with complex multisystem injuries.[33,37–39]

Chest radiographs (CXR) have traditionally been recommended as a good initial screening test[37]; however, recent studies have shown that a significant TAI can occur in the presence of a normal study (**Fig. 2**).[30] If a patient has an abnormal CXR consistent with TAI (**Box 4**),[37] CT angiography (CTA) of the chest should urgently be performed. When the study is normal, the decision to proceed with CTA should be considered in the context of the overall patient condition, associated injuries (**Box 5**),[31,35,39–41] and symptoms. However, many patients with TAI present with no symptoms and minimal to no signs of injury, thus underscoring the importance of a high index of suspicion based on mechanism.[37]

Given the increasing focus on radiation exposure for patients with trauma, routine screening of all patients for TAI with CTA is impractical. However, given that there are no highly sensitive tests available, liberal use of CTA for screening patients who are severely injured with high-risk mechanisms has been advocated. Patients with symptoms (substernal chest pain or significant thoracic back pain) or signs (thoracic seatbelt sign, pseudocoarctation, pulse deficit, new cardiac murmur, interscapular murmur)[37] of potential TAI should undergo urgent CTA of the chest. Although invasive contrast arterography historically has been considered the gold standard for diagnosis of TAI, it has largely been replaced by the use of CTA because of the ease of obtaining CTA and its comparable sensitivity and specificity.[30,37,39] Other imaging modalities including transesophageal echocardiography (TEE) and magnetic resonance imaging are rarely used for initial screening.[39] TEE is generally reserved for unstable patients who cannot undergo CTA.[37]

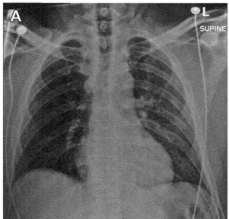
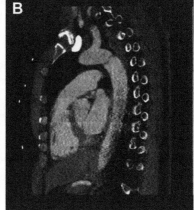

Fig. 2. Unremarkable chest radiograph in a patient with major aortic injury. Chest radiographs do not reliably exclude major aortic injury, as shown in this example. This chest radiograph is from a 45-year-old man involved in a head-on motorcycle collision and the aorta is unremarkable (*A*). At the time of initial evaluation, CT angiography (CTA) was obtained of his chest secondary to mechanism and he was found to have an aortic transection (*B*).

Box 4
CXR findings suggestive of blunt TAI

Widen mediastinum

Indistinct aortic knob

Massive hemothorax

Left mainstem bronchus displacement

Tracheal deviation to the right

Nasogastric tube deviation to the right

Left apical cap

With the increasing popularity of CTA evaluation following major trauma mechanisms, subtle injuries of the aorta termed minimal aortic injury have increased the overall incidence of TAI. Minimal injury has no uniformly accepted definition or management.[42] In an effort to standardize the approach to TAI, the Society of Vascular Surgery (SVS) recently suggested that intimal or periadventitial defects represent minimal aortic injury that initially can be managed nonoperatively.[33] Hallmarks of nonoperative management include rapid impulse and blood pressure control. Impulse control is achieved with beta-blockade and blood pressure control usually with nitroprusside or nitroglycerine infusions initially.[37,43–45] The optimum heart rate and blood pressure goals are based on clinical judgment rather than substantial clinical evidence; however, generally a heart rate less than 80 beats per minute and systolic blood pressure less than 100 to 120 mm Hg have been advocated.[45]

Recent studies have been published justifying the initial nonoperative management of minimal aortic injury given that, in short-term follow-up, few patients went on to require operative therapy because of progression of injury. Most studies have estimated the rate of progression to operative therapy to be 10% to 11%.[45,46] In contrast, other studies have shown a high rate (50%) of progression to pseudoaneurysm formation in follow-up.[47] The studies have used varying definitions of minimal injury, which likely contributes to the variability in outcome. All patients with minimal aortic injury

---

Box 5
Injuries associated with blunt TAI

Severe traumatic brain injury

Other blunt thoracic trauma

   Multiple rib fractures/flail chest

   Sternal fracture

   Pulmonary contusion

   Cardiac contusion

   Diaphragmatic injury

Major intra-abdominal solid organ injury

Major long bone extremity fracture

Significant pelvic fractures

who do not undergo repair should have repeat imaging to assess for healing or progression. The optimum time frame for initial follow-up is poorly defined, with imaging generally performed at 1 to 8 weeks after injury.

Several investigators have attempted to develop grading criteria of injuries.[33,48] Type I (intimal tears) represent minimal aortic injury (detailed earlier). All other grades of injury according to the SVS recommendations should be considered for operative intervention. Type II injuries are intramural hematomas, type III represent pseudoaneurysms, and type IV are various types of rupture defined as free rupture, contained rupture, or periaortic hematomas. The SVS provides a level 2, class C recommendation that repair be considered within the first 24 hours for patients stable enough to undergo repair.[33] If patients cannot have immediate repair because of concomitant injury, "repair [should occur] immediately after other [life threatening] injuries have been treated."[33] This recommendation is in contrast with the most recent American Association for the Surgery of Trauma (AAST) multicenter outcome study, which suggested a mortality benefit in stable patients repaired after the first 24 hours of care.[49]

For patients requiring operative repair, survival has improved as endovascular treatment has largely supplanted open repair in most major trauma centers (**Fig. 3**). In the latest AAST multicenter trial (known as AAST 2007) published in 2009, nearly two-thirds of all injuries were repaired with an endovascular technique.[39,49] This is in contrast with the 1997 study by the same group in which 100% were repaired open.[35] The emergence of endovascular repair as the preferred approach is caused by the marked reported reduction in mortality and major morbidity including spinal

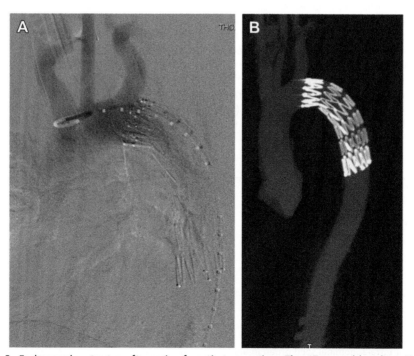

Fig. 3. Endovascular stent graft repair of aortic transection. The 45-year-old male patient underwent endovascular repair of his aortic transection. The intraoperative stent placement is shown (*A*). One month follow-up CTA shows appropriate graft placement without migration or endoleak (*B*).

cord ischemia and perioperative strokes. Some studies have suggested a reduction of mortality as high as 35% to 45% with endovascular repair.[33,39,49–51] The mortality and major morbidity rates with open repair have traditionally been variable, reflecting differences in center experience levels with these complex repairs. Large national databases have estimated that modern-day mortalities range from 15% to 20%, paraplegia rates 2% to 10%, and stroke rates 4% to 6% with open repair.[33,35,50] However, high-volume single-center studies and 1 study based on the National Inpatient Sample have reported lower rates that approach the rates of endovascular repair.[32,34,52,53] In a recent meta-analysis and the 2007 AAST study, endovascular repair had a mortality of 8% to 13%, a 0% to 3% paraplegia rate, and less than 1% risk of stroke.[39,49,50,54]

Initial reluctance with adopting endovascular repair was caused by several factors including graft limitations, young demographic of the typical trauma patient, and lack of long-term follow-up data. Graft limitations have been improved with the development of specific aortic grafts for aortic injury and several types are now commercially available. These grafts are made in smaller aortic diameters and with conforming technology necessary to accommodate the aortic size and shape of young patients with trauma.[30] Despite initial improved survival, long-term survival has not been different between open and endovascular techniques and reintervention rate has been higher for the endovascular repairs.[33] In the recent AAST study, early graft-related complications increased from 0.5% in 1997 to more than 18% in 2007.[39,49]

Younger patients with trauma still present management challenges because long-term data on outcome are limited. Stent migration and late endoleak remain potential concerns because the aorta is known to increase in size over the lifetime of patients.[30,53] Follow-up data on more than 600 procedures were recently reported by Hoffer and colleagues[51] and showed an early endoleak rate of 4.2% and a late endoleak rate of 0.9%. Although low complication rates were reported, 1 in 10 deaths were attributed to early endoleak in the study.[51] Given the small, but measurable, risk of late complications, patients must also be followed for a lengthy period of time, which presents unique challenges in young patients with trauma who are known to have particularly high loss to follow-up.

There are important ethical considerations in placing a graft in a potentially unreliable patient. In addition, lifetime radiation exposure and imaging costs are substantial factors in young patients. Questions remain as to the length of follow-up and frequency with which grafts should be evaluated in the youngest patients. Despite these concerns and limitations, endovascular repair is now generally the accepted standard of care for injuries amenable to this operative approach.[33]

PERIPHERAL ARTERIAL INJURIES

Peripheral arterial injuries (PAIs) are the most common vascular injuries encountered in patients with trauma. Although BCVI and blunt TAI are rarer and more lethal, PAIs account for approximately 40% to 70% of all vascular injuries and death is uncommon in the civilian population.[1,55] Despite lower associated direct mortality from PAI, the potential for significant morbidity is high, especially when lower extremity vessels are involved.[56,57] In the past, limb loss was substantial for lower extremity blunt injuries, ranging between 28% and 71%.[58,59] Given advances in diagnosis, operative technique, damage control options, and better resuscitation, the modern-day amputation rates have decreased to 6.5% to 20% for blunt lower extremity injuries and 0.4% to 4% for penetrating injuries.[1,58] Limb loss is less common in the upper extremity[60,61] because there is a lower likelihood of delayed recognition.

Delay in diagnosis or time to revascularization are the most critical factors in poor outcome[1,58] and delays typically occur when evaluation or management is complicated by other life-threatening injuries.[56] Delay in diagnosis frequently occurs when signs of injury are present and go unrecognized.[56,58] A complete neurovascular physical examination is mandated in all patients with significant multisystem or extremity trauma, including a clear documentation of the distal pulse examination.

For patients who present with significant soft tissue loss with likely injury, direct emergent operative exploration of the involved vessel should be performed.[56] For those with less extensive soft tissue loss, if any hard signs of injury are found (**Box 6**),[1,2,58,62] they should rapidly be transported to the operating room.[56,58,62,63] In hemodynamically stable patients with absent pulses in the upper extremity, nearly all have an injury requiring repair and, in the case of absent lower extremity pulses, most need repair. Vasospasm is more common in the lower extremity and is often present when there is an abnormal pulse examination but no definitive injury is found in the operating room.[64] Definitive repair should be the goal for stable patients with injury and damage control techniques (shunt insertion) should be used in unstable multi-injured patients.

If there is presence of a pulse but the examination is asymmetric or the pulse waxes/wanes, an ankle-brachial index (ABI) should be performed. If the ABI is abnormal (<0.9 in a healthy patient or difference of >0.1 in patients with preexisting vascular disease[1,56]), further imaging is warranted.[1,56,63] For patients with one or more soft signs (**Box 7**)[1,2,62] in conjunction with an associated high-risk orthopedic injury (**Box 8**), imaging should also be pursued.[63] Routine vascular imaging is no longer recommended for patients with isolated posterior knee dislocations with normal pulse examinations.[56,64,65] When pulses are absent and an associated fracture-dislocation is present, the fracture should be reduced and the pulse examination repeated.[66] Studies have estimated the risk of an arterial injury to be as low as 3% with a single soft sign to as high as 25% with multiple findings present.[1,2,62]

Invasive arteriography has traditionally been the gold standard when imaging is warranted and data support improved outcome secondary to reduction in time to revascularization when the arteriography is performed in the operating room.[56] Patients who require another emergent operative procedure, are unstable with high-risk associated orthopedic injuries, those with a high pretest probability of arterial injury (for example, multiple soft signs), or those in whom hard signs are present but better localization of the injury is necessary (ie, multiple gunshot wounds to a single extremity) should also go directly to the operating room for intraoperative arteriography.[1,56]

With the emergence and refinement of noninvasive CTA techniques for extremity evaluation, those in whom there is a lower index of suspicion of injury but an abnormal pulse examination, multidetector row helical (minimum 16 slice, 64 slice preferred)

Box 6
Hard signs of arterial extremity trauma

No distal pulse

Active, external bleeding

Rapidly expanding contained hematoma

Signs of distal ischemia (5 Ps: pallor, paresthesias, pain, paralysis, poikilothermia)

Palpable thrill or audible bruit over the suspected area of injury

---

Box 7
Soft signs of arterial extremity trauma

Delayed capillary refill

Abnormal pulse examination

    Waxing or waning pulse

    Pulse present but diminished compared with contralateral extremity

    ABI of less than 0.9 in otherwise healthy young patient

    ABI difference of greater than 0.1 in patients suspected of underlying vascular disease

Neurologic deficit in a nerve that travels with known artery

Small, nonexpanding hematoma over a vascular distribution

History of arterial bleeding at scene or in transport

Wound immediately proximal to vascular distribution

CTA has been shown to have equal sensitivity and specificity for diagnosis compared with invasive arteriography.[1,63,67,68] Extremity diagnostic usefulness is diminished in cases in which there are multiple retained foreign metallic bodies next to the vessels of interest or in cases of external compression of a vessel from hematoma.[1] If patients have a normal pulse examination associated with a single soft sign, the need for further imaging is controversial. Recently published practice guidelines from the WTA advocate for clinical observation in these cases.[1]

Although vascular injuries, especially in cases of penetrating trauma, can occur in isolation, they are often present in patients with severely compromised extremities (**Fig. 4**). Extensive soft tissue loss or bony involvement complicates the decision to attempt vascular repair and is a major factor in the probability of long-term success.[58] The Mangled Extremity Severity Score (MESS)[69] was originally developed as a guide for practitioners when faced with a significantly injured extremity. Patients with MESS scores of 8 or higher were traditionally considered nonsalvagable.[56]

This definitive cut-off has been recently challenged in the literature, in which functional limb salvage rates of greater than 50% were achieved with rapid revascularization (<5 hours after injury) and liberal use of fasciotomy in patients with a MESS greater than or equal to 8.[56] Although a high MESS is associated with a 10-fold greater risk of amputation,[56] salvage is still possible and an initial attempt at limb salvage has been found to be cost-effective.[70] Selective salvage should be attempted in patients with soft tissue and bony injury amenable to possible repair and who are otherwise hemodynamically stable enough to tolerate repair.[71] Repair should not be attempted in cases in which there is major nerve damage rendering the limb paralyzed. For those who are unstable from complex multisystem injuries, life prevails over limb.

Box 8
High-risk orthopedic injuries associated with vascular arterial injury

Posterior knee dislocation	Popliteal artery injury
Tibial plateau fracture	Popliteal artery injury
Femur fracture	Superficial femoral artery injury
Shoulder dislocation	Axillary artery injury
Supracondylar humerus fracture	Brachial artery injury

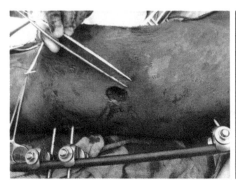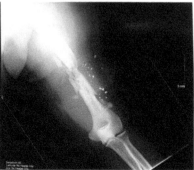

Fig. 4. Penetrating injury to the upper extremity. Extremity vascular injuries are often associated with major skeletal and soft tissue injury. The penetrating wound in the upper extremity of this patient is associated with significant bony destruction. (*Courtesy of* Timothy Pritts, MD, PhD, and Warren Dorlac, MD, Cincinnati, OH.)

Functional outcome is the primary objective in peripheral arterial trauma. Multiple modifiable factors contribute to a good recovery with the most significant predictor being the warm ischemia time.[58,71] Liberal usage of fasciotomies has also contributed to lower amputation rates[58,71] and fasciotomies should be a prophylactic maneuver.[58,72] The development of compartment syndrome in the already compromised extremity is particularly problematic[73] and leads to greater risk of amputation and mortality.[74] Fasciotomies should be considered in all severely injured extremities (MESS≥8), those in whom repair is not complete within 6 hours of injury, those requiring significant resuscitation or transfusion, or those with a high risk of development of compartment syndrome secondary to orthopedic fractures including complex open fractures.[2,56,58,74]

In addition to the potential modifiable risk factors discussed earlier, several nonmodifiable risk factors contribute to poor outcome. The presence of an associate venous injury in the same limb, extensive soft tissue loss leading to infection, extensive bony injury requiring complex bony reconstruction, delayed presentation to the hospital, preexisting vascular disease, major nerve injury, and the peripheral artery injury all are major factors.[1,58,62,73] Popliteal injuries occur in less than 0.2% of all traumas; however, they have the highest risk of limb loss of any peripheral arterial injury.[56,58]

For the multi-injured patient, the presence of prolonged shock caused by other causes of hemorrhage is particularly problematic. Melton and colleagues[75] showed that limb salvage was greater in patients who had no factors that precluded early initiation of anticoagulation. For that reason, early treatment with heparin or aspirin is often initiated unless contraindicated.[58,73] Thrombosis of repair is catastrophic and patients should be carefully observed in a unit where expeditious recognition of a change in pulse examination is possible.

Although open repair remains the standard of care (**Box 9**),[56,58,62] there is a growing interest in the application of less invasive options for treatment of select injuries. The WTA advocates for endovascular embolization of isolated vascular injuries in which the limb is not threatened.[1] For example, embolization is an option with a viable foot if there is a pseudoaneurysm, extravasation, or arteriovenous fistula in an isolated lower extremity vessel such as the anterior tibial or tibioperoneal system. In addition, if a single vessel below the trifurcation is injured with a viable foot, repair is not required.

Box 9
Principles of peripheral vascular arterial repair

1. Prompt recognition of injury and transport to the operating room.

2. Administer preoperative antibiotics against gram-positive organisms at a minimum. If gross contamination of the wound, broad-spectrum antibiotics should be used.

3. Prep and drape widely. Vein graft is often needed from the contralateral uninjured limb.

4. Timing of repair versus orthopedic stabilization is controversial. In general, blood flow should be restored first or a shunt inserted if repair is to follow a lengthy orthopedic intervention.

5. Achieve proximal and distal control before exploring hematomas.

6. Use systemic heparin if it is not contraindicated.

7. Debride back to healthy tissue on the injured vessel. Primary anastomosis is preferred if it is possible without tension, especially in contaminated wounds. If loss of length is present, vein graft is preferred rather than synthetic grafts.

8. Vein grafts traditionally were taken from contralateral limbs, but this is not always necessary. Outcomes in recent studies have been equivalent.

9. Liberal use of fasciotomy is the standard of care.

10. Cover exposed vessels in complex soft tissue loss immediately.

11. Considered completion arteriography and always check pulses before leaving the operating room.

For patients with small nonocclusive arterial injuries on CTA or invasive arteriography with no symptoms (no ischemia) amenable to systemic heparinization, nonoperative repair has been successful.[58]

DAMAGE CONTROL STRATEGIES IN VASCULAR EXTREMITY TRAUMA

The use of temporary vascular shunts and tourniquets in the treatment of limb-threatening or life-threatening arterial injuries has gained renewed interest because of lessons learned in the Iraq and Afghanistan conflicts. Neither is a new concept. Shunts were first described for use in extremity trauma in the early 1970s.[76] Use in civilian trauma centers was infrequent over the last 3 decades. However, for military patients injured in austere environments with longer transport times to definitive care, shunts have proved invaluable for limb and life salvage.

Major extremity injury has been one of the most frequent injuries in the recent military conflicts because of improvised explosive devices (IEDs) and accounts for up to 75% of all combat injuries.[77,78] Military research has suggested improved outcomes with shunts because of the increased time available to achieve a definitive repair, and rates of early limb salvage have been reported to be as high as 95% to 100%.[79–81] Long-term lower extremity amputation- free rates have approached 79% to 85%.[79,82]

Shunts have been particularly valuable in patients with complex multisystem injury or those with complex extremity injuries (**Fig. 5**).[83] Shunt placement in severely injured patients helps preserve limb salvage opportunities while allowing for the rewarming and resuscitation necessary for treatment of concomitant life-threatening injuries.[61] Routine shunting has become the standard of care in the military, especially in

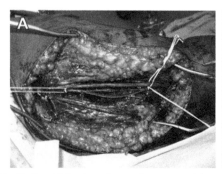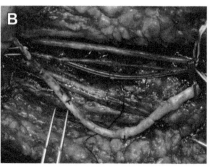

Fig. 5. Brachial artery shunt placement. A brachial artery shunt was placed into the vessel to allow for orthopedic fixation (*A*). Following orthopedic external fixation and soft tissue debridement, a reverse saphenous vein graft was placed (*B*). (*Courtesy of* Timothy Pritts, MD, PhD, and Warren Dorlac, MD, Cincinnati, OH.)

complex contaminated wounds.[76,84] Results have also been favorable even when systemic heparinization is not possible.[85] Complications from the shunts have been rare.[82] The use of shunts in civilian patients with trauma remains generally confined to either situations in which other life-threatening injuries preclude immediate definitive operative vascular repair, for limb replantation, or for complex orthopedic stabilization before vascular repair.[61,71]

In combat casualty care, loss of life from exsanguinating extremity trauma historically has accounted for nearly 10% of preventable deaths.[86] Since 2004, tourniquets have been issued to all military personnel. Battlefield tourniquet usage has saved considerable lives, especially when applied before the development of shock.[87] In comparison, survival was dismal for those who met indications for tourniquet placement but did not have it applied.[87]

Tourniquets have been feared in the civilian world because of concern that application would lead to nerve and muscle injury.[87] In general, tourniquet time should be minimized and ideally not exceed 2 hours.[78] In the military, the risk of complications was less than 2%.[86] In a large study of 862 tourniquet applications, no limbs were lost as a result of the tourniquet.[88] The usefulness for civilian use (**Box 10**) is still being defined, but enthusiasm for tourniquets has been renewed.[1,78]

Box 10
Principles of proper tourniquet application

1. Set at the lowest effective pressure to stop hemorrhage

2. Minimize time of tourniquet (<2 hours)

3. Apply the tourniquet early in significant hemorrhage, before the development of shock

4. Closely monitor hemorrhage control and viability of extremity

5. Keep meticulous record of tourniquet time

6. Wide tourniquets or side-by-side tourniquets minimize tissue damage and may be more effective in large wounds

From Sambasivan CN, Schreiber MA. Emerging therapies in traumatic hemorrhage control. Curr Opin Crit Care 2009;15(6):560–8.

NEW HORIZONS IN ENDOVASCULAR APPROACHES FOR VASCULAR TRAUMA

Until recently, endovascular approaches for vascular trauma were largely limited to blunt thoracic aortic injuries and an occasional carotid injury. With the increase in endovascular experience and graft options, the approach to other vascular injuries is evolving to include multiple case reports and clinical series of successful endovascular treatment of nearly every arterial system.[89–91] A recent report using the National Trauma Databank (NTDB) showed an increase in endovascular procedures for vascular trauma from 1% of cases in 2002 to nearly 11% in 2008.[92] This same study also showed an independent risk reduction in mortality for subclavian injuries treated with endovascular techniques when analysis was controlled for major confounders. Additional recent work has shown that nearly 6% of all peripheral vascular injuries from 2007 to 2009 reported to the NTDB were approached with an endovascular technique as the initial procedure of choice.[93] Injuries were also able to be addressed early (<24 hours) in the hospital course even in more severely injured patients.[92]

Beyond uses in thoracic aortic trauma, the most literature exists for extension of endovascular repair for subclavian and axillary artery injuries (**Fig. 6**). These injuries are typically difficult to assess open and endovascular options may provide opportunity for reduced mortality and morbidity. The largest single-center study to date examined 57 patients with a 100% immediate technical success and a 5% early graft failure.[92] A recent systematic review of the available literature from 1996 to 2012 found a total of 160 cases reported. Short-term success was 96% with long-term graft patency of 84%.[94] Although potentially promising, further study of the application of endovascular techniques for subclavian, axillary, peripheral arterial trauma, and major venous injuries is warranted before widespread adoption.

Balloon occlusion for temporary vascular control is also gaining renewed interest. Use has been described recently for penetrating arterial injuries, inferior vena cava control, major hepatic vascular injury, and pelvic exsanguination.[95,96] The breadth of experience is limited but proponents advocate that it results in reduced blood

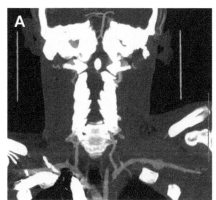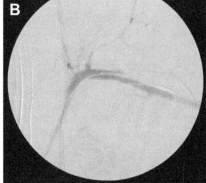

Fig. 6. Endovascular repair of subclavian artery injury. An 18-year-old man who sustained multiple gunshot wounds to the extremities, thorax, and abdomen presented hemodynamically stable with markedly diminished upper extremity pulse. CT angiogram showed a pseudoaneurysm of the left subclavian artery (*A*). The patient had additional complex injuries in multiple extremities and major neck injuries requiring operative repair. The subclavian was successfully stented (*B*).

loss, especially in difficult exposures, avoids entering the hematoma without proximal control, reduces operative time, and, in select cases, can be paired with endovascular covered stent repairs. A 10-year retrospective experience of externally placed balloon catheters published in 2011 examined outcomes in 44 patients. Most of the patients presented in extremis. Survival rates were 50% to 67% for those requiring placement for abdominal injuries.[96] Initial bleeding control was successful in 93% of the patients.[96] Given the success with external balloon control, the concept of endovascular application of occlusion has grown.[95] Most of the current literature is single case reports, but the technique has attractive potential. As in the case of endovascular repair, endovascular control of hemorrhage requires further study.

REFERENCES

1. Feliciano DV, Moore FA, Moore EE, et al. Evaluation and management of peripheral vascular injury. Part 1. Western Trauma Association/critical decisions in trauma. J Trauma 2011;70(6):1551–6.
2. Asensio JA, Kuncir EJ, Garcia-Nunez LM, et al. Femoral vessel injuries: analysis of factors predictive of outcomes. J Am Coll Surg 2006;203(4):512–20.
3. Burlew CC, Biffl WL. Imaging for blunt carotid and vertebral artery injuries. Surg Clin North Am 2011;91(1):217–31.
4. Callcut RA, Hanseman DJ, Solan PD, et al. Early treatment of blunt cerebrovascular injury with concomitant hemorrhagic neurologic injury is safe and effective. J Trauma Acute Care Surg 2012;72(2):338–45 [discussion: 345–6].
5. Cothren CC, Moore EE. Blunt cerebrovascular injuries. Clinics (Sao Paulo) 2005; 60(6):489–96.
6. Fabian TC, Patton JH Jr, Croce MA, et al. Blunt carotid injury. Importance of early diagnosis and anticoagulant therapy. Ann Surg 1996;223(5):513–22 [discussion: 522–5].
7. DiCocco JM, Emmett KP, Fabian TC, et al. Blunt cerebrovascular injury screening with 32-channel multidetector computed tomography: more slices still don't cut it. Ann Surg 2011;253(3):444–50.
8. Berne JD, Cook A, Rowe SA, et al. A multivariate logistic regression analysis of risk factors for blunt cerebrovascular injury. J Vasc Surg 2009;51(1):57–64.
9. Bromberg WJ, Collier BC, Diebel LN, et al. Blunt cerebrovascular injury practice management guidelines: the Eastern Association for the Surgery of Trauma. J Trauma 2010;68(2):471–7.
10. Biffl WL. Diagnosis of blunt cerebrovascular injuries. Curr Opin Crit Care 2003; 9(6):530–4.
11. Cothren CC, Moore EE, Ray CE Jr, et al. Screening for blunt cerebrovascular injuries is cost-effective. Am J Surg 2005;190(6):845–9.
12. Stein DM, Boswell S, Sliker CW, et al. Blunt cerebrovascular injuries: does treatment always matter? J Trauma 2009;66(1):132–43 [discussion: 143–4].
13. Biffl WL, Cothren CC, Moore EE, et al. Western Trauma Association critical decisions in trauma: screening for and treatment of blunt cerebrovascular injuries. J Trauma 2009;67(6):1150–3.
14. Miller PR, Fabian TC, Croce MA, et al. Prospective screening for blunt cerebrovascular injuries: analysis of diagnostic modalities and outcomes. Ann Surg 2002;236(3):386–93.
15. Burlew CC, Biffl WL, Moore EE, et al. Blunt cerebrovascular injuries: redefining screening criteria in the era of noninvasive diagnosis. J Trauma Acute Care Surg 2012;72(2):330–5 [discussion: 336–7]; [quiz: 539].

16. Callcut RA, Spain DA. Implications of applying adult BCVI screening criteria in pediatric patients. J Trauma 2011;71(3).

17. Berne JD, Reuland KS, Villarreal DH, et al. Sixteen-slice multi-detector computed tomographic angiography improves the accuracy of screening for blunt cerebrovascular injury. J Trauma 2006;60(6):1204–9 [discussion: 1209–10].

18. Biffl WL, Egglin T, Benedetto B, et al. Sixteen-slice computed tomographic angiography is a reliable noninvasive screening test for clinically significant blunt cerebrovascular injuries. J Trauma 2006;60(4):745–51.

19. Mayberry JC, Brown CV, Mullins RJ, et al. Blunt carotid artery injury: the futility of aggressive screening and diagnosis. Arch Surg 2004;139(6):609–12 [discussion: 612–3].

20. Wei CW, Montanera W, Selchen D, et al. Blunt cerebrovascular injuries: diagnosis and management outcomes. Can J Neurol Sci 2010;37(5): 574–9.

21. Kleindienst A, Harvey HB, Mater E, et al. Early antithrombotic prophylaxis with low molecular weight heparin in neurosurgery. Acta Neurochir (Wien) 2003; 145(12):1085–90 [discussion: 1090–1].

22. Thumbikat P, Poonnoose PM, Balasubrahmaniam P, et al. A comparison of heparin/warfarin and enoxaparin thromboprophylaxis in spinal cord injury: the Sheffield experience. Spinal Cord 2002;40(8):416–20.

23. Romualdi E, Micieli E, Ageno W, et al. Oral anticoagulant therapy in patients with mechanical heart valve and intracranial haemorrhage. A systematic review. Thromb Haemost 2009;101(2):290–7.

24. Cothren CC, Biffl WL, Moore EE, et al. Treatment for blunt cerebrovascular injuries: equivalence of anticoagulation and antiplatelet agents. Arch Surg 2009;144(7):685–90.

25. Biffl WL, Moore EE, Offner PJ, et al. Blunt carotid arterial injuries: implications of a new grading scale. J Trauma 1999;47(5):845–53.

26. DiCocco JM, Fabian TC, Emmett KP, et al. Optimal outcomes for patients with blunt cerebrovascular injury (BCVI): tailoring treatment to the lesion. J Am Coll Surg 2011;212(4):549–57.

27. Biffl WL, Moore EE, Elliott JP, et al. Blunt cerebrovascular injuries. Curr Probl Surg 1999;36(7):505–99.

28. Cothren CC, Moore EE, Ray CE Jr, et al. Carotid artery stents for blunt cerebrovascular injury: risks exceed benefits. Arch Surg 2005;140(5):480–5 [discussion: 485–6].

29. Biffl WL, Ray CE Jr, Moore EE, et al. Treatment-related outcomes from blunt cerebrovascular injuries: importance of routine follow-up arteriography. Ann Surg 2002;235(5):699–706 [discussion: 706–7].

30. Propper BW, Clouse WD. Thoracic aortic endografting for trauma: a current appraisal. Arch Surg 2010;145(10):1006–11.

31. Arthurs ZM, Starnes BW, Sohn VY, et al. Functional and survival outcomes in traumatic blunt thoracic aortic injuries: an analysis of the National Trauma Databank. J Vasc Surg 2009;49(4):988–94.

32. Yamane BH, Tefera G, Hoch JR, et al. Blunt thoracic aortic injury: open or stent graft repair? Surgery 2008;144(4):575–80.

33. Lee WA, Matsumura JS, Mitchell RS, et al. Endovascular repair of traumatic thoracic aortic injury: clinical practice guidelines of the Society for Vascular Surgery. J Vasc Surg 2011;53(1):187–92.

34. Hong MS, Feezor RJ, Lee WA, et al. The advent of thoracic endovascular aortic repair is associated with broadened treatment eligibility and decreased

overall mortality in traumatic thoracic aortic injury. J Vasc Surg 2011;53(1): 36–42 [discussion: 43].

35. Fabian TC, Richardson JD, Croce MA, et al. Prospective study of blunt aortic injury: multicenter trial of the American Association for the Surgery of Trauma. J Trauma 1997;42(3):374–80 [discussion: 380–3].

36. Teixeira PG, Inaba K, Barmparas G, et al. Blunt thoracic aortic injuries: an autopsy study. J Trauma 2011;70(1):197–202.

37. Nagy K, Fabian T, Rodman G, et al. Guidelines for the diagnosis and management of blunt aortic injury: an EAST Practice Management Guidelines Work Group. J Trauma 2000;48(6):1128–43.

38. Azizzadeh A, Charlton-Ouw KM, Chen Z, et al. An outcome analysis of endovascular versus open repair of blunt traumatic aortic injuries. J Vasc Surg 2013; 57(1):108–14.

39. Demetriades D, Velmahos GC, Scalea TM, et al. Diagnosis and treatment of blunt thoracic aortic injuries: changing perspectives. J Trauma 2008;64(6): 1415–8.

40. Demetriades D, Velmahos GC, Scalea TM, et al. Operative repair or endovascular stent graft in blunt traumatic thoracic aortic injuries: results of an American Association for the Surgery of Trauma multicenter study. J Trauma 2008;64(3): 561–70.

41. Nikolic S, Atanasijevic T, Mihailovic Z, et al. Mechanisms of aortic blunt rupture in fatally injured front-seat passengers in frontal car collisions: an autopsy study. Am J Forensic Med Pathol 2006;27(4):292–5.

42. Paul JS, Neideen T, Tutton S, et al. Minimal aortic injury after blunt trauma: selective nonoperative management is safe. J Trauma 2011;71(6):1519–23.

43. Reed AB, Thompson JK, Crafton CJ, et al. Timing of endovascular repair of blunt traumatic thoracic aortic transections. J Vasc Surg 2006;43(4):684–8.

44. Fabian TC, Davis KA, Gavant ML, et al. Prospective study of blunt aortic injury: helical CT is diagnostic and antihypertensive therapy reduces rupture. Ann Surg 1998;227(5):666–76 [discussion: 676–7].

45. Caffarelli AD, Mallidi HR, Maggio PM, et al. Early outcomes of deliberate nonoperative management for blunt thoracic aortic injury in trauma. J Thorac Cardiovasc Surg 2010;140(3):598–605.

46. Kidane B, Abramowitz D, Harris JR, et al. Natural history of minimal aortic injury following blunt thoracic aortic trauma. Can J Surg 2012;55(6):377–81.

47. Malhotra AK, Fabian TC, Croce MA, et al. Minimal aortic injury: a lesion associated with advancing diagnostic techniques. J Trauma 2001;51(6): 1042–8.

48. Azizzadeh A, Keyhani K, Miller CC 3rd, et al. Blunt traumatic aortic injury: initial experience with endovascular repair. J Vasc Surg 2009;49(6):1403–8.

49. Demetriades D, Velmahos GC, Scalea TM, et al. Blunt traumatic thoracic aortic injuries: early or delayed repair–results of an American Association for the Surgery of Trauma prospective study. J Trauma 2009;66(4):967–73.

50. Tang GL, Tehrani HY, Usman A, et al. Reduced mortality, paraplegia, and stroke with stent graft repair of blunt aortic transections: a modern meta-analysis. J Vasc Surg 2008;47(3):671–5.

51. Hoffer EK, Forauer AR, Silas AM, et al. Endovascular stent-graft or open surgical repair for blunt thoracic aortic trauma: systematic review. J Vasc Interv Radiol 2008;19(8):1153–64.

52. Amabile P, Collart F, Gariboldi V, et al. Surgical versus endovascular treatment of traumatic thoracic aortic rupture. J Vasc Surg 2004;40(5):873–9.

53. Patel HJ, Hemmila MR, Williams DM, et al. Late outcomes following open and endovascular repair of blunt thoracic aortic injury. J Vasc Surg 2011;53(3): 615–20.

54. Murad MH, Rizvi AZ, Malgor R, et al. Comparative effectiveness of the treatments for thoracic aortic transection [corrected]. J Vasc Surg 2011;53(1):193–9.e1–21.

55. Dorlac WC, DeBakey ME, Holcomb JB, et al. Mortality from isolated civilian penetrating extremity injury. J Trauma 2005;59(1):217–22.

56. Callcut RA, Acher CW, Hoch J, et al. Impact of intraoperative arteriography on limb salvage for traumatic popliteal artery injury. J Trauma 2009;67(2):252–7 [discussion: 257–8].

57. Tan TW, Joglar FL, Hamburg NM, et al. Limb outcome and mortality in lower and upper extremity arterial injury: a comparison using the National Trauma Data Bank. Vasc Endovascular Surg 2011;45(7):592–7.

58. Frykberg ER. Popliteal vascular injuries. Surg Clin North Am 2002;82(1):67–89.

59. Mullenix PS, Steele SR, Andersen CA, et al. Limb salvage and outcomes among patients with traumatic popliteal vascular injury: an analysis of the National Trauma Data Bank. J Vasc Surg 2006;44(1):94–100.

60. Padayachy V, Robbs JV, Mulaudzi TV, et al. A retrospective review of brachial artery injuries and repairs–is it still a "training artery"? Injury 2010;41(9): 960–3.

61. Kauvar DS, Sarfati MR, Kraiss LW. National trauma databank analysis of mortality and limb loss in isolated lower extremity vascular trauma. J Vasc Surg 2011; 53(6):1598–603.

62. Rowe VL, Salim A, Lipham J, et al. Shank vessel injuries. Surg Clin North Am 2002;82(1):91–104.

63. Peng PD, Spain DA, Tataria M, et al. CT angiography effectively evaluates extremity vascular trauma. Am Surg 2008;74(2):103–7.

64. Klineberg EO, Crites BM, Flinn WR, et al. The role of arteriography in assessing popliteal artery injury in knee dislocations. J Trauma 2004;56(4):786–90.

65. Hollis JD, Daley BJ. 10-year review of knee dislocations: is arteriography always necessary? J Trauma 2005;59(3):672–5 [discussion: 675–6].

66. Barnes CJ, Pietrobon R, Higgins LD. Does the pulse examination in patients with traumatic knee dislocation predict a surgical arterial injury? A meta-analysis. J Trauma 2002;53(6):1109–14.

67. Patterson BO, Holt PJ, Cleanthis M, et al. Imaging vascular trauma. Br J Surg 2012;99(4):494–505.

68. Inaba K, Branco BC, Reddy S, et al. Prospective evaluation of multidetector computed tomography for extremity vascular trauma. J Trauma 2011;70(4): 808–15.

69. Helfet DL, Howey T, Sanders R, et al. Limb salvage versus amputation. Preliminary results of the Mangled Extremity Severity Score. Clin Orthop Relat Res 1990;(256):80–6.

70. Chung KC, Saddawi-Konefka D, Haase SC, et al. A cost-utility analysis of amputation versus salvage for Gustilo type IIIB and IIIC open tibial fractures. Plast Reconstr Surg 2009;124(6):1965–73.

71. Huynh TT, Pham M, Griffin LW, et al. Management of distal femoral and popliteal arterial injuries: an update. Am J Surg 2006;192(6):773–8.

72. Bechara C, Huynh TT, Lin PH. Management of lower extremity arterial injuries. J Cardiovasc Surg (Torino) 2007;48(5):567–79.

73. Guerrero A, Gibson K, Kralovich KA, et al. Limb loss following lower extremity arterial trauma: what can be done proactively? Injury 2002;33(9):765–9.

74. Branco BC, Inaba K, Barmparas G, et al. Incidence and predictors for the need for fasciotomy after extremity trauma: a 10-year review in a mature level I trauma centre. Injury 2011;42(10):1157–63.

75. Melton SM, Croce MA, Patton JH Jr, et al. Popliteal artery trauma. Systemic anticoagulation and intraoperative thrombolysis improves limb salvage. Ann Surg 1997;225(5):518–27 [discussion: 527–9].

76. Hancock H, Rasmussen TE, Walker AJ, et al. History of temporary intravascular shunts in the management of vascular injury. J Vasc Surg 2010;52(5):1405–9.

77. Borut LT, Acosta CJ, Tadlock LC, et al. The use of temporary vascular shunts in military extremity wounds: a preliminary outcome analysis with 2-year follow-up. J Trauma 2010;69(1):174–8.

78. Sambasivan CN, Schreiber MA. Emerging therapies in traumatic hemorrhage control. Curr Opin Crit Care 2009;15(6):560–8.

79. Dua A, Patel B, Kragh JF Jr, et al. Long-term follow-up and amputation-free survival in 497 casualties with combat-related vascular injuries and damage-control resuscitation. J Trauma Acute Care Surg 2012;73(6):1515–20.

80. Taller J, Kamdar JP, Greene JA, et al. Temporary vascular shunts as initial treatment of proximal extremity vascular injuries during combat operations: the new standard of care at Echelon II facilities? J Trauma 2008;65(3):595–603.

81. Fox CJ, Gillespie DL, Cox ED, et al. Damage control resuscitation for vascular surgery in a combat support hospital. J Trauma 2008;65(1):1–9.

82. Gifford SM, Aidinian G, Clouse WD, et al. Effect of temporary shunting on extremity vascular injury: an outcome analysis from the Global War on Terror vascular injury initiative. J Vasc Surg 2009;50(3):549–55 [discussion: 555–6].

83. Percival TJ, Rasmussen TE. Reperfusion strategies in the management of extremity vascular injury with ischaemia. Br J Surg 2012;99(Suppl 1):66–74.

84. Burkhardt GE, Rasmussen TE, Propper BW, et al. A national survey of evolving management patterns for vascular injury. J Surg Educ 2009;66(5):239–47.

85. Rasmussen TE, Clouse WD, Jenkins DH, et al. The use of temporary vascular shunts as a damage control adjunct in the management of wartime vascular injury. J Trauma 2006;61(1):8–12 [discussion: 12–5].

86. D'Alleyrand JC, Dutton RP, Pollak AN. Extrapolation of battlefield resuscitative care to the civilian setting. J Surg Orthop Adv 2010;19(1):62–9.

87. Kragh JF Jr, Walters TJ, Baer DG, et al. Survival with emergency tourniquet use to stop bleeding in major limb trauma. Ann Surg 2009;249(1):1–7.

88. Kragh JF Jr, O'Neill ML, Walters TJ, et al. Minor morbidity with emergency tourniquet use to stop bleeding in severe limb trauma: research, history, and reconciling advocates and abolitionists. Mil Med 2011;176(7):817–23.

89. Zimmerman P, d'Audiffret A, Pillai L. Endovascular repair of blunt extremity arterial injury: case report. Vasc Endovascular Surg 2009;43(2):211–4.

90. Joglar F, Kabutey NK, Maree A, et al. The role of stent grafts in the management of traumatic tibial artery pseudoaneurysms: case report and review of the literature. Vasc Endovascular Surg 2010;44(5):407–9.

91. Stewart DK, Brown PM, Tinsley EA Jr, et al. Use of stent grafts in lower extremity trauma. Ann Vasc Surg 2011;25(2):264.e9–13.

92. Avery LE, Stahlfeld KR, Corcos AC, et al. Evolving role of endovascular techniques for traumatic vascular injury: a changing landscape? J Trauma Acute Care Surg 2012;72(1):41–6.

93. Worni M, Scarborough JE, Gandhi M, et al. Use of endovascular therapy for peripheral arterial lesions: an analysis of the National Trauma Data Bank from 2007 to 2009. Ann Vasc Surg 2013;27(3):299–305.

94. DuBose JJ, Rajani R, Gilani R, et al. Endovascular management of axillo-subclavian arterial injury: a review of published experience. Injury 2012; 43(11):1785–92.

95. Bui TD, Mills JL. Control of inferior vena cava injury using percutaneous balloon catheter occlusion. Vasc Endovascular Surg 2009;43(5):490–3.

96. Ball CG, Wyrzykowski AD, Nicholas JM, et al. A decade's experience with balloon catheter tamponade for the emergency control of hemorrhage. J Trauma 2011;70(2):330–3.

Superficial Venous Disease

Kellie R. Brown, MD*, Peter J. Rossi, MD

KEYWORDS

- Superficial venous disease • Thrombosis • Varicose veins • Venous reflux

KEY POINTS

- Superficial venous disease is common and can cause significant disability.
- The concerning disease states of the superficial venous system are venous reflux, varicose veins, and superficial venous thrombosis (SVT).
- Superficial venous reflux can be a significant contributor to chronic venous stasis wounds of the lower extremity, the treatment of which can be costly both in terms of overall health care expenditure and lost working days for affected patients.
- Although commonly thought of as a benign process, SVT is associated with several underlying pathologic processes, including malignancy and deep venous thrombosis (DVT).
- Most treatments of superficial disease are carried out in the office setting, allowing for both patient and physician convenience.

INTRODUCTION

Superficial venous disease is a common clinical problem. The concerning disease states of the superficial venous system are venous reflux, varicose veins, and SVT. Superficial venous reflux can be a significant contributor to chronic venous stasis wounds of the lower extremity, the treatment of which can be costly both in terms of overall health care expenditure and lost working days for affected patients. Although commonly thought of as a benign process, SVT is associated with several underlying pathologic processes, including malignancy and DVT. Additionally, SVT can lead to serious clinical consequences when it evolves into DVT.

EPIDEMIOLOGY

The incidence of superficial venous disease increases with age, and women are more commonly affected overall than men.[1–3] The San Diego Population Study[1] prospectively collected data from an ethnically diverse population of 2211 women and men.

Division of Vascular Surgery, The Medical College of Wisconsin, 9200 West Wisconsin Avenue, Milwaukee, WI 53226, USA
* Corresponding author.
E-mail address: krbrown@mcw.edu

Surg Clin N Am 93 (2013) 963–982
http://dx.doi.org/10.1016/j.suc.2013.04.007
0039-6109/13/$ – see front matter Published by Elsevier Inc.

surgical.theclinics.com

The investigators determined that incidence of superficial venous disease was the most common in Hispanic patients (3.6%), followed by non-Hispanic white patients (2.6%), Asians (1.5%), and African Americans (0.9%). The incidence of disease increased with age, and overall venous disease was found more common in women (2.8% vs 1.5%). Although individual patient risk factors were not evaluated in this study, a retrospective study from the Netherlands found that in patients treated for SVT, at-risk patients had a personal history of phlebitis (33%), family history of phlebitis (31%), immobilization in the last 3 months (11%), trauma in the past 3 months (13%), surgery in the past 3 months (8%), or underlying malignancy (7%).[1]

The Framingham Study likewise provided information regarding the prevalence of varicose veins; 3822 patients were evaluated.[2] Although age was not related to the incidence of varicose veins, women were more commonly affected than men. Among women, patients with varicose veins were more likely to be obese, hypertensive, and have a sedentary lifestyle. Among men, patients with varicose veins were more likely to smoke cigarettes and have lower levels of physical activity than their counterparts without varicose veins. The investigators suggested that overall control of cardiovascular risk factors would not only prevent heart disease but also potentially reduce the incidence of varicose veins.[2]

Another population-based study[3] showed that lifestyle (smoking, alcohol consumption, dietary fiber intake, social class, and intestinal transit time) had no significant association with development of venous reflux but did show a decreased incidence of superficial venous reflux in women with a history of oral contraceptive use (odds ratio [OR] 0.71). In men, however, increasing height (OR 1.13) and chronic straining at stool (OR 1.94) were positively associated with the development of superficial venous reflux.[3]

ANATOMY, PHYSIOLOGY, AND PATHOPHYSIOLOGY
Saphenous Veins and Tributaries

The greater (or long) saphenous vein courses from its position anterior to the medial malleolus, where it collects venous drainage from the dorsal venous arch of the foot, along the medial leg and thigh to its termination at the saphenofemoral junction in the groin. The term, *saphenous*, may be derived from the Arabic *al safin* (concealed) or from the Greek *safaina* (evident).[4] This is relevant in that the greater saphenous vein is actually a deep superficial vein, the only visible portion in the distal leg in a person of normal size. The greater saphenous vein in the thigh runs within the saphenous fascia, which gives the characteristic appearance of the saphenous eye on gray scale ultrasonographic imaging. The saphenous nerve runs within the saphenous fascia with the vein, with obvious implications to surgical therapy. Many collateral veins contribute flow to the greater saphenous vein, including pelvic collaterals and the anterior and posterior accessory saphenous veins.[4] The saphenous veins have bicuspid valves that prevent reflux in the undiseased state. These valves are able to withstand a pressure of 200 mm Hg to 300 mm Hg under normal circumstances. Anatomic studies have documented that the greater saphenous vein has generally between 7 and 9 valves from the ankle to the saphenofemoral junction, with valves more numerous below the knee.[5,6] The greater saphenous vein can be duplicated, with obvious implications to surgical therapy.[7]

The short (small) saphenous vein runs on the posterior aspect of the leg from the foot, diving between the heads of the gastrocnemius muscle to drain into the popliteal vein. The sural nerve travels in close proximity to the small saphenous vein. The small saphenous vein is duplicated much less often (4%) than the greater saphenous vein.[4] The small saphenous vein may terminate in numerous areas but in 80% of the population terminates in the popliteal fossa into either the popliteal vein or a gastroc-nemius vein.[8]

A posterior thigh communicating vein, known as the Giacomini vein, has been thought to contribute to superficial venous insufficiency.[8] This vein is a proximal exten-sion of the small saphenous vein and connects to the proximal greater saphenous vein, thigh muscular veins, or femoral vein. A study of 301 limbs found, however, that 70.4% of limbs had a Giacomini vein identified on duplex scan and that this vein had no effect on the severity of venous reflux in symptomatic patients. The inves-tigators suggested that the Giacomini vein should be investigated in cases of patients having small saphenous reflux or when significant symptoms are present in patients with a competent greater saphenous vein on duplex imaging.[8]

Calf Muscle Pump and Valve System

The large veins of the lower extremity receive blood from the action of the calf muscle pump. The components of this pump are the skeletal muscle, intramuscular venous sinusoids, and the superficial and deep veins. As the muscles of the leg contract, blood is forced from the intramuscular veins toward the heart. A normally functioning calf muscle pump system reduces the pressure in the greater saphenous vein at the ankle from 80 mm Hg to 100 mm Hg at rest (standing) to 20 mm Hg to 30 mm Hg with only modest activity. With vigorous exercise, a pressure of 300 mm Hg can be reached.[6] Valves open during muscle contraction and close quickly (normally 0.5–1.0 s) in response to retrograde flow.[9] Perforating veins connect the superficial and deep venous systems, and these perforators have bidirectional flow under normal physiologic conditions. These perforators become pathologic when either the deep or superficial system develops insufficiency, which then allows unidirectional flow from an incompetent system. As the longest continuous vein in the human body, it logically follows that the greater saphenous vein is commonly affected by superficial venous disorders. Incompetent venous valves are likely the primary problem leading to the majority of all venous disease.[10]

The calf muscle pump is implicated in superficial venous insufficiency. Conditions that lead to altered muscle contraction (trauma, immobility, and paralysis) can result in stasis of blood in the soleal blood pools, leading to destruction of the gastrocnemius and soleal veins. These conditions are often chronic, with few good treatment options available.[6]

Varicose Veins

Primary varicose veins likely develop as the result of valvular incompetence and ulti-mately reflux. Primary varicose veins develop de novo, and secondary varicose veins are the result of another underlying pathophysiologic process, such as superficial venous thrombosis (discussed later) or malignancy. Varicose veins are at best un-sightly and at worst lead to chronic ulceration, usually in the gaiter area of the leg prox-imal to the medial malleolus. The treatment of this disease spectrum may account for up to 3% of US health care expenditures on a yearly basis.[1]

The underlying cause of primary varicose veins and venous insufficiency is not well understood. As noted by Lim and Davies,[11] several studies have documented abnor-malities in matrix metalloproteinase activity, specifically isozymes 1, 2, 3, 7, and 9. The conclusions of multiple studies, however, are inconsistent and this remains an area of ongoing research.[11]

Hyperlipidemia has been detected in several patients with varicose veins.[12] Recently, altered phospholipid metabolism has been postulated as having an effect on the development of varicose veins. Using mass spectroscopy, Tanaka and colleagues[13] determined that several phospholipids were detected in abnormal distributions around the valves of saphenous veins with demonstrated reflux. One of the phospholipids included phosphatadiylcholine, which is a chemokine for macrophages and could result in an inflammatory process leading to valve damage. This process seems, however, independent of serum lipid levels, and what incites these peculiar distributions of phosopholipids around saphenous vein valves is currently unknown.[13] In a follow-up study, Tanaka and colleageus also demonstrated an abnormally low number of lymphatic channels in the adventitia of varicose veins on D2-40 staining compared with control veins, hypothesizing that abnormal lipid transport may lead to some of the cellular derangements found in varicose vein walls.[14]

Microscopic arteriovenous shunting has been proposed as a mechanism for varicose vein formation. A 2008 study[15] examined 39 patients with varicose veins and compared them with 10 control patients. Greater saphenous veins were cannulated, and venous pressures and oxygen tensions were measured. There was no demonstrated difference between the control group and the varicosity group, which makes significant arteriovenous shunting unlikely.[15]

In addition to valve abnormalities, primary defects in the saphenous vein wall have been implicated as a cause of varicose veins and venous insufficiency. Varicose veins can develop in the absence of valvular incompetence.[16,17] Elsharawy[18] examined 70 greater saphenous veins from 35 patients (24 patients with varicose veins and 11 patients without). Although a significant increase in collagen and elastin was demonstrated in varicose veins compared with controls, there was no difference in the makeup of the vein wall in varicose veins with and without valvular insufficiency. This supports the theory that a wall weakness allows dilation of the vein and progressive separation of the valve cusps rather than a primary valve defect leading to reflux.[18]

Coagulation disorders are an often under-recognized risk factor for superficial venous disease. Up to two-thirds of patients with varicose veins may have at least one inherited thrombophilia, and patients with chronic venous ulceration may have an underlying clotting disorder in up to 75% of cases.[19] Women with multiple pregnancies have likewise been thought to have a predisposition to developing superficial venous reflux, and this has been shown to be true for lower extremity nonsaphenous venous reflux disease.[20]

Regardless of the cause of the valvular dysfunction, valvular abnormalities are present in up to 70% of patients with superficial venous insufficiency.[6,21,22]

Superficial Venous Thrombophlebitis

Superficial thrombophlebitis has previously been thought by many physicians to be a fairly benign clinical entitity. SVT, however, has important clinical consequences. The Prospective Observational Superficial Thrombophlebitis[23] study evaluated 844 consecutive patients with SVT identified on compression ultrasonography. Of these patients, 24.9% also were diagnosed with either DVT or pulmonary embolism. Of the 600 patients that had no DVT or pulmonary embolism at initial evaluation, 10.2% developed complications within the 3 months of diagnosis, despite the majority (540/600) treated with anticoagulation. Complications included DVT, pulmonary embolism, extension of SVT, and recurrence of SVT. Male gender and patients with a history of DVT or pulmonary embolus, history of cancer, and absence of varicose veins were significant predictors of complications.[23] Superficial thrombophlebitis can ultimately lead to valvular incompetence, resulting in secondary venous insufficiency.

Telangiectasias and Reticular Veins

Dilated small cutaneous veins (telangiectasias and reticular veins) are commonly thought the result of venous insufficiency of either the deep or superficial system.[24] These veins are often a cosmetic concern. Dilated small cutaneous veins have been shown to be present in 25% of women and 6% of men with an increasing incidence with age.[25] Although a majority of patients are asymptomatic, symptoms, including leg heaviness, limb swelling, and fatigue, develop in up to 39% of patients, with women more commonly afflicted.[25] These findings are corroborated by other investigators.[26] Although the pathology behind these small cutaneous veins is poorly understood, incompetence of reticular veins on duplex scanning has been detected in up to 89% of examined telangiectasias, and 15% of these reticular veins had an incompetent perforator connected to the deep venous system.[27] Multiple patterns of greater and small saphenous vein reflux have been reported in more than 40% of patients with telangiectasias, including short-segment saphenous reflux with a competent saphenofemoral junction.[28] It is unclear, however, if correction of the reflux improves the overall ability to treat small cutaneous veins and prevent recurrences.

CEAP CLASSIFICATION

First reported in 1996,[29] the clinical, etiologic, anatomic, pathologic (CEAP) classification of lower extremity venous disease has been used to allow uniform classification of lower extremity venous disease. The clinical classification ranges from 0 (no visible or palpable changes) to 6 (active ulceration). An A or S is added to the class to signify asymptomatic or symptomatic status, respectively.

- $C0$—symptoms of leg heaviness, edema, or pruritis with no skin changes
- C_1—stage at which first signs appear, including telangiectasias or reticular veins (**Fig. 1**)
- C_2—development of varicose veins (**Fig. 2**)
- C_3—presence of venous edema (**Fig. 3**)
- C_4—skin trophic changes of venous origin (**Fig. 4**)
- C_5—healed ulcer with trophic changes (**Fig. 5**)
- C_6—active ulceration (**Fig. 6**)
- A—asymptomatic
- S—symptomatic

The etiologic classification describes the cause of the venous disease.

- E_c—congenital
- E_p—primary
- E_s—secondary
- E_n—no venous cause identified

The anatomic classification describes the anatomy of the venous disease.

- A_s—superficial
- A_p—perforator
- A_d—deep
- A_n—no location identified

The pathologic classification identifies the pathophysiology of the disease.

- P_r—reflux
- P_o—obstruction

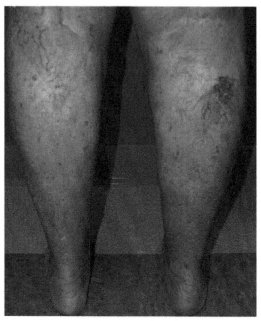

Fig. 1. The CEAP classification of lower extremity venous disease. C_1—stage at which first signs appear, including telangiectasias or reticular veins.

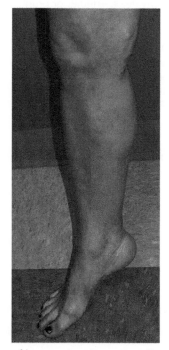

Fig. 2. The CEAP classification of lower extremity venous disease. C_2—development of varicose veins.

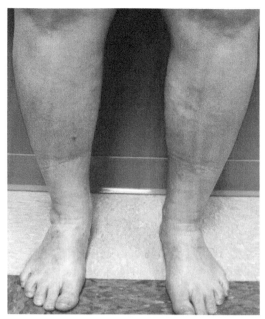

Fig. 3. The CEAP classification of lower extremity venous disease. C_3—presence of venous edema.

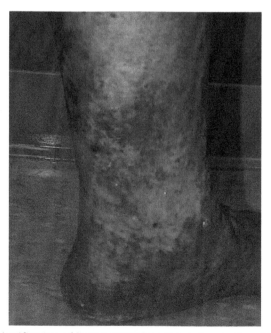

Fig. 4. The CEAP classification of lower extremity venous disease. C_4—skin trophic changes of venous origin.

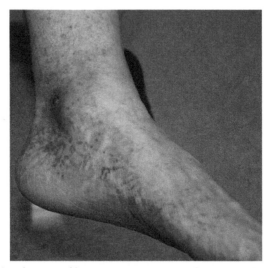

Fig. 5. The CEAP classification of lower extremity venous disease. C₅—healed ulcer with trophic changes.

- $P_{r,o}$—reflux and obstruction
- P_n—no pathophysiology identified

The clinical classification is the most commonly used part of the CEAP classification. The other parts of CEAP are most useful in research.

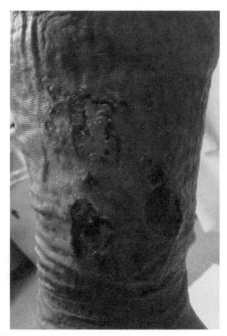

Fig. 6. The CEAP classification of lower extremity venous disease. C₆—active ulceration.

EVALUATION
History

The evaluation of a venous patient begins with an accurate history. Pertinent factors in the history include type and duration of symptoms, exacerbating and alleviating factors, history of DVT or other clotting disorders, and previous treatments.

Typical symptoms of superficial venous disease include

- Aching
- Heaviness
- Fatigue
- Restless legs
- Cramping
- Itching
- Swelling

Most patients describe an increase in symptoms with prolonged standing or sitting and alleviation with elevation. Many patients deny pain but acknowledge a more subtle dull ache or fatigue. Often these symptoms have been present for many years and have been attributed to age or other factors. The symptoms are typically less noticeable in the morning or with elevation but get worse throughout the day and are often exacerbated in women by the menstrual cycle. Nighttime cramping and restless legs also may be due to venous disease and often are noticeable after a particularly long or active day. Patients often experience itching in the area of their varicose veins. Sometimes this is accompanied by venous stasis dermatitis but often itching alone is the symptom. Some patients notice an increase in symptoms after exercise, particularly after vigorous exercise such as distance running, although during exercise, the symptoms are often improved. Many of these symptoms are significantly or completely relieved with treatment of the superficial venous reflux.

It is important to ask patients about history of blood clots or clotting disorders. Patients who have a history of DVT are at risk for deep as well as superficial venous insufficiency, and particular attention must be paid to the patency of the deep system prior to treatment of their superficial disease. Patients with a history of superficial thrombophlebitis meet the criteria for varicose vein treatment. If there is a history of more than one episode of thrombophlebitis, a hypercoagulable work up is warranted prior to treatment.

Varicose vein recurrence after treatment is common, so it is important to ask about prior treatments. Saphenous veins are duplicated in the calf in 25% of patients and in the thigh in 8% of patients, so even in the setting of previous saphenous ablation or stripping there may be a patent, refluxing saphenous vein.[30]

Physical Examination

On physical examination, it is important to note the location and size of the varicose veins and whether there is any evidence of thrombophlebitis or superficial venous occlusion. A preponderance of telangiectasias (spider veins) in the ankle region, called corona phlebectatica, is a sign of superficial venous disease (**Fig. 7**). In addition, a thorough skin evaluation is important. Cutaneous manifestations of superficial venous disease may include

- Venous ulceration (see **Fig. 6**)
- Atrophe blanche (**Fig. 8**)
- Lipodermatosclerosis (see **Fig. 4**)
- Venous stasis dermatitis (**Fig. 9**)

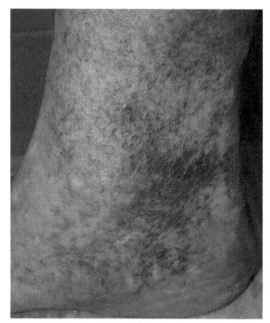

Fig. 7. A preponderance of telangiectasias (spider veins) in the ankle region, which is called corona phlebectatica, is a sign of superficial venous disease.

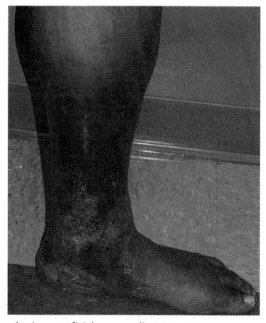

Fig. 8. Atrophe blanche in superficial venous disease.

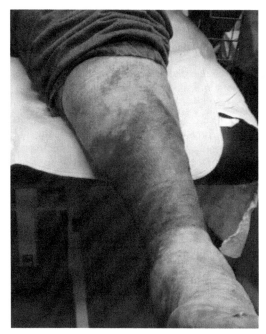

Fig. 9. Venous stasis dermatitis in superficial venous disease.

Stasis dermatitis is manifest as skin pigmentation, induration, or eczema. Presence of edema is also important to note.

The pattern of varicosities can also be a clue to the cause of the venous disease. Varicose veins in the medial thigh and calf are often related to the great saphenous vein, and varicosities in the anterolateral thigh and knee are often related to anterior saphenous insufficiency. Ulceration in the lateral ankle is suspicious for small saphenous vein insufficiency. Despite these clues, physical examination is not the best way to determine the anatomy and cause of superficial venous disease. For this, duplex ultrasound is necessary.

Ultrasound Examination

Formal ultrasound examination of the venous system includes evaluation of both the deep and superficial systems. The study should focus on documenting venous patency as well as presence or absence of normal valvular function. The common femoral, femoral, profunda femoris, popliteal, and tibial veins are the deep veins that are typically interrogated. The great saphenous vein, anterior accessory saphenous vein, small saphenous vein, and any visible perforators are typically evaluated in the superficial system. The sources of reflux for visible varicosities should be mapped out by an ultrasonographer. The location, duration, and patency of reflux should be documented. If superficial venous reflux is found, the size of the abnormal veins should be documented.

Patency is assessed by compressing the vein, and reflux is assessed by distal augmentation or retrograde compression. Distal augmentation is accomplished by compression of the leg below the ultrasound probe, directing flow proximally. This compression should be done sharply and quickly. Reflux is defined as reversal of flow on release of compression for more than 0.5 seconds in duration. Reflux for less than 0.5 seconds for veins in the superficial system, less than 1 second for the femoral or popliteal veins, and 350 milliseconds for perforating veins is considered normal valvular closing time.[31] Retrograde compression is accomplished by direct compression above the ultrasound probe. This propels blood toward the feet if the valve is incompetent. The Valsalva maneuver can be used to assess the saphenofemoral junction but is less reliable distally, and a competent terminal valve in the saphenofemoral junction renders the maneuver useless.[32]

Other Studies

The combination of history, physical, and ultrasound is generally both necessary and sufficient to determine the source of superficial venous insufficiency and to formulate a treatment plan. There are times, however, when these are not enough.

Pelvic congestion syndrome is a condition that is caused by incompetent pelvic and ovarian veins. Patients with this condition can present with pelvic pain, aching, fullness, and/or dyspareunia. These symptoms are often accompanied by vulvar and lower extremity varicosities. These veins are evaluated by transvaginal ultrasound, magnetic resonance venogram, or CT venogram, and the presence or absence of pelvic varicosities is documented.[31] If they are present, definite diagnosis and treatment is achieved with catheter-directed venography.

Congenital vascular malformation is another condition that is generally not completely evaluated by ultrasound and examination alone. In any patient who has had varicose veins since birth or early childhood, congenital venous malformation should be suspected. In addition, patients who have extremity port-wine stains or other birthmarks or significant limb size or length discrepancies should be evaluated for vascular malformation. This is best done by MRI of the affected extremity.[33]

TREATMENT
Axial Reflux

Acceptable treatments for reflux in the great saphenous vein, small saphenous, or anterior accessory saphenous veins include

- Conservative therapy
- Thermal ablation
- Sclerotherapy
- Surgical stripping

Conservative therapy
Conservative therapy for venous insufficiency primarily consists of compression therapy. Weight loss, exercise, and limb elevation are also encouraged. Conservative therapy is inexpensive (compared with more invasive treatments) and safe. Compression stockings are uncomfortable, however, and patient compliance with consistent use is low.[34] The same is true for weight loss and exercise. In addition, although conservative therapy often helps control symptoms of superficial venous disease, it does nothing to correct the underlying problem. For this reason, conservative therapy is not typically chosen for long-term treatment of superficial venous insufficiency in most cases.

Thermal ablation
Thermal ablation, using either laser or radiofrequency as the heat generator, has become increasingly commonplace as the primary treatment of axial reflux. Thermal ablation has been found safe and effective, with few side effects and no hospital stay.[35–40] These techniques allow for closure of the axial vein without surgery and in most cases improve or eliminate patients' symptoms.

Thermal ablation is typically done in a procedure room in an office setting. The patient's leg is prepped and draped, and the course of the vein to be treated is marked out using ultrasound. Local anesthetic is placed, and ultrasound-guided access to the saphenous vein is accomplished. Using the Seldinger technique, a wire is passed into the vein, over which a sheath is placed. The laser or radiofrequency catheter is then placed into the vein and position is confirmed using ultrasound. Tumescent anesthesia is induced, which consists of injecting a dilute local anesthetic solution under ultrasound guidance around the entire length of the vein to be treated. The heat source is then activated, and the catheter is withdrawn at appropriate levels and speeds to adequately treat the vein.

Laser ablation works by heat induced injury to the vein wall. The laser energy generates heat that results in the formation of steam bubbles at the tip of the laser fiber. The bubbles emanate from the end of the catheter to thermally injure the venous endothelium. The bubbles dissipate quickly and pose no systemic risk of embolization. The volume of steam generated is directly related to the amount of laser energy produced. It is generally accepted that a range of 60 J/cm to 80 J/cm is safe resulting in successful ablation.[41]

Radiofrequency ablation works by generating an elective current with the radiofrequency generator and catheter that flows through the vein wall. This results in heat generation through a phenomenon called resistive heating. Histologically, resistive heating causes the collagen fibrils primarily in the subendothelial layer of the vein wall to denature and shorten. The venous diameter decreases and blood proteins remaining in the lumen congeal to obliterate the residual lumen.[41] Venous fibrosis ensues and the vein becomes less visible on duplex ultrasonography.[42]

Outcomes after laser or radiofrequency ablation are comparable. Laser ablation has been shown to result in a 97% successful occlusion at 1-year follow-up and 93% at 3-year follow-up.[36,37] Radiofrequency ablation has been shown to result in an 87% successful occlusion at 5 years.[39] Several randomized controlled trials have failed to show a significant difference in outcome between the 2 modalities.[43–46]

Complications of thermal ablation include[31]

- DVT (1%–3%)
- Paresthesias (1%–3%)
- Skin injury/ulceration (<1%)
- Thrombophlebitis (1%–2%)
- Skin discoloration (1%–2%)

Many of these complications are uncommon and require supportive care. In cases of ulceration or skin burn, wound care is necessary. With DVT, which is also referred to as endovenous heat-induced thrombosis, anticoagulation is required. As long as the thrombosis does not fill the entire lumen of the common femoral vein at the saphenofemoral junction, the anticoagulation with low-molecular-weight heparin and weekly repeat ultrasound is the treatment of choice. The heparin is continued until the thrombus retracts and the entire lumen of the femoral vein is clear. If the thrombus fills the lumen of the femoral vein, 3 months of anticoagulation is generally recommended.[47] Paresthesias are uncommon, but ablation of the below-knee saphenous vein should be avoided to prevent saphenous nerve injury; and ablation of the SSV below mid-calf should be avoided to prevent sural nerve injury.

Sclerotherapy

Sclerotherapy, either liquid or foam, is another available modality to treat axial reflux. Typically, a foam sclerosant is used for the larger axial veins, because this provides for improved contact of the sclerosant to the vein wall for a longer period of time, which allows for more effective treatment.[41] There is no currently Food and Drug Administration (FDA)-approved foam sclerosant available in the United States, and the creation of a foam from one of the FDA-approved liquid sclerosants generates a novel drug preparation in the eyes of the FDA and is not approved.

To perform sclerotherapy of the major axial veins, the patient is placed in Trendelenburg position, and the vein to be treated is accessed under ultrasound guidance. Generally, 5 cm^3 or less of sclerosant is injected while firm pressure is applied to the saphenofemoral junction with the ultrasound probe to occlude the common femoral vein. The extremity is then elevated to 45° and an additional 3 mL of sclerosant injected to fill the incompetent veins distally. Competent valves should prevent migration of the foam into the deep system. At the conclusion of the procedure, duplex ultrasonography interrogation of the deep system is required to evaluate for migration of foam. If foam bubbles are found within the deep system, aggressive ankle flexion-extension maneuvers dissipate the foam.[41]

The results of foam sclerotherapy have generally not been as good as with thermal ablation, resulting in a successful occlusion rate of 77% at 3 years.[46]

Complications of foam sclerotherapy include[31,48]

- Transient visual disturbances (<2%)
- Headache (<2%)
- DVT (<1%)
- Superficial thrombophlebitis (<1%)
- Skin discoloration/staining (1%–30%)
- Skin necrosis (<0.1%)
- Anaphylaxis (<0.01%)

Stroke has been reported in the literature after foam sclerotherapy, but this is rare.[49]

High ligation and stripping

High ligation and stripping, which has been the standard of care for great and small saphenous insufficiency for more than 100 years, has been largely replaced with less invasive techniques. In general, the results of surgical therapy are comparable to thermal ablation, but the complication rate is higher, as is the amount of postoperative pain and recovery time.[31] There are still times, however, when surgical stripping is indicated. These indications include thermal ablation or sclerotherapy failure, superficial location of the treatment vein just below the skin, large diameter of the axial vein (>1.5–2 cm), and patient preference. In general, thermal ablation is contraindicated in veins that are less than 1 cm below the skin (or those that cannot be pushed >1 cm below the skin with tumescent anesthesia) and in veins that are large.

Tributary Reflux

Most visible varicose veins are tributaries of the main axial veins. In many cases, once treatment of the larger axial veins in completed, the varicose veins regress. Only approximately 40% of patients require a second procedure to treat their varicose veins once the saphenous vein is treated.[50] Therefore, thermal ablation of the saphenous system is often completed first, and secondary procedures are performed as necessary.

There are 3 main treatments available for treatment of the remaining varicose veins:

- Microphlebectomy
- Powered phlebectomy
- Sclerotherapy

Microphlebectomy

Microphlebectomy, or ambulatory phlebectomy, is a term now generally used rather than varicose vein stripping. This refers to the removal of tributary varicosities through small incisions in the skin. This procedure has evolved significantly in the past several years. It is now generally completed in the office, under local tumescent anesthesia, and with no hospital stay. Typically, patients are awake or have light sedation. After marking the varicosities with the patient standing, the patient is placed on the bed, and the leg is prepped and draped. A small incision is made over each varix, using a small blade, such as a Beaver blade or an 11 blade, or some operators use an 18-gauge needle. A vein hook is advanced through the incision and the varix is brought out through the incision. A hemostat is placed on the varix and, with gentle retraction, the varix is removed. The skin dimpling often indicates where the next incision should be placed. Hemostasis is maintained with pressure. Once all of the varices are addressed, the incisions are reapproximated using Steri-Strips, and a dressing is placed. A compression hose or bandage is typically placed over the treatment area to maintain hemostasis.

Powered phlebectomy

Transilluminated power phlebectomy is another technique for treatment of tributary reflux. This procedure is done in the operating room under regional or general anesthetic. If the varicosities are limited, it may be done under local anesthetic with sedation. The instrumentation for powered phlebectomy includes a power unit that controls an irrigation pump and resection oscillation speeds, an illuminator hand piece, and a resector hand piece. The instruments are placed through small incisions near the veins to be removed, and the light is used to transilluminate the varicosities. Tumescent anesthetic is introduced, and the resector is used to dissect and suction out the varicosities. Small punch incisions in the skin overlying the area of treatment are placed to allow for any collected blood to be flushed out with an irrigator.

This technique allows for decreased number of incisions, but is otherwise not different in outcome from microphlebectomy.[31]

Complications of powered phlebectomy include[31]

- Ecchymosis/hematoma (5%–95%)
- Paresthesias/nerve injury (9%–39%)
- Skin perforation (1%–5%)
- Superficial thrombophlebitis (2%–10%)
- Swelling (5%–17%)
- Hyperpigmentation (1%–3%)
- DVT (1%)
- Cellulitis (1%)

Powered phlebectomy is generally reserved for those patients who have many large varicosities and in whom microphlebectomy would be long and involved.[31]

Sclerotherapy

Another method of treatment of tributary varicosities is sclerotherapy. Sclerotherapy is performed with patients supine, in Trendelenburg position. The sclerosant is drawn up in small tuberculin syringes, and a 30-gauge needle is used. Treatment should proceed from large veins to small veins, and from proximal limb to distal limb. Gentle injection is done after a flash of blood in the hub of the needle confirms that the needle is intraluminal. Typically only 1 mL or less is injected per access site. Multiple injections are generally necessary and not more than 10 to 20 injections are recommended.[31]

The operator should watch carefully for any sign of extravasation, such as a wheal or significant pain. Once the injections are completed, the patient is placed in compression hose for several days after treatment.[31]

Perforator Reflux

Incompetent perforator veins are often the cause of persistent symptoms after treatment of saphenous and tributary reflux has been treated, and isolated perforator reflux may also be responsible for venous stasis ulceration. Therefore, it is important to identify these on ultrasound and incorporate perforator treatment into the entire treatment plan. Perforator treatment is indicated in patients with persistent, severe venous insufficiency as well as those with venous stasis ulcers (C_{4-6}).[31] The most common ways to treat perforator reflux include

- Thermal ablation (laser or radiofrequency ablation)
- Ultrasound-guided sclerotherapy
- Subfascial endoscopic perforator surgery (SEPS)

Thermal ablation

Thermal ablation of incompetent perforators is similar to thermal ablation of axial veins. The perforator vein is accessed under ultrasound guidance, and the ablation catheter is advanced into the perforator and located at or just below the fascia. Tumescent anesthetic is then induced, and ablation is carried out. The outcomes of perforator ablation are promising, resulting in an up to 80% 5-year closure rate and an increased rate of ulcer healing.[51,52]

Ultrasound-guided sclerotherapy

Ultrasound-guided sclerotherapy is another minimally invasive method to treat incompetent perforators. Again, the perforator is accessed using ultrasound guidance, and the sclerosant is injected with ultrasound confirmation of intraluminal injection. The leg is elevated during injection to help decrease risk of flow into the deep system. Often foam sclerotherapy is used in these veins. Usually only 0.5 cm^3 to 1 cm^3 of sclerosant is injected. The outcome of perforator sclerotherapy is not as good as with thermal ablation, but it is technically easier to perform. This treatment results in up to 75% closure rate at 2 years.[53]

Subfascial endoscopic perforator surgery

SEPS is a more invasive method of perforator ablation, but the success rate is high and results in an 80% ulcer healing rate and a 13% 2-year ulcer recurrence rate.[31,54] This is accomplished in the operating room under regional or general anesthetic with tourniquet control of bleeding. A laparoscope is placed beneath the fascia of the medial leg, and balloon dissection and carbon dioxide insufflation are established. Paratibial fasciotomy to enter the deep posterior compartment is necessary for visualization of the medial leg perforators. The visible perforating veins are then divided, either with the harmonic scalpel or with endoscopic clips. Once completed, the leg is wrapped with a compressive bandage and patients are allowed to recover. This is typically an outpatient surgery.

Complications of SEPS include[54]

- Infection (6%)
- Hematoma (9%)
- Neuralgia (7%)
- DVT (1%)

In general, percutaneous less-invasive methods of treatment have become common, and SEPS is reserved for those with severe deep or superficial venous disease with recalcitrant ulceration.

SUMMARY

Superficial venous disease is common and can cause significant disability. Treatments have become less invasive, have lower complication rates and decreased recovery time, and are more cosmetic. Most treatments for superficial disease are carried out in the office setting, allowing for both patient and physician convenience.

REFERENCES

1. Criqui MH, Jamosmos M, Fronek A, et al. Chronic venous disease in an ethnically diverse population: the San Diego population study. Am J Epidemiol 2003;158:448–56.
2. Brand FN, Dannenberg AL, Abbott RD, et al. The epidemiology of varicose veins: the Framingham study. Am J Prev Med 1988;4:96–101.
3. Fowkes FG, Lee AJ, Evans CJ, et al. Lifestyle risk factors for lower limb venous reflux in the general population: Edinburgh vein study. Int J Epidemiol 2001;30: 846–52.
4. Caggiati A, Bergan JJ. The saphenous vein: derivation of its name and its relevant anatomy. J Vasc Surg 2002;35:172–5.
5. Lajos TZ, Espersen C. Anatomical considerations of the venous drainage of the lower extremities: clinical implications. J Surg Res 1983;34:1–6.
6. Wakefield TW, Dalsing MC. Venous Disease. In: Mulholland MW, Lillemoe KD, Doherty GM, et al, editors. Greenfield's Surgery: Scientific Principles and Practice. Philadelphia: Lippincott, Williams & Wilkins; 2011.
7. Kockaert M, de Roos KP, van Dijk L, et al. Duplications of the great saphenous vein: a definition problem and implications for therapy. Dermatol Surg 2012;38: 77–82.
8. Delis KT, Knaggs AL, Khodabkahsh P. Prevalence, anatomic patterns, valvular competence, and clinical significance of the Giacomini vein. J Vasc Surg 2004;40:1174–83.
9. van Bemmelen PS, Bedford G, Beach K, et al. Quantitative segmental evaluation of venous valvular reflux with duplex ultrasound scanning. J Vasc Surg 1989;10: 425–31.
10. Bergan JJ, Pascarella L, Schmid-Schonbein GW. Pathogenesis of primary chronic venous disease: insights from animal models of venous hypertension. J Vasc Surg 2008;47:183–92.
11. Lim CS, Davies AH. Pathogenesis of primary varicose veins. Br J Surg 2009;96: 1231–42.
12. Iannuzzi A, Panico S, Ciardullo AV, et al. Varicose veins of the lower limbs and venous capacitance in postmenopausal women: relationship with obesity. J Vasc Surg 2002;36:965–8.
13. Tanaka H, Zaima N, Yamamoto N, et al. Imaging mass spectroscopy reveals unique lipid distribution in primary varicose veins. Eur J Vasc Endovasc Surg 2010;657:657–63.
14. Tanaka H, Zaima N, Sasaki T, et al. Loss of lymphatic vessels and regional lipid accumulation is associated with great saphenous vein incompetence. J Vasc Surg 2012;55:1440–8.

15. Murphy MA, Hands L. Is arteriovenous shunting involved in the development of varicosities? A study of the intraluminal pressure and oxygen content in varicose veins. Phlebology 2008;23:137–41.

16. Cooper DG, Hillman-Cooper CS, Barker SG, et al. Primary varicose veins: the saphenofemoral junction, distribution of varicosities and pattern of incompetence. Eur J Vasc Endovasc Surg 2003;25:53–90.

17. Wong JK, Duncan JL, Nichols DM. Whole-leg duplex mapping for varicose veins: observations on patterns of reflux in recurrent and primary legs, with clinical correlation. Eur J Vasc Endovasc Surg 2003;25:267–75.

18. Elsharawy MA, Naim MM, Abdelmaguid EM, et al. Role of saphenous vein wall in the pathogenesis of primary varicose veins. Interact Cardiovasc Thorac Surg 2007;6:219–24.

19. Darvall KA, Sam RC, Adam DJ, et al. Higher prevalence of thrombophilia in patients with varicose veins and venous ulcers than controls. J Vasc Surg 2009;49: 1235–41.

20. Labropoulos N, Tiongson J, Pryor L, et al. Nonsaphenous superficial vein reflux. J Vasc Surg 2001;34:872–7.

21. O'Donnell TF Jr. Chronic venous insufficiency: an overview of epidemiology, classification, and anatomic considerations. Semin Vasc Surg 1998;1:60.

22. Eklof BG, Kistner RL, Masuda EM. Venous bypass and valve reconstruction: long-term efficacy. Vasc Med 1998;3:157–64.

23. Decousus H, Quere I, Presles E, et al. Superficial venous thrombosis and venous thromboembolism: a large, prospective epidemiologic study. Ann Intern Med 2010;152:218–24.

24. Bihari I, Muranyi A, Bihari P. Laser-doppler examination shows high flow in some common telangiectasias of the lower limb. Dermatol Surg 2005;31:388–90.

25. Kroger K, Ose C, Roesener J, et al. Symptoms individuals with small cutaneous veins. Vasc Med 2002;7:13–7.

26. Chiesa R, Marone EM, Limoni C, et al. Chronic venous disorders: correlation between visible signs, symptoms, and presence of functional disease. J Vasc Surg 2007;46:322–30.

27. Somjen GM, Ziegenbein R, Johnston AH, et al. Anatomical examination of leg telangiectasias with duplex scanning. J Dermatol Surg Oncol 1993;10: 940–5.

28. Engelhorn CA, Engelhorn AL, Cassou MF, et al. Patterns of saphenous venous reflux in women presenting with lower extremity telangiectasias. Dermatol Surg 2007;33:282–8.

29. Kistner RL, Eklof B, Masuda EM. Diagnosis of chronic venous disease of the lower extremities: the "CEAP" classification. Mayo Clin Proc 1996;71:338–45.

30. Thompson H. The surgical anatomy of the superficial and perforating veins of the lower limb. Ann R Coll Surg Engl 1979;61(3):198–205.

31. Gloviczki P, Comerota AJ, Dalsing MC, et al. The care of patients with varicose veins and associated chronic venous diseases: clinical practice guidelines of the Society for Vascular Surgery and the American Venous Forum. J Vasc Surg 2011;53:2S–48S.

32. Hamper UM, DeJong MR, Scoutt LM. Ultrasound evaluation of the lower extremity veins. Radiol Clin North Am 2007;45:525–47.

33. Rutherford RB. Noninvasive evaluation for congenital arteriovenous fistulas and malformations. Semin Vasc Surg 2012;25(1):49–57.

34. Raju S, Hollis K, Neglen P. Use of compression stockings in chronic venous disease: patient compliance and efficacy. Ann Vasc Surg 2007;21(6):790–5.

35. Navarro L, Min R, Boné C. Endovenous laser: a new minimally invasive method of treatment of varicose veins—preliminary observations using an 810mm diode laser. Dermatol Surg 2001;27:117–22.
36. Proebstle TM, Moehler T, Herdemann S. Reduced recanalization rates of the great saphenous vein after endovenous laser treatment with increased energy dosing: definition of a threshold for the endovenous fluence equivalent. J Vasc Surg 2006;44(4):834–9.
37. Min RJ, Khilnani N, Zimmet SE. Endovenous laser treatment of saphenous vein reflux: long-term results. J Vasc Interv Radiol 2003;14:991–6.
38. Marston WA, Brabham VW, Mendes R, et al. The importance of deep venous reflux velocity as a determinant of outcome in patients with combined superficial and deep venous reflux treated with endovenous saphenous ablation. J Vasc Surg 2008;48(2):400–6.
39. Merchant RF, Pinchot O. Long-term outcomes of endovenous radiofrequency obliteration of saphenous reflux as a treatment for superficial venous insufficiency. J Vasc Surg 2005;42(3):502–9.
40. Merchant RF, Pichot O, Mayers KA. Four year follow-up on endovascular radiofrequency obliteration of saphenous reflux. Dermatol Surg 2005;31:129–34.
41. Brown KR, Moore CJ. Update on the treatment of saphenous reflux: laser, RFA or foam? Perspect Vasc Surg Endovasc Ther 2009;21(4):226–31.
42. Pichot O, Kabnick LS, Creton D, et al. Duplex ultrasound scan findings two years after great saphenous vein radiofrequency endovenous obliteration. J Vasc Surg 2004;39:189–95.
43. Goode SD, Chowdhury A, Crockett M, et al. Laser and radiofrequency ablation study (LARA study): a randomised study comparing radiofrequency ablation and endovenous laser ablation (810 nm). Eur J Vasc Endovasc Surg 2010;40:246–53.
44. Rasmussen LH, Lawaetz M, Bjoern L, et al. Randomized clinical trial comparing endovenous laser ablation, radiofrequency ablation, foam sclerotherapy and surgical stripping for great saphenous varicose veins. Br J Surg 2011;98:1079–87.
45. Nordon IM, Hinchcliffe RJ, Brar R, et al. A prospective double-blind randomized controlled trial of radiofrequency versus laser treatment of the great saphenous vein in patients with varicose veins. Ann Surg 2011;254(6):876–81.
46. van den Bos R, Arends L, Kockaert M, et al. Endovenous therapies of lower extremity varicosities: a meta-analysis. J Vasc Surg 2009;49:230–9.
47. Lawrence PF, Chandra A, Wu M, et al. Classification of proximal endovenous closure levels and treatment algorithm. J Vasc Surg 2010;52(2):388–93.
48. Guex JJ, Allaert FA, Gillet JL, et al. Immediate and midterm complications of sclerotherapy: report of a prospective multicenter registry of 12,173 sclerotherapy sessions. Dermatol Surg 2005;31:123–8.
49. Forlee MV, Grouden M, Moore DJ, et al. Stroke after varicose vein foam injection sclerotherapy. J Vasc Surg 2006;43:162–4.
50. Schanzer H. Endovenous ablation plus microphlebectomy/sclerotherapy for the treatment of varicose veins: single or two-stage procedure? Vasc Endovascular Surg 2010;44(7):545–9.
51. Bacon JL, Dinneen AJ, Marsh P, et al. Five-year results of incompetent perforator vein closure using trans-luminal occlusion of perforator. Phlebology 2009;24(2):74–8.
52. Lawrence PF, Alktaifi A, Rigberg D, et al. Endovenous ablation of incompetent perforating veins is effective treatment for recalcitrant venous ulcers. J Vasc Surg 2011;54:737–42.

53. Masuda EM, Kessler DM, Lurie F, et al. The effect of ultrasousnd-guided sclerotherapy of incompetent perforator veins on venous clinical severity and disability scores. J Vasc Surg 2006;43(3):551–6.

54. Tenbrook JA Jr, Iafrati MD, O'donnell TF Jr, et al. Systematic review of outcomes after surgical management of venous disease incorporating subfascial endoscopic perforator surgery. J Vasc Surg 2004;39:583–9.

Venous Thromboembolic Disease

Pasithorn A. Suwanabol, MD, John R. Hoch, MD*

KEYWORDS

- Thromboembolism • Post-thrombotic syndrome • Thrombectomy • Thrombolysis

KEY POINTS

- Venous thromboembolic disease and its complications are a significant cause of morbidity and mortality.
- Clinical diagnosis is challenging, and providers should utilize risk assessment tools to aid in determining which patients should undergo additional imaging studies.
- The vast majority of patients with venous thromboembolism can be treated with standard therapy.
- Operative intervention should be considered in all patients with ileofemoral thrombosis who have symptoms lasting less than 14 days, low bleeding risk, and adequate life expectancy.

INTRODUCTION

Venous thromboembolic (VTE) disease is a significant cause of morbidity and mortality worldwide. Annual incidence of VTE is estimated to be as high as 1 million cases per year in the United States alone,[1] and with the increase in the elderly and obese populations, this number is expected to rise.[2] Traditionally, VTE has been treated with systemic anticoagulation, with the primary goals of preventing propagation of thrombus, development of pulmonary embolism (PE), and recurrence of VTE. However, the late manifestations of VTE, notably post-thrombotic syndrome (PTS), are being increasingly recognized. Subsequently, the management of VTE in preventing its long-term sequelae is being scrutinized. Much data exist that demonstrate the ineffectiveness of conventional anticoagulation in preventing such sequelae. As such, there has been an effort to evaluate the use of catheter-directed thrombolysis and reintroduce surgical thrombectomy for the treatment of VTE.

Simply put, thrombus develops as a result of stasis, endothelial injury, and an imbalance between the coagulation and fibrinolytic systems, collectively known as Virchow

Division of Vascular Surgery, Department of Surgery, University of Wisconsin School of Medicine and Public Health, 600 Highland Avenue, Madison, WI 53792, USA
* Corresponding author. BX7375 Clinical Science Center – H4, 600 Highland Avenue, Madison, WI 53792-3284.
E-mail address: hoch@surgery.wisc.edu

Surg Clin N Am 93 (2013) 983–995
http://dx.doi.org/10.1016/j.suc.2013.05.003
0039-6109/13/$ – see front matter © 2013 Elsevier Inc. All rights reserved.

triad.[3] Emerging data have demonstrated that the development of VTE is much more complex; however, the exact mechanisms are far beyond the scope of this article. Despite this complexity, it should be recognized that the vast majority of VTE is preventable, and early recognition is essential for good patient outcomes.

PTS is a common finding following VTE; the incidence of PTS is as high as 50% in patients with ileofemoral deep vein thrombosis (DVT) who are treated with anticoagulation alone.[2,4,5] Risk factors for the development of PTS are proximal vein involvement, thrombus extent, history of ipsilateral thrombosis, obesity, advanced age, and female sex.[3,6,7] PTS develops in part as a result of thrombotic damage to venous valves causing valvular incompetency or reflux. The combination of reflux coupled with possible residual thrombotic obstruction causes venous hypertension in the limb, leading to symptoms of PTS. This is manifested as chronic pain in the form of aching, swelling, fatigue, and paresthesias. Additionally, skin changes can result in chronic dermatitis or at its most severe, ulceration.[1,2,5] Patients with PTS have been found to demonstrate quality of life measures as low as those with other chronic diseases such as diabetes or congestive heart failure.[1,2,4,5] In addition to the adverse effects on quality of life, the burden on health care costs as a result of PTS is substantial. In the United States alone, it is estimated that annual cost of VTE diagnosis and treatment may exceed $3.2 to $15.5 billion, and this does not include the cost of its complications such as PTS or that of society.[8,9]

CLINICAL PRESENTATION

Clinical diagnosis of VTE is incredibly challenging due to the lack of sensitive or specific physical examination findings; only half of patients present with the classic findings of pain, swelling, and tenderness.[10,11] In fact, the most current American College of Chest Physicians evidence-based clinical practice guidelines (CHEST guidelines) argue for the use of objective testing for DVT given the unreliability of clinical assessment as well as the consequences of missed diagnosis.[12] Nonetheless, a comprehensive history and physical examination are critical in the initial evaluation of a patient with suspected VTE. Additionally, risk factors can be identified at this time, which may aid in determining which patients should be evaluated further. Known risk factors of VTE include advanced age, malignancy, history of VTE, pregnancy, obesity, tobacco use, and acute medical illness or surgery (**Fig. 1**).[13–15]

DIAGNOSTIC PROCEDURES

An essential tool in predicting the pretest probability of VTE is the Wells model, which stratifies patients as having low, moderate or high probability of DVT based on signs and symptoms as well as risk factors (see **Fig. 1**).[10,12,16] The prevalence rates of having DVT within each group are 5% (95% confidence interval [CI], 4%–8%), 17% (95% CI, 13%–23%), and 53% (95% CI, 44%–61%), respectively based on validation (see **Fig. 1**).[12,16,17]

Using a D-dimer assay as a screening tool is helpful but not always reliable in diagnosing DVT, as this degradation product of cross-linked fibrin is often elevated in surgical patients as well as those with infection, atrial fibrillation, and pregnancy.[12] Thus, D-dimer may be sensitive in diagnosing VTE, but it is not specific. It is worthwhile mentioning that there are variations in D-dimer assays available, with the most sensitive tests being the enzyme-linked immunosorbent assays (ELISAs) (sensitivity 94%, 95% CI, 89%–95%) and the latex semiquantitative assays (sensitivity 85%, 95% CI, 68%–93%). The whole-blood D-dimer assay is the most specific (specificity 71%, 95% CI, 57%–83%).[12,18]

- Active cancer (treatment within 6 months or palliation) → + 1 point
- Paralysis, paresis, or recent immobilization of lower extremity → + 1 point
- Bedridden for > 3 days or major surgery within past 4 weeks → + 1 point
- Localized tenderness along distribution of deep veins → + 1 point
- Entire leg swollen → + 1 point
- Unilateral calf swelling with > 3 cm difference from unaffected calf (below tibial tuberosity) → + 1 point
- Pitting edema confined to symptomatic leg → + 1 point
- Collateral superficial veins (non-varicose) → + 1 point
- Alternative diagnosis as likely as or more likely than DVT → - 2 points

Score (total points): _____

Clinical Risk Score Interpretation (probability of DVT):

>/= 3 points	High clinical probability (75%)
1-2 points	Moderate clinical probability (17%)
< 1 point	Low clinical probability (3%)

Fig. 1. Wells clinical Prediction rule for DVT. (*Adapted from* Wells PS, Anderson DR, Bormanis J, et al. Value of assessment of pretest probability of deep-vein thrombosis in clinical management. Lancet 1997;350(9094):1795–8; with permission.)

Doppler ultrasonography (DUS) is typically the first and most frequently used imaging modality. Although DUS is widely available, inexpensive, and noninvasive, its interpretation is subject to variability within and between patients and operators.[19] Diagnosis is based on the ability to visualize thrombus, noncompressibility of the vein(s), and abnormal blood flow patterns.[20,21] Mean sensitivity and specificity of venous ultrasonography for diagnosis of symptomatic proximal DVT are 97% and 94%, respectively.[22] The sensitivity and specificity of detecting distal DVT such as tibial vein exceeds 90% in technically adequate studies.[23]

The authors utilize the algorithm in **Fig. 2** based largely on the most recent CHEST guidelines.[12,24] Briefly, in those with suspected DVT, a D-dimer is obtained, and the Wells Clinical Risk Score is calculated. In those patients with low clinical probability and negative D-dimer, DVT can be excluded. In those with low clinical probability but positive D-dimer, the authors perform duplex ultrasound. Patients who have a moderate-to-high clinical probability of DVT, regardless of D-dimer status, should undergo DUS evaluation. If DUS is unavailable, one should initiate systemic anticoagulation if the clinical suspicion is high and the patient carries a low risk of bleeding complications. This is because the risk of bleeding in such patients is low, while the complications and cost of delayed diagnosis are not considered acceptable.[24]

If there is uncertainty in the diagnosis or extent of disease, further imaging should be performed with computed tomography (CT) or magnetic resonance imaging (MRI). CT and MRI both have sensitivities and specificities for detection of VTE greater than 95%, and allow for the visualization of deeper structures such as the inferior vena cava (IVC) or pelvic veins.[10,19] CT can also identify extrinsic compression but requires the use of intravenous iodinated contrast agent and exposure to radiation. MRI has the ability to differentiate between acute and chronic thrombus, and detects movement of blood. However, MRI is time-consuming and expensive.[10,12,19]

In those found to have VTE, determining full extent of thrombus and detecting the presence of PE are necessary, as is identifying any potential underlying etiologies. Those who require additional laboratory testing to evaluate underlying etiologies

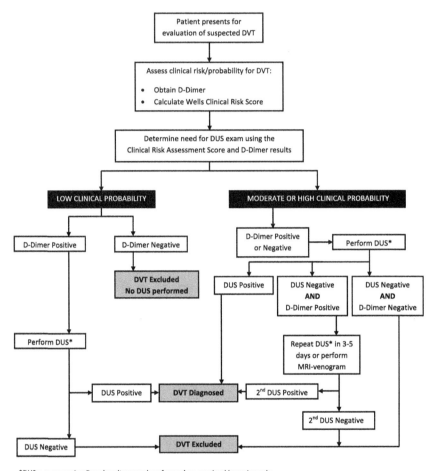

Fig. 2. University of Wisconsin algorithm for DUS evaluation of suspected DVT.

include individuals younger than 50 years and those without risk factors for VTE, family history of thromboembolic disorders, unusual thrombus location, or history of recurrent DVT.[20,24] Laboratory studies of fibrinogen, antithrombin III, proteins C and S, factor V Leiden, prothrombin gene mutation, antiphospholipid/anticardiolipin antibody, factor VIII levels, and homocysteine should be obtained. Hematology consultation is recommended in those with positive laboratory findings, those with unprovoked DVT, or those without risk factors.[12]

Contrast venography is considered the gold standard in the diagnosis of VTE. However, challenges in technique, interpretation, and invasive nature have helped drive the development of noninvasive diagnostic imaging modalities.[12] This technique is performed by injecting contrast into the dorsal foot vein and imaging the lower extremity venous system using fluoroscopy. This allows for visualization of a filling defect suggestive, but not diagnostic, for DVT. Advantages of contrast venography are high sensitivity and specificity, and the ability to perform therapeutic maneuvers. Disadvantages to contrast venography are the expense, lack of availability in some centers, and its limited use in patients with renal insufficiency and/or allergies to contrast agents. Thus, contrast venography is not routinely used and is reserved for patients in whom other imaging modalities cannot definitively make the diagnosis, or for therapeutic interventions.[12,19]

PREVENTION

Although as many as 64% of surgical patients are at risk for developing venous thromboembolism, only 59% of these patients receive thromboprophylaxis.[25] Individual risk assessment for the development of venous thromboembolism for both surgical and nonsurgical patients can be achieved by utilizing the Caprini Risk Assessment Model (RAM), which has been validated in a large retrospective trial of general, vascular, and urological surgery patients (**Fig. 3**). Based on this score, risk of VTE can be estimated, and appropriate prophylaxis can be initiated.[15,26] The most current CHEST guidelines have made recommendations with regard to the Caprini score (**Table 1**).[13]

1 Point

    Age 41-60 years
    Procedure with local anesthesia
    Prior major surgery (< 1 month)
    History of inflammatory bowel disease
    Obesity (BMI > 25 kg/m^2)
    Acute myocardial infarction (< 1 month)
    Heart failure exacerbation (< 1 month)
    Swollen legs/Varicose veins (current)
    Sepsis (< 1 month)
    Serious lung disease (< 1 month)

1 Point (women only)

    Oral contraceptives or hormone replacement therapy
    Pregnancy or postpartum (< 1 month)
    History of unexplained stillborn infant, spontaneous abortion (>/= 3), premature birth with toxemia or growth restricted infant

2 Points

    Age 61-74 years
    History of malignancy
    Major surgery > 45 minutes
    Central venous access
    Laparoscopic surgery > 45 minutes
    Arthroscopic surgery
    Immobility > 72 hours
    Leg plaster cast or brace
    Morbid obesity (BMI 40-49 kg/m^2)

3 Points

    Age > 75 years
    History of SVT, DVT/PE
    Present cancer or chemotherapy
    Family history of thrombosis
    Established thrombophilia

5 Points

    Elective major lower extremity arthroplasty
    Hip, pelvis or leg fracture (< 1 month)
    Stroke (< 1 month)
    Multiple trauma (< 1 month)
    Acute spinal cord injury (< 1 month)

Check all that apply and add for total risk score.

Total Risk Factor Score: _____

Recommended prophylaxis regimen:

Total Risk Factor Score	Risk Level	Prophylaxis Regimen
0-1	Very low	No specific measures, early and frequent ambulation
2	Low	Sequential compression devices
3-4	Moderate	Pharmacologic agent (heparin or enoxaparin)
5 or more	High	Pharmacologic agent (heparin or enoxaparin) AND sequential compression devices
> 2	High BLEED risk	Sequential compression devices

Fig. 3. Venous thromboembolism risk assessment. (*Adapted from* Caprini JA, Arcelus JI, Reyna JJ. Effective risk stratification of surgical and nonsurgical patients for venous thromboembolic disease. Semin Hematol 2001;38(2 Suppl 5):12–9; with permission.)

Table 1
VTE prophylaxis in nonorthopedic surgery patients

Risk of Symptomatic VTE	Caprini Score	Risk of Major Bleeding Complications	
		Average Risk (1%)	High Risk (2%)
Very low (<0.5%)	0	No specific prophylaxis	
Low (1.5%)	1–2	Mechanical prophylaxis, preferably with IPC	
Moderate (3%)	3–4	LDUH, LMMH, or mechanical prophylaxis, preferably with IPC	Mechanical prophylaxis, preferably with IPC
High (6%)	≥5	LDUH or LMWH plus mechanical prophylaxis with ES or IPC	Mechanical prophylaxis, preferably with IPC, until risk of bleeding diminishes and pharmacologic prophylaxis can be added
High-risk cancer surgery	≥5	LDUH or LMWH plus mechanical prophylaxis with ES or IPC and extended duration prophylaxis with LMWH after discharge	Mechanical prophylaxis, preferably with IPC, until risk of bleeding diminishes and pharmacologic prophylaxis can be added
High risk, LDUH and LMWH contraindicated or not available	≥5	Fondaparinux or low-dose aspirin (160 mg); mechanical prophylaxis, preferably with IPC; or both	Mechanical prophylaxis, preferably with IPC, until risk of bleeding diminishes and pharmacologic prophylaxis can be added

Abbreviations: ES, elastic stockings; IPC, intermittent pneumatic compression; LDUH, low-dose unfractionated heparin; LMWH, low molecular weight heparin.

Data from Gould MK, Garcia DA, Wren SM, et al. Prevention of VTE in nonorthopedic surgical patients: antithrombotic therapy and prevention of thrombosis, 9th edition. American College of Chest Physicians evidence-based clinical practice guidelines. Chest 2012;141(Suppl 2):e227S–77S.

TREATMENT
Nonoperative Therapy

Current CHEST guidelines advocate the use of anticoagulation without operative intervention in patients with acute proximal DVT, superficial vein thrombosis greater than 5 cm in length, or in symptomatic or clinically significant hepatic vein thrombosis. Removal of catheters associated with upper extremity DVT is not necessary if the catheter is functional or needed.[12]

Patients with acute isolated distal (peroneal, anterior tibial, and posterior tibial veins) DVT without severe symptoms may be managed with 2 weeks of serial imaging and no anticoagulation if the thrombus does not demonstrate extension. Approximately 15% of symptomatic distal DVT extends proximally to the popliteal veins if untreated, although this rarely occurs beyond the first 2 weeks.[12,27–30] Those identified to be most at risk of extension include thrombus greater than 5 cm in length or greater than 7 mm in diameter, multiple vein involvement, no identifiable provoking factor, history of malignancy, history of VTE, and inpatient status.[12,18,28–31]

Conventional treatment of venous thromboembolism consists of an initial systemic anticoagulant such as intravenous unfractionated heparin, low molecular weight heparin, or fondaparinux. This is then followed by 3 to 6 months of systemic anticoagulation with an oral vitamin K antagonist (VKA) and a goal therapeutic range of 2.0 to 3.0 international normalized ratio (INR). Those requiring extended anticoagulation include those with unprovoked and/or proximal VTE or those with malignancy, as long as they have a low risk of bleeding. Serial assessments are necessary to follow prolonged anticoagulant use. Early ambulation and the use of graduated compression hose (30–40 mm Hg) are essential.[24]

The unstable nature of VKA and its need for frequent monitoring have led to the development of novel oral anticoagulants: rivaroxaban and dabigatran. Rivaroxaban directly inhibits factor Xa, whereas dabigatran directly inhibits thrombin. Both anticoagulants have demonstrated more predictable pharmacokinetic and pharmacodynamic profiles and require less frequent monitoring. However, reversal of both agents is challenging, with hemodialysis being the only effective method of removing and thus reversing dabigatran, and prothrombin complex concentrate only recently demonstrating potential for reversal of both.[32–34] Both rivaroxaban and dabigatran have been tested in phase 3 clinical trials that have demonstrated safety and at least noninferiority when compared with warfarin in the treatment of VTE.[35,36] Currently, the US Food and Drug Administration has approved the use of rivaroxaban for DVT prophylaxis. Dabigatran has been used off-label for thromboprophylaxis.

Operative Therapy

Evidence has suggested that reducing clot burden improves both the short- and long-term outcomes in patients with VTE disease. Residual thrombus is associated with an increased risk of recurrence,[3,37–39] and PTS syndrome is known to develop in veins with residual thrombus.[40] Additionally, rapid thrombus clearance is correlated with decreased valve reflux.[41–43] This is thought to be a result of decreased venous hypertension as well as newer thrombus being more responsive to thrombolytic therapy. Therefore, prompt and complete removal of clot has been strongly advocated by some groups to provide early restoration of vein patency and prevent valve dysfunction.[3,5,6,44] Currently, there is no evidence to support an exact time frame for initiation of therapy.

Although standard anticoagulation therapy achieves the goal of preventing clot propagation, recurrence, and the development of PE, alone it has been found to be ineffective at completely reducing clot burden. It has been argued that acute proximal DVT requires more aggressive therapy, and because 80% of symptomatic DVTs affect the popliteal and more proximal veins, invasive interventions are more feasible.[45,46] Thus, the use of operative intervention in addition to conventional treatment has been endorsed by many. In a systematic review and meta-analysis performed by Casey and colleagues,[5] the authors found that both thrombectomy and catheter-directed thrombolysis (CDT) were associated with a decrease in PTS (95% CI), venous reflux (95% CI), and obstruction (95% CI) when compared with systemic anticoagulation alone.

Open thrombectomy

Poor initial outcomes, advances in endovascular interventions, and the perception that specialized centers and/or surgeons are required have made open surgical thrombectomy a seldom-utilized technique.[1,47–49] Nonetheless, the technique should be understood and mastered, as it can be used in conjunction with minimally invasive techniques as well as in those with contraindications to thrombolytic therapy.

Modern open thrombectomy has been found to be effective in thrombus removal, with up to 75% patency at 60-month follow-up. Additionally, contemporary thrombectomy has been associated with very low morbidity and mortality.[50] However, few reports exist, and these are primarily single-center experiences with few patients. A prospective randomized study out of Sweden published in 1997 demonstrated that patients who underwent thrombectomy compared with standard anticoagulation alone trended toward less severe sequelae such as leg swelling and ulceration.[51] A retrospective review of data from the American College of Surgeons National Surgical Quality Improvement Program (ACS NSQIP) has demonstrated that thrombectomy is indeed infrequently utilized. However, the authors report an associated 30-day morbidity rate of 25% and a mortality rate of 8.8%. Despite this, the authors acknowledge that the patients undergoing thrombectomy versus CDT or systemic anticoagulation alone are likely to have more significant comorbidities, and when CDT fails or there are contraindications to CDT, thrombectomy remains a viable option.[1]

Briefly, the technique involves making a longitudinal incision over the femoral vein, creating a venotomy, elevating and wrapping the affected limb with an Esmark bandage, and manually compressing the limb to milk the thrombus proximally. Incomplete removal of thrombus can be remedied by passing a #3 or #4 Fogerty balloon catheter into a venotomy created in the posterior tibial vein and advanced proximally. The infrainguinal venous system of the affected limb is then perfused with recombinant tissue plasminogen activator. Completion venography is then performed, and the venotomies are closed with fine monofilament suture.[52] Patients are then transitioned from systemic anticoagulation to oral vitamin K antagonist for 3 to 6 months, and a minimum of 2 years of graduated compression.

Catheter-directed thrombolysis

Systemic thrombolysis for the treatment of VTE disease has been examined in multiple trials. A Cochrane review has demonstrated that thrombolysis (mainly systemic) has demonstrated enhanced clot lysis and a reduction in the incidence of PTS when compared with standard anticoagulation alone.[2,53] However, the high risk of serious bleeding complications with systemic thrombolysis was found to be unacceptable,[2,54–56] and additional studies have demonstrated that lysis is incomplete.[6,57,58]

Catheter-directed thrombolysis provides localized delivery of thrombolytic agents that is more concentrated yet provides an overall lower systemic dose. This has been found to be a more effective method of reducing clot burden while at the same time decreasing risk of bleeding complications such as intracranial hemorrhage (<1%), retroperitoneal hematoma (1%), and musculoskeletal, urogenital, and gastrointestinal bleeds (3% combined). Success rates as defined by vein patency and preservation of valve function have been reported to be as high as 80% to 90%, with bleeding complications of approximately 5% to 10%.[59]

Most bleeding complications are minor and associated with the venous access site.[52] Additional reported disadvantages to CDT include long duration of infusion times of 1 to 3 days, its high cost, and its lack of being widely available. A small but significant risk of PE following CDT exists,[2,60,61] with some authors advocating the use of IVC filters (IVCFs) in a select group of patients.[52] Current CHEST guidelines recommend IVCF placement only in those who have contraindications to anticoagulation, and that anticoagulation should be initiated once bleeding resolves.[12]

The Catheter-directed Venous Thrombolysis (CaVenT) study represented 1 of the first randomized controlled trials that demonstrated the safety and efficacy of CDT compared with standard treatment alone in patients with acute ileofemoral DVT. At 6-month follow-up, 64% of patients who had undergone CDT demonstrated iliofemoral patency by DUS and air-plethysmography versus 35.8% of patients treated with standard anticoagulation alone. Ten of the 49 patients who underwent CDT had bleeding complications, with major bleeding in 2 patients.[62] A follow-up study at 24 months demonstrated an absolute risk reduction (14.4%) for the development of PTS in patients treated with anticoagulation and CDT compared with anticoagulation alone.[45]

A current trial in progress, Thrombus Obliteration by Rapid Percutaneous Endo-vascular Intervention in Deep Venous Occlusion (TORPEDO), aims to evaluate the superiority of endovascular intervention over anticoagulation alone. Midterm results recently published demonstrate a decrease in recurrent VTE (2.3% vs 14.8%, $P = .003$) as well as PTS (3.4% vs 27.2%, $P<.001$) in patients undergoing CDT at 6-month follow-up.[63,64]

Finally, the acute venous thrombosis: thrombus removal with adjunctive catheter-directed thrombolysis (ATTRACT) trial is a randomized controlled trial funded by the National Heart Lung and Blood Institute (NHLBI)/National Institutes of Health (NIH) currently open for enrollment. Its primary goal is determining whether the addition of CDT as an adjunct to standard anticoagulation reduces PTS by one-third over a 2-year follow-up period. The study will also provide information related to quality of life and cost-effectiveness analysis. It has the potential to completely transform the standard of care in those with acute ileofemoral DVT.[65]

CLINICAL PRACTICE GUIDELINES

Based in large part by the previously mentioned systematic review and meta-analysis performed by Casey and colleagues, the Society of Vascular Surgery and the American Venous Forum developed practice guidelines for early thrombus removal for acute ileofemoral DVT. Grade 1 recommendations demonstrate the highest level of confidence that the intervention will provide more benefit than harm. Grade A recommendations designate the highest level of evidence such as randomized trials. In summary, early thrombus removal is suggested in those with first acute ileofemoral DVT with symptoms less than 14 days and low bleeding risk (Grade 2C), and those with limb-threatening venous ischemia (Grade 1A). Percutaneous catheter-based techniques are suggested for these patients (Grade 2C), and open thrombectomy for those in whom thrombolytic therapy is contraindicated (Grade 2C).[6]

THE UNIVERSITY OF WISCONSIN EXPERIENCE

In the authors' practice, if there is a high level of clinical suspicion, parenteral unfractionated heparin is initiated. The authors then proceed with duplex ultrasound, and once the diagnosis has been made, if the extent of thrombus cannot be clearly delineated, adjunctive imaging is performed with computed tomography venogram (CTV) or magnetic resonance venogram (MRV). The authors advocate for early thrombus removal in patients with ileofemoral thrombosis who have: symptoms lasting less than 14 days, low bleeding risk, and adequate life expectancy. Catheter-directed thrombolysis is the authors' first-line technique for thrombus extraction. If patients have a contraindication to thrombolysis, the authors then elect to perform open thrombectomy. Following initiation of CDT, serial and completion venographies are performed. Adjunctive procedures such as ultrasound acceleration or pharmacomechanical thrombolysis are used at the discretion of the surgeon. These procedures have been argued to further reduce the dose of thrombolytic used as well as infusion time.[12,24,66] Iliac vein stent placement is used in those with external venous compression such as in those with May-Thurner[67] or when there is a residual venous stenosis greater than 50%. After the procedure, patients are transitioned to oral anticoagulation with VKA. Early ambulation and graduated compression stockings are also used consistently in the authors' practice. The authors do not routinely place IVCF with the exception of thrombus that extends into the inferior vena cava. Although current CHEST guidelines do not advocate the widespread use of CDT, they do recognize that certain patient populations may benefit, including those with ileofemoral DVT and those who value the prevention of PTS.

SUMMARY

Thromboembolic disease is the third most common vascular disease following coronary artery disease and cerebrovascular disease,[2] with 1 in 20 Americans developing acute venous thromboembolism at some point in their lives.[68] Conventional treatment with anticoagulation alone aims to impede the progression of thrombus and prevent recurrence and the development of PE. This is appropriate for the majority of patients. However, in certain patient populations, this alone does not address the long-term complications of VTE, namely PTS and skin ulcerations that bring a tremendous financial and personal burden. Surgeons should be familiar with the surgical techniques that have been demonstrated to improve outcomes with low risk. Recent studies of catheter-directed thrombolysis have demonstrated its safety, efficacy, and possibly the superiority over standard treatment alone. Ongoing studies may ultimately determine the standard by which VTE disease is treated in the future.

REFERENCES

1. Davenport DL, Xenos ES. Early outcomes and risk factors in venous thrombectomy: an analysis of the American College of Surgeons NSQIP dataset. Vasc Endovascular Surg 2011;45(4):325–8.
2. Patterson BO, Hinchliffe R, Loftus IM, et al. Indications for catheter-directed thrombolysis in the management of acute proximal deep venous thrombosis. Arterioscler Thromb Vasc Biol 2010;30(4):669–74.
3. Popuri RK, Vedantham S. The role of thrombolysis in the clinical management of deep vein thrombosis. Arterioscler Thromb Vasc Biol 2011;31(3):479–84.
4. Kahn SR, Ginsberg JS. The post-thrombotic syndrome: current knowledge, controversies, and directions for future research. Blood Rev 2002;16(3):155–65.
5. Casey ET, Murad MH, Zumaeta-Garcia M, et al. Treatment of acute iliofemoral deep vein thrombosis. J Vasc Surg 2012;55(5):1463–73.
6. Meissner MH, Gloviczki P, Comerota AJ, et al. Early thrombus removal strategies for acute deep venous thrombosis: clinical practice guidelines of the Society for Vascular Surgery and the American Venous Forum. J Vasc Surg 2012;55(5): 1449–62.
7. Kahn SR, Shrier I, Julian JA, et al. Determinants and time course of the post-thrombotic syndrome after acute deep venous thrombosis. Ann Intern Med 2008;149(10):698–707.
8. Mahan CE, Holdsworth MT, Welch SM, et al. Deep-vein thrombosis: a United States cost model for a preventable and costly adverse event. Thromb Haemost 2011;106(3):405–15.
9. Cundiff DK. Anticoagulation therapy for venous thromboembolism. MedGenMed 2004;6(3):5.
10. Bounameaux H, Perrier A, Righini M. Diagnosis of venous thromboembolism: an update. Vasc Med 2010;15(5):399–406.
11. Hildner FJ, Ormond RS. Accuracy of the clinical diagnosis of pulmonary embolism. JAMA 1967;202(7):567–70.
12. Bates SM, Jaeschke R, Stevens SM, et al. Diagnosis of DVT: antithrombotic therapy and prevention of thrombosis, 9th edition. American College of Chest Physicians evidence-based clinical practice guidelines. Chest 2012;141(Suppl 2): e351S–418S.

13. Gould MK, Garcia DA, Wren SM, et al. Prevention of VTE in nonorthopedic surgical patients: antithrombotic therapy and prevention of thrombosis, 9th edition. American College of Chest Physicians evidence-based clinical practice guidelines. Chest 2012;141(Suppl 2):e227S–77S.
14. Gangireddy C, Rectenwald JR, Upchurch GR, et al. Risk factors and clinical impact of postoperative symptomatic venous thromboembolism. J Vasc Surg 2007;45(2):335–41 [discussion: 341–2].
15. Caprini JA, Arcelus JI, Reyna JJ. Effective risk stratification of surgical and nonsurgical patients for venous thromboembolic disease. Semin Hematol 2001;38(2 Suppl 5):12–9.
16. Wells PS, Anderson DR, Bormanis J, et al. Value of assessment of pretest probability of deep-vein thrombosis in clinical management. Lancet 1997;350(9094): 1795–8.
17. Wells PS, Owen C, Doucette S, et al. Does this patient have deep vein thrombosis? JAMA 2006;295(2):199–207.
18. Di Nisio M, Squizzato A, Rutjes AW, et al. Diagnostic accuracy of D-dimer test for exclusion of venous thromboembolism: a systematic review. J Thromb Haemost 2007;5(2):296–304.
19. Perry JT, Statler JD. Advances in vascular imaging. Surg Clin North Am 2007; 87(5):975–93.
20. Murphy EH, Ilves M, Arko FR. Endovascular interventions for deep venous thrombosis. Fischer's mastery of surgery. 6th edition. Philadelphia: Lippincott Williams & Wilkins; 2012. p. 2400–8.
21. Goldhaber SZ, Bounameaux H. Pulmonary embolism and deep vein thrombosis. Lancet 2012;379(9828):1835–46.
22. Zierler BK. Ultrasonography and diagnosis of venous thromboembolism. Circulation 2004;109(12 Suppl 1):I9–14.
23. Bradley MJ, Spencer PA, Alexander L, et al. Colour flow mapping in the diagnosis of the calf deep vein thrombosis. Clin Radiol 1993;47(6):399–402.
24. Kearon C, Akl EA, Comerota AJ, et al. Antithrombotic therapy for VTE disease: antithrombotic therapy and prevention of thrombosis, 9th edition. American College of Chest Physicians evidence-based clinical practice guidelines. Chest 2012;141(Suppl 2):e419S–94S.
25. Cohen AT, Tapson VF, Bergmann JF, et al. Venous thromboembolism risk and prophylaxis in the acute hospital care setting (ENDORSE study): a multinational cross-sectional study. Lancet 2008;371(9610):387–94.
26. Bahl V, Hu HM, Henke PK, et al. A validation study of a retrospective venous thromboembolism risk scoring method. Ann Surg 2010;251(2):344–50.
27. Bell WR, Simon TL. Current status of pulmonary thromboembolic disease: pathophysiology, diagnosis, prevention, and treatment. Am Heart J 1982;103(2): 239–62.
28. Büller HR, Ten Cate-Hoek AJ, Hoes AW, et al. Safely ruling out deep venous thrombosis in primary care. Ann Intern Med 2009;150(4):229–35.
29. Penaloza A, Laureys M, Wautrecht JC, et al. Accuracy and safety of pretest probability assessment of deep vein thrombosis by physicians in training using the explicit Wells clinical model. J Thromb Haemost 2006;4(1):278–81.
30. Oudega R, Hoes AW, Moons KG. The Wells rule does not adequately rule out deep venous thrombosis in primary care patients. Ann Intern Med 2005;143(2):100–7.
31. Kearon C, Julian JA, Newman TE, et al. Noninvasive diagnosis of deep venous thrombosis. McMaster Diagnostic Imaging Practice Guidelines Initiative. Ann Intern Med 1998;128(8):663–77.

32. Galanis T, Thomson L, Palladino M, et al. New oral anticoagulants. J Thromb Thrombolysis 2011;31(3):310–20.
33. Eerenberg ES, Kamphuisen PW, Sijpkens MK, et al. Reversal of rivaroxaban and dabigatran by prothrombin complex concentrate: a randomized, placebo-controlled, crossover study in healthy subjects. Circulation 2011;124(14):1573–9.
34. Weitz JI, Eikelboom JW, Samama MM, et al. New antithrombotic drugs: antithrombotic therapy and prevention of thrombosis, 9th edition. American College of Chest Physicians evidence-based clinical practice guidelines. Chest 2012;141(Suppl 2):e120S–51S.
35. Bauersachs R, Berkowitz SD, Brenner B, et al. Oral rivaroxaban for symptomatic venous thromboembolism. N Engl J Med 2010;363(26):2499–510.
36. Schulman S, Kearon C, Kakkar AK, et al. Dabigatran versus warfarin in the treatment of acute venous thromboembolism. N Engl J Med 2009;361(24):2342–52.
37. Hull RD, Marder VJ, Mah AF, et al. Quantitative assessment of thrombus burden predicts the outcome of treatment for venous thrombosis: a systematic review. Am J Med 2005;118(5):456–64.
38. Comerota AJ. Thrombolysis for deep venous thrombosis. J Vasc Surg 2012;55(2):607–11.
39. Aziz F, Comerota AJ. Quantity of residual thrombus after successful catheter-directed thrombolysis for iliofemoral deep venous thrombosis correlates with recurrence. Eur J Vasc Endovasc Surg 2012;44(2):210–3.
40. Prandoni P, Frulla M, Sartor D, et al. Vein abnormalities and the post-thrombotic syndrome. J Thromb Haemost 2005;3(2):401–2.
41. Meissner MH, Caps MT, Bergelin RO, et al. Propagation, rethrombosis and new thrombus formation after acute deep venous thrombosis. J Vasc Surg 1995;22(5):558–67.
42. Meissner MH, Manzo RA, Bergelin RO, et al. Deep venous insufficiency: the relationship between lysis and subsequent reflux. J Vasc Surg 1993;18(4):596–605 [discussion: 606–8].
43. Prandoni P, Lensing AW, Cogo A, et al. The long-term clinical course of acute deep venous thrombosis. Ann Intern Med 1996;125(1):1–7.
44. Comerota AJ, Throm RC, Mathias SD, et al. Catheter-directed thrombolysis for iliofemoral deep venous thrombosis improves health-related quality of life. J Vasc Surg 2000;32(1):130–7.
45. Enden T, Haig Y, Kløw NE, et al. Long-term outcome after additional catheter-directed thrombolysis versus standard treatment for acute iliofemoral deep vein thrombosis (the CaVenT study): a randomised controlled trial. Lancet 2012;379(9810):31–8.
46. Kearon C. Natural history of venous thromboembolism. Circulation 2003;107(23 Suppl 1):I22–30.
47. Comerota AJ, Gale SS. Technique of contemporary iliofemoral and infrainguinal venous thrombectomy. J Vasc Surg 2006;43(1):185–91.
48. Büller HR, Agnelli G, Hull RD, et al. Antithrombotic therapy for venous thromboembolic disease: the Seventh ACCP Conference on Antithrombotic and Thrombolytic Therapy. Chest 2004;126(Suppl 3):401S–28S.
49. Lansing AM, Davis WM. Five-year follow-up study of iliofemoral venous thrombectomy. Ann Surg 1968;168(4):620–8.
50. Lindow C, Mumme A, Asciutto G, et al. Long-term results after transfemoral venous thrombectomy for iliofemoral deep venous thrombosis. Eur J Vasc Endovasc Surg 2010;40(1):134–8.

51. Plate G, Eklöf B, Norgren L, et al. Venous thrombectomy for iliofemoral vein thrombosis—10-year results of a prospective randomised study. Eur J Vasc Endovasc Surg 1997;14(5):367–74.

52. Comerota AJ. The current role of operative venous thrombectomy in deep vein thrombosis. Semin Vasc Surg 2012;25(1):2–12.

53. Watson LI, Armon MP. Thrombolysis for acute deep vein thrombosis. Cochrane Database Syst Rev 2004;(4):CD002783.

54. Welkie JF, Comerota AJ, Katz ML, et al. Hemodynamic deterioration in chronic venous disease. J Vasc Surg 1992;16(5):733–40.

55. Kahn SR, Hirsch A, Shrier I. Effect of postthrombotic syndrome on health-related quality of life after deep venous thrombosis. Arch Intern Med 2002;162(10):1144–8.

56. Kahn SR, Ducruet T, Lamping DL, et al. Prospective evaluation of health-related quality of life in patients with deep venous thrombosis. Arch Intern Med 2005;165(10):1173–8.

57. Goldhaber SZ, Buring JE, Lipnick RJ, et al. Pooled analyses of randomized trials of streptokinase and heparin in phlebographically documented acute deep venous thrombosis. Am J Med 1984;76(3):393–7.

58. Schwieder G, Grimm W, Siemens HJ, et al. Intermittent regional therapy with rt-PA is not superior to systemic thrombolysis in deep vein thrombosis (DVT)—a German multicenter trial. Thromb Haemost 1995;74(5):1240–3.

59. Comerota AJ, Grewal N, Martinez JT, et al. Postthrombotic morbidity correlates with residual thrombus following catheter-directed thrombolysis for iliofemoral deep vein thrombosis. J Vasc Surg 2012;55(3):768–73.

60. Mewissen MW, Seabrook GR, Meissner MH, et al. Catheter-directed thrombolysis for lower extremity deep venous thrombosis: report of a national multicenter registry. Radiology 1999;211(1):39–49.

61. Bjarnason H, Kruse JR, Asinger DA, et al. Iliofemoral deep venous thrombosis: safety and efficacy outcome during 5 years of catheter-directed thrombolytic therapy. J Vasc Interv Radiol 1997;8(3):405–18.

62. Enden T, Kløw NE, Sandvik L, et al. Catheter-directed thrombolysis vs. anticoagulant therapy alone in deep vein thrombosis: results of an open randomized, controlled trial reporting on short-term patency. J Thromb Haemost 2009;7(8):1268–75.

63. Sharifi M, Mehdipour M, Bay C, et al. Endovenous therapy for deep venous thrombosis: the TORPEDO trial. Catheter Cardiovasc Interv 2010;76(3):316–25.

64. Sharifi M, Bay C, Mehdipour M, et al. Thrombus Obliteration by Rapid Percutaneous Endovenous Intervention in Deep Venous Occlusion (TORPEDO) trial: midterm results. J Endovasc Ther 2012;19(2):273–80.

65. Comerota AJ. The ATTRACT trial: rationale for early intervention for iliofemoral DVT. Perspect Vasc Surg Endovasc Ther 2009;21(4):221–4 [quiz: 224–5].

66. Jaff MR, McMurtry MS, Archer SL, et al. Management of massive and submassive pulmonary embolism, iliofemoral deep vein thrombosis, and chronic thromboembolic pulmonary hypertension: a scientific statement from the American Heart Association. Circulation 2011;123(16):1788–830.

67. Suwanabol PA, Tefera G, Schwarze ML. Syndromes associated with the deep veins: phlegmasia cerulea dolens, May-Thurner syndrome, and nutcracker syndrome. Perspect Vasc Surg Endovasc Ther 2010;22(4):223–30.

68. Goldhaber SZ. Venous thromboembolism: epidemiology and magnitude of the problem. Best Pract Res Clin Haematol 2012;25(3):235–42.

Hemodialysis Access

David A. Rose, MD[a],*, Emmanuel Sonaike, MD[b],
Kakra Hughes, MD[a]

KEYWORDS

- Hemodialysis • Arteriovenous fistula • DOQI • Complications

KEY POINTS

- The number of patients requiring dialysis is increasing, in particular those patients over the age of 75.
- The arteriovenous (AV) fistula is the preferred access for hemodialysis due to fewer complications and decreased mortality.
- A multidisciplinary approach, including access to surgeons, nephrologists, and interventionalists, is important to ensure optimal patient care.
- Access complications are common and require early recognition and treatment.
- Postoperative access surveillance is important to ensure timely diagnosis and treatment of access-related complications.
- There is a continued need for high-quality data to assist in determining the best access for each patient.

BACKGROUND

According to the United States Renal Data System, more than 106,000 patients began hemodialysis in 2009. The end-stage renal disease (ESRD) population in 2009 included 370,274 patients on hemodialysis; 27,522 on peritoneal dialysis; and 172,553 with a functioning kidney transplant. Racial and ethnic differences persist, with African Americans and Native Americans representing a higher incidence of patients with ESRD. The cost of ESRD is significant, accounting for 6% of the Medicare budget in 2009, which equated to $29 billion.[1] Complications of hemodialysis access represent a tremendous burden on patients and a significant cost to the health care system. The most rapidly growing segment of the ESRD population is those aged 75 and older. This elderly population introduces special challenges in the placement, maintenance, and management of complications of hemodialysis access.

Disclosures: None.
[a] Department of Surgery, Howard University Hospital, Howard University College of Medicine, 2041 Georgia Avenue, Northwest, Suite 4B04, Washington, DC 20060, USA; [b] Department of Surgery, Howard University Hospital, Howard University College of Medicine, 2041 Georgia Avenue, Northwest, Suite 4B17, Washington, DC 20060, USA
* Corresponding author.
E-mail address: darose@howard.edu

Surg Clin N Am 93 (2013) 997–1012
http://dx.doi.org/10.1016/j.suc.2013.05.002
0039-6109/13/$ – see front matter © 2013 Elsevier Inc. All rights reserved.

DIALYSIS OUTCOMES QUALITY INITIATIVE GUIDELINES

Hemodialysis access remains one of the most common vascular procedures in the United States performed by general, vascular, and transplant surgeons alike. Unfortunately, in many areas related to dialysis access, there is a lack of high-quality evidence to guide access surgeons.[2] In 1997, the Dialysis Outcomes Quality Initiative (DOQI) published guidelines with respect to vascular access and established national goals for the creation of AV fistulae. Several of these guidelines have been selected as clinical performance measures by regulatory agencies to drive quality improvement, and the Fistula First project most recently has been at the forefront of this effort.[3] Fistula First, recognized by the Centers for Medicare and Medicaid Services in 2005, established a goal of 66% (autogenous) AV fistula prevalent use in the United States. As of April 2012, the national rate of autogenous AV fistula prevalence was 60%.[4]

THE IDEAL HEMODIALYSIS ACCESS

In a perfect world, the best access would be long lasting, be able to deliver adequate flow rates, and have a low rate of complications. Several studies and consensus articles have documented the autogenous AV fistula as having longer patency, having fewer complications, requiring fewer interventions, and less costly than AV grafts or catheters, thus becoming the primary choice for hemodialysis access.[2,5–7] In addition, epidemiologic studies have demonstrated lower mortality rates for patients who use AV fistulae compared with patients using prosthetic grafts or catheters.[8] The role of the access surgeon is to select the proper patient and the appropriate procedure and to use sound clinical judgment to gain the best possible outcome. Ideally, patients should have a functioning autogenous access at the time of initiation of dialysis; unfortunately, the majority of patients begin dialysis with a catheter.[1]

Although this article focuses on the role of the access surgeon, what cannot be overemphasized is the critical role of the nephrologist in timely referral of patients and the multidisciplinary role of nurses, dialysis technicians, and interventionalists in the care of the access patient. Patients seen by a nephrologist are more likely to undergo access surgery before initiating dialysis and are less likely to initiate dialysis with a catheter.[1,9]

This article reviews the steps involved in providing a timely, functioning hemodialysis access and managing potential complications in a patient population typically characterized by significant comorbidities. Particular emphasis is placed on the creation of an autogenous AV fistula.

PATIENT EVALUATION
History

In preparing patients for placement of an AV access, there is no substitute for a careful history and physical examination. A history of diabetes mellitus, peripheral vascular arterial disease, and severe congestive heart failure may all increase the risk of access-related complications.[10–12] Of particular importance is a history of prior failed accesses, the presence of a pacemaker or defibrillator, peripherally inserted central catheters (PICCs), central venous lines, and multiple prior intravenous catheters.[3,12] Although the nondominant extremity is typically chosen as the first site of access placement, an adequate vein in the dominant arm in favor of a prosthetic access in the nondominant arm should not be overlooked.

Physical Examination

Arterial

The physical examination should document bilateral arm systolic pressures. The brachial, radial, and ulnar pulses are palpated, paying attention to compressibility. An Allen test is performed to document a patent palmar arch.[2,13] A calcified artery may not necessarily exclude access in that extremity but usually warrants further evaluation with duplex ultrasound and/or angiography to verify unobstructed inflow. Lower extremity femoral and distal pulses should be documented because some patients may eventually exhaust upper extremity options and require lower extremity access placement/surgery.

Venous

The forearm cephalic and basilic veins and the upper arm cephalic veins are examined typically with a tourniquet in place. The veins should be soft throughout their length. Areas of thickening are suggestive of prior phlebitis mostly from intravenous catheters. Limb edema or the presence of enlarged superficial chest wall veins suggest the presence of central venous stenosis (CVS) or occlusion, which may require venography because duplex sonography typically has limitations in imaging the subclavian and innominate veins.

Duplex ultrasound venous mapping

Although a normal clinical arterial examination (including equal arm pressures) may not require any further preoperative evaluation of the arterial system, the presence of obesity, multiple prior catheterizations, and an inability to visualize the deep veins often prevents an adequate clinical venous examination. Thus, the duplex ultrasound has become an integral part of the venous evaluation of the hemodialysis access patient. Duplex sonography determines the presence and size of veins not visible on clinical examination, in particular the upper arm basilic vein that lies deep to the fascia. It also identifies areas of stenosis or occlusion not readily apparent on clinical examination. Studies have shown ultrasound increases the chances of placing an AV fistula.[6,14] What is considered an adequate vein diameter to create a successful AV fistula varies in the literature from 2.5 mm to 4 mm.[14,15] For patients with suspected CVS or occlusion, venography offers better visualization compared with ultrasound and may additionally also provide the opportunity to address the lesion with angioplasty and/or stenting, often at the same setting.

Patients with arterial occlusive disease presents a particular challenge not only with respect to poor inflow but also with the dilemma of using contrast dye in patients with already compromised nephrons. Options to mitigate the effects of dye include hydration, the use of bicarbonate or N-acetylcysteine, and limiting contrast.[16] Duplex ultrasound and magnetic resonance angiography without gadolinium (due to its association with nephrogenic systemic fibrosis) are other options to provide additional anatomic information, thus limiting the use of contrast. Certainly the information gained from the use of contrast must be weighed against hastening the progression to dialysis-dependent renal failure.

SURGICAL ACCESS CREATION

In preparation for placement of a patient's first access, some important guiding principles established by DOQI, as well as clinical practice guidelines developed by the Society for Vascular Surgery (SVS), are worth noting.[2,3]

- Place an autogenous fistula whenever possible.
- Begin distally in the forearm to preserve proximal sites.
- Upper extremity accesses are preferred over lower extremity.

Patients should typically be referred for hemodialysis access once a diagnosis of chronic kidney disease (CKD) stage 4 has been made with a glomerular filtration rate less than 20 mL/min to 25 mL/min or at least 6 months before anticipated dialysis. This allows sufficient time for access placement, maturation, and possible revision. If the evaluation of a patient suggests that an autogenous access is not possible, then prosthetic graft placement should be delayed until just before the need for dialysis.[2,3]

Forearm Options

Several options exist in the forearm to provide patients with an autogenous access. The DOQI guidelines recommend the first 2 of the following as preferential before proceeding to a forearm prosthetic or upper arm autogenous fistula. The SVS clinical practice guidelines suggest the use of the proximal radial artery and the forearm transposed basilic vein as options to maintain the access in the forearm.

1. Radiocephalic (wrist AV fistula) or posterior radial branch–cephalic (snuffbox AV fistula)
2. Brachiocephalic (elbow AV fistula)
3. Proximal radial artery fistula
4. Forearm transposed basilic vein fistula

The full range of options in the upper extremity is shown in **Table 1**.

A decision that has to be made frequently is the choice of access when all forearm autogenous options are exhausted. Both the DOQI and SVS guidelines suggest placing a forearm prosthetic access, thus satisfying the premise of staying distally first. It is also acceptable to move to the upper arm transposed brachial basilic vein fistula to maintain an all autogenous algorithm; this has been the preference in the authors' practice and there is support in the literature for lower complications with use of autogenous basilic vein over a forearm graft.[17] The advantage of the forearm prosthetic access first lies in the preservation of upper arm veins for future use. In addition, a functioning forearm access over time may enlarge upper arm veins that would have been borderline for use as a primary fistula. If the prosthetic forearm

Table 1		
Upper extremity autogenous arteriovenous fistula options		
Upper extremity forearm	Posterior radial branch–cephalic vein (snuffbox)	Radial artery–cephalic vein (wrist)
	Radial artery–transposed cephalic vein	Brachial/proximal radial artery–cephalic vein loop
	Radial artery–basilic vein transposition (straight or looped)	Ulnar artery–basilic vein transposition
Upper extremity upper arm	Brachial/proximal radial–cephalic direct access	Brachial–cephalic transposition
	Brachial–basilic transposition	Brachial artery–brachial vein transposition
	Proximal radial–median antebrachial/cephalic vein bidirectional flow	

Data from Sidawy AN, Spergel LM, Besarab A, et al. The Society for Vascular Surgery: clinical practice guidelines for the surgical placement and maintenance of arteriovenous hemodialysis access. J Vasc Surg 2008;48:2S–25S.

access is chosen first, it is critical to follow the patient closely to appropriately time the placement of the upper arm autogenous access and to ensure that heroic attempts at salvaging the forearm prosthetic access do not eliminate upper arm veins for future use. This may occur if stents are placed across the elbow joint, resulting in upper arm veins plagued by intimal hyperplasia and too short for easy transposition.

Upper Arm Options

With older patients presenting for hemodialysis access creation, forearm options are increasingly limited. This may be reflective of a population subjected to multiple prior hospital admissions and intravenous catheterizations: thus, the need for viable upper arm options (**Table 2**). The upper arm cephalic vein is the first choice. This vein is located superficially and lateral along the upper arm and can be anastomosed to the brachial artery just distal to the antecubital crease or to the proximal radial artery. In some cases, the vein may not reach the forearm brachial artery; in such instances, the cephalic vein can be transposed to the upper arm brachial artery. The second choice in the upper arm is the transposed basilic vein AV fistula. This vessel in its upper portion lies deep to the fascia and is usually spared from prior cannulation. The procedure may be accomplished in a 1- or a 2-staged fashion. In the former, the transposition and anastomosis are performed in a single operation, whereas in the latter, the anastomosis is done first and, after a period of vein maturation, the transposition is performed in a second operation.[18] The transposed brachial vein is also an option when the cephalic and basilic veins are not suitable. This vein is somewhat more tedious to harvest due to its location next to the brachial artery and the presence of several side branches. It has, nonetheless, been shown a viable alternative.[19] Although the saphenous and femoral veins have been described for use in the upper extremity, the authors suspect that this is not commonly undertaken and that most access surgeons move on to a prosthetic upper arm access. This is usually accomplished between the brachial artery and the basilic or axillary vein, in a straight or looped manner.

Upper extremity access sites should be exhausted before resorting to lower extremity access placement. The lower extremities are less desirable due to higher rates of infection, steal, and poorer patency.[20,21] When considering lower extremity hemodialysis access, careful attention should be paid to examination of the pulses because many of these patients may have concomitant peripheral arterial disease, and steal syndrome is of concern. For patients with prior femoral vein catheterization, a duplex ultrasound can verify patency before access placement. For the lower extremity, the more common choices are shown in **Table 3**.

Table 2
Upper extremity prosthetic access options

Upper extremity forearm	Radial to antecubital straight	Brachial-antecubital loop
Upper extremity upper arm	Brachial artery–axillary vein	
Lower extremity	Femoral artery–femoral vein loop	
Body wall	Axillary artery–axillary vein (necklace) Axillary artery–jugular vein	Axillary artery–axillary vein (loop)

Data from Sidawy AN, Spergel LM, Besarab A, et al. The Society for Vascular Surgery: clinical practice guidelines for the surgical placement and maintenance of arteriovenous hemodialysis access. J Vasc Surg 2008;48:2S–25S.

Table 3	
Lower extremity access options	
Autogenous	**Prosthetic**
Saphenous vein transposed to the superficial femoral artery	Femoral artery to femoral vein loop configuration
Femoral vein transposed to superficial femoral artery	

Data from Sidawy AN, Spergel LM, Besarab A, et al. The Society for Vascular Surgery: clinical practice guidelines for the surgical placement and maintenance of arteriovenous hemodialysis access. J Vasc Surg 2008;48:2S–25S.

Body wall access grafts are options after upper and lower extremity sites are no longer available. These include primarily the axillary artery as inflow, with the axillary vein, internal jugular, and femoral veins serving as outflow. Prior to establishing a body wall access, central venous evaluation is necessary.[22]

TECHNICAL CONSIDERATIONS

The following are technical considerations common to most hemodialysis access procedures:

- Gentle handling of tissues, minimizing trauma to artery and vein
- Use of magnifying loupes for anastomosis
- Careful creation of subcutaneous tunnels
- Vein assessment with gentle heparin distention
- Clinical assessment of patency

The following description of the transposed basilic vein AV fistula illustrates several points applicable to most dialysis access procedures. The transposed basilic vein fistula was described by Dagher and colleagues[23] in 1976 and has been shown a viable alternative to prosthetic grafts when suitable forearm veins are not available.

- The procedure may be accomplished under intravenous sedation or regional or general anesthesia.
- Almost routinely, the authors repeat the preoperative ultrasound on the table to verify the size and patency of the vein. With the patient relaxed and vasodilated, it is not unusual to occasionally find a vein of good caliber that was deemed inadequate preoperatively.
- The basilic vein may be accessed beginning in the axilla with a longitudinal incision and tracing distally along the medial aspect of the upper arm.
- Alternatively, the exposure may be done just proximal to the antecubital crease, tracing the vein proximally.
- The exposure may be accomplished with a single or skip incisions.
- Careful attention is paid to identifying and preserving the medial antebrachial cutaneous nerve, which crosses the basilic vein.
- Side branches are ligated with silk ligatures and the vein is transected distally.
- At the distal upper arm, the basilic vein normally gives off the medial antecubital branch before continuing onto the forearm. The authors generally trace the larger vessel to gain additional length.
- The basilic vein is transected distally and gently distended with heparinized saline to check for side branch leaks and reassess the size of the vessel (**Fig. 1**).

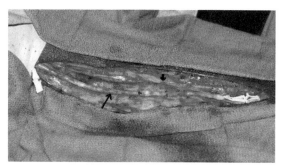

Fig. 1. Basilic vein distended (*long arrow*). Medial antebrachial cutaneous nerve (*short arrow*).

- At this point, the vein is marked to prevent twisting during the tunneling portion of the procedure.
- In the distal aspect of the incision, the brachial artery is dissected out deep to the fascia and controlled with vessel loops.
- Creation of the subcutaneous tunnel may be accomplished with several commercial devices; shown in **Fig. 2** is the Scanlan tunneling device with a 6-mm plastic sleeve. Care should be taken to ensure that the tunnel is not too deep, because this makes access difficult for dialysis nurses. It is recommended that the vein be no deeper than 6 mm from the skin surface.[14]
- Once the tunnel is created, the patient is given systemic heparin, typically 70 U/kg to 100 U/kg unfractionated heparin. The vein is pulled through the tunnel using the marked side to prevent twisting, and then it is flushed with heparinized saline, ensuring there is no resistance.
- Care should be taken to ensure there is a smooth transition between the exit point from the tunnel in the upper aspect of the arm as the vein returns to its anatomic position (the so-called swing segment), because this has been a location noted for subsequent stenosis.[24]
- The anastomosis is created in an end of vein to side of artery fashion, with a running nonabsorbable monofilament suture of 6-0 or 7-0.
- It is recommended that the anastomosis not exceed 4 mm to 6 mm to minimize occurrence of steal syndrome.[2]

Probably the best predictor of a successful anastomosis is the presence of a continuous thrill. A pulsatile fistula should prompt the surgeon to investigate for outflow

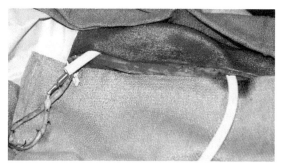

Fig. 2. A Scanlan tunneling device with a 6-mm plastic sleeve.

obstruction, which may take the form of a technical issue, such as a twist of the vein or an unrecognized CVS or occlusion.

POSTOPERATIVE SURVEILLANCE

Once the access is successfully created, the goal is to achieve functional patency defined as the ability to deliver a flow rate of at least 350 mL/min to 400 mL/min and maintaining a treatment time of less than 4 hours. The rule of 6s is helpful in this regard, referring to a fistula with a diameter of 6 mm, no deeper than 6 mm, and with a flow rate of 600 mL/min.[3,14]

Unfortunately, access failures are common with thrombosis resulting from venous anastomotic stenosis, CVS/occlusion, or poor inflow. In addition, a significant number of autogenous fistulae fail to mature to functional patency. The most sobering results came from the Dialysis Access Consortium Study Group, which was designed to study the effects of clopidogrel on early failure of dialysis fistulas. Although clopidogrel was shown to decrease the frequency of early thrombosis, the number of fistulae that were suitable for dialysis only approached 40%.[25]

Salvaging access after thrombosis is usually more difficult and costly than intervening before thrombosis and, as such, methods for detecting a failing graft are important.

Clinical Monitoring

A well-functioning autogenous fistula has a soft pulsation and a continuous low-pitched bruit and collapses with elevation of the arm.[2] In contrast, a pulsatile fistula, the presence of high-pitched bruit, prolonged bleeding after dialysis, and a fistula that does not collapse with arm elevation suggest venous outflow obstruction and access dysfunction prompting evaluation.

Measurement of Access Flow

Access blood flow is one of the best determinants of access function, with studies showing flow rates of less than 600 mL/min predictive of a significant stenosis.[26]

Static Venous Dialysis Pressures

Static venous pressures are more useful for prosthetic accesses when performed in a standardized fashion normalized for systemic blood pressure and trended over time. Prepump arterial dialysis pressures can be used to assess arterial inflow and have utility in evaluating autogenous accesses.[2,27]

Although studies have documented the ability to intervene before graft thrombosis with various surveillance methodologies and address stenotic lesions, it is unclear if this prolongs the life of the dialysis access. What is clear is that early intervention before thrombosis leads to decreased morbidity and is less costly to the health care system.[1,3,28]

MANAGEMENT OF ACCESS COMPLICATIONS
The Nonmaturing Fistula

Despite being the preferred access for hemodialysis, the AV fistula is plagued by primary failure rates, ranging from 20% to 60%.[25,29] This puts a premium on prudent decision making in the initial choice of vessels and close follow-up in the perioperative period. The ability to predict maturation of the fistula has been difficult with all of the following described in the literature as possible methods to anticipate successful access functionality.[30,31]

- Preoperative arterial and venous diameters
- Preoperative venous compliance
- Postoperative doppler blood flow

If an autogenous fistula does not show clinical signs of enlargement in the first 4 to 6 weeks, the differential diagnosis includes

- Access that is placed too deeply
- Nonligated venous side branches
- Venous stenosis
- Insufficient arterial inflow

It is not unreasonable to begin the evaluation of a nonmaturing fistula with duplex ultrasonography, which can identify the size and depth of the fistula as well as side branches and areas of stenosis. Obtaining a contrast fistulogram, however, that includes imaging of the inflow artery all the way to the central veins, provides the opportunity to diagnose and treat several of the etiologies of a failing fistula. Arterial and venous stenosis may be addressed with angioplasty; patent side branches may be coil embolized. There is support in the literature for aggressive attempts at salvaging the failing fistula, and small veins may be augmented, as described by Garcia and colleagues,[32] with balloon-assisted angioplasty, who achieved a greater than 90% salvage rate for fistulas with less than 3-mm veins.[33]

Venous Outflow Stenosis/Occlusion

Venous anastomotic stenosis

Venous anastomotic stenosis is the main cause of prosthetic graft thrombosis typically occurring in the first year. The primary cause is intimal hyperplasia. Clinical detection of venous stenosis may be difficult in that minor lesions can be asymptomatic; however, this may not be of consequence because treatment of asymptomatic stenosis has not been associated with prolonged graft survival. A pulsatile access, prolonged bleeding after decannulation, or abnormal surveillance pressures suggests outflow obstruction. Not infrequently, graft thrombosis may be the presenting symptom of an outflow venous lesion.

Management may be accomplished by endovascular or open surgery. Endovascular methods include percutaneous balloon angioplasty with or without stenting. Studies suggest that stenting may add no advantage in venous anastomotic lesions.[34,35] A recent small study demonstrated, however, improved results with nitinol stenting.[36] Surgical options include patch angioplasty of the venous anastomosis or bypass grafts.[37]

Managing the thrombosed graft requires clot removal and, most importantly, addressing the underlying culprit lesion. Endovascular methods include thrombolysis, mechanical lysis, or combination.[2] Alternatively, patients may undergo surgical thrombectomy with revision. Both are considered effective therapies for the treatment of AVG thrombosis with associated stenosis.[3,38,39]

Central venous stenosis

CVS is an important problem because recognizing its presence before access creation may prohibit the use of the ipsilateral extremity unless the lesion can be treated. CVS is associated with venous hypertension, which, in the face of a functioning access, can lead to severe edema and discoloration of the ipsilateral upper extremity and, in advanced cases, neuralgias and ulcerations of the fingertips.[40] This problem may be avoided by limiting the use of central venous catheters. When central venous access is required, the internal jugular, as opposed to the subclavian, vein is preferable.

Previous subclavian vein access is associated with a CVS or thrombosis rate of 10% to 40%.[41] In approximately 10% of cases, CVS occurs in patients who have not had previous central venous catheterization.[42] Due to limitations in physical examination and duplex ultrasound, contrast venography is required to fully evaluate the central veins. In contradistinction to venous anastomotic lesions, the literature suggests a benefit to the use of stents in the superior vena cava.[43] The use of covered stents has been safely used in the treatment of central venous lesions; however, it is unclear whether they offer a significant long-term patency advantage.[44] Surgical management may include bypass of subclavian lesions to the internal jugular vein, contralateral bypass, or atrial bypass for SVC occlusion.[45,46]

For patients with occluded central veins, the Hemodialysis Reliable Outflow vascular access device has recently become an option for maintaining an upper extremity access. The device combines a prosthetic graft combined with a catheter designed to traverse an occluded or stenotic central vein and provide atrial access.[47]

Graft Infection

Dialysis access infection has an incidence of 0.5% to 5% per year for autogenous AV fistulae and 4% to 20% per year for prosthetic AV grafts.[48] Infection ranks second only to cardiovascular disease as a cause of death for hemodialysis patients and is responsible for 20% of loss of vascular access.[49] Infection is classified as early (<30 days) and late (>30 days) after access creation. The most common organism is *Staphylococcus aureus* (accounting for 50%–70% of infections), followed by coagulase-negative staphylococci, followed by polymicrobial infections involving gram-negative organisms.[50] The pathophysiology includes uremia-induced immunologic dysfunction, characterized by impaired neutrophil chemotaxis and phagocytosis, as well as impaired lymphocyte-mediated cellular immunity.[51]

Treatment considerations for dialysis access infection include type of access (prosthetic vs autogenous), type of presentation (ie, bleeding or pus), site of infection (ie, para-anastomotic or mid-AV access), extent of infection, access patency, and bacteria etiology.

Diagnosis

Diagnosis is usually clinical with local manifestation of cellulitis, abscess, or pseudoaneurysm. Duplex imaging may be helpful in determining the extent of involvement and in distinguishing pseudoaneurysm from noninfectious perigraft fluid collections. Occasionally, indium In 111–tagged leukocyte scan may be required to diagnose subclinical infection in unexpected sites, such as abandoned grafts.[52]

Management

Autogenous AV fistulae may occasionally respond to 4 to 6 weeks of parenteral broad-spectrum antibiotics.[53] In para-anastomotic cases or in patients presenting with bleeding, sacrifice of the access is often required. In prosthetic grafts, systemic antibiotics are successful only if the infection is simple cellulitis without actual involvement of the graft. Total or subtotal graft excision is usually required for infections involving the entire graft or when there is systemic sepsis or infection caused by a virulent organism, such as *Pseudomonas*. Subtotal excision is when a small cuff of graft is left at the arterial end and oversewn, in situations when the arterial anastomosis is intact and uninfected.[54] Segmental graft excision with construction of a new jump graft through an uninfected field may be accomplished in cases of localized graft infection. When necessary, radial artery or distal brachial artery (ie, below the profunda brachii) ligation can typically be accomplished and is well tolerated in the presence of adequate collateral circulation.[48]

Noninfectious fluid collections

Noninfectious fluid collections, such as seromas, hematomas, and lymphoceles, may often be treated with observation alone and do not typically require access excision. Although interventions may occasionally be needed for these diagnoses, interventions, such as aspiration, may also lead to the introduction of infection.

Aneurysms/Pseudoaneurysms

Diffuse aneurysmal dilation of long-standing autogenous AV fistulae rarely requires intervention. The cause of these true aneurysms may involve increased venous pressure from central stenosis and immunosuppression. Indications for intervention include compromise of the overlying skin, rapid expansion, and intraluminal thrombus, leading to compromised dialysis.

Pseudoaneurysms occur in approximately 2% to 10% of polytetrafluoroethylene grafts.[53] These may be infectious or noninfectious and may be anastomotic or related to repeated puncture. Infectious pseudoaneurysms are treated as graft infections (discussed previously). A small puncture site pseudoaneurysm may be treated with observation alone, in the absence of rapid expansion. Pseudoaneurysms resulting from repeated puncture and graft material deterioration and pseudoaneurysms resulting from anastomotic disruption, however, typically require surgical revision. Segmental resection and jump graft reconstruction are often successful.[53] Endovascular grafting (ie, placement of a covered stent) provides an alternative to traditional surgical approaches for pseudoaneurysms.[55]

Arterial Steal Syndrome

Arterial steal syndrome is characterized by unilateral neurologic symptoms associated with signs of distal ischemia, such as tissue loss and cyanosis. Risk factors include female gender, diabetes mellitus, and brachial artery origin. Incidence ranges from a low of 0.25% to 2% in forearm AV access to a high of 4% to 9% in access involving the brachial artery.[56] More than half of reported cases involve diabetes mellitus and female gender. Arterial steal is more pronounced in lower extremity AV access.[57] Between half and two-thirds of patients who develop arterial steal do so less than 1 month after access construction.[58]

Differential diagnosis

Differential diagnosis includes nerve entrapment, ischemic monomelic neuropathy (IMN), regional venous hypertension, and distal arteriosclerosis (which may coexist with arterial steal syndrome). Regional venous hypertension often is characterized by associated edema and ulceration whereas IMN and nerve entrapment manifests as isolated neurologic symptoms. Patients with IMN and nerve entrapment typically have a palpable pulse distal to the access.

Management

When significant neurologic symptoms occur, prompt correction of ischemia is indicated to prevent permanent nerve injury. Patients with untreated steal can develop persistent chronic pain. Management options include banding, ligation, and revision of the arterial inflow (ie, distal revascularization and interval ligation [DRIL]).

Inflow arterial occlusive disease is more common in lower extremity AV access but can also occur in the upper extremity. Diagnosis may be made by contrast angiography, and endovascular therapeutic techniques may be used at the time of angiography.[59,60]

Simple ligation of an access is the most effective way to control access-related ischemia. The obvious disadvantage is loss of the existing access and the need to create an alternative access.

Banding of an AV access involves narrowing the venous outflow to decrease blood flow through the fistula, thus diverting more blood flow distally to the ischemic extremity. Unfortunately, the extent of banding needed to eliminate steal while maintaining continued access patency is difficult to quantify, and banding can often lead to thrombosis of the fistula, particularly for low-flow fistulae.[61]

DRIL involves a bypass from the artery proximal to the access anastomosis to the artery distally, followed by ligation of the artery distal to the AV access. DRIL led to a full resolution of ischemic symptoms in more than 80% of patients in one small study.[62,63]

Revision using distal inflow, which involves revision of the arterial inflow to a more distal site, and proximalization of the arterial inflow, which entails rerouting of the arterial inflow to a larger and more proximal site, are both described in small case series.[64,65]

Ischemic Monomelic Neuropathy

Ischemic monomelic neuropathy, although a rare occurrence, carries such devastating consequences that it is worthwhile describing. It represents a diffuse ischemic insult to the forearm nerves after creation of an AV access. The pathophysiology is not well understood. The typical presenting symptoms are severe pain and weakness of the arm and hand in the setting of palpable pulses and a warm hand. According to the DOQI guidelines, older patients with diabetes and an elbow or upper arm access are at risk for this complication. The treatment is immediate closure of the fistula/graft. Despite this, some patients may suffer permanent neurologic deficits.[66]

SUMMARY

Establishing a reliable access for patients with ESRD remains a significant challenge. The procedures offered are plagued by several access-related complications (discussed previously) and overall limited durability. Diligence is required to survey and maintain a functioning access in an aging dialysis population to prevent access thrombosis.

REFERENCES

1. US Renal Data System, USRDS 2011 Annual Data Report: Atlas of Chronic Kidney Disease and End-Stage Renal Disease in the United States, National Institutes of Health, National Institute of Diabetes and Digestive and Kidney Diseases. Bethesda (MD); 2011.
2. Sidawy AN, Spergel LM, Besarab A, et al. The Society for Vascular Surgery: clinical practice guidelines for the surgical placement and maintenance of arteriovenous hemodialysis access. J Vasc Surg 2008;48:2S–25S.
3. National Kidney Foundation. KDOQI clinical practice guidelines and clinical practice recommendations for 2006 updates: hemodialysis adequacy, peritoneal dialysis adequacy and vascular access. Am J Kidney Dis 2006;48(Suppl 1): S1–322.
4. Arteriovenous fistula first breakthrough coalition. Available at: http://www.fistulafirst.org. Accessed November 20, 2012.

5. Murad MH, Elamin MB, Sidawy AN, et al. Autogenous vs prosthetic vascular access for hemodialysis: a systematic review and meta-analysis. J Vasc Surg 2008;48(Suppl 5):34S–47S.
6. Ascher E, Gade P, Hingorani A, et al. Changes in the practice of angioaccess surgery: impact of dialysis outcome and quality initiative recommendation. J Vasc Surg 2000;31:84–92.
7. Huber T, Carter J, Carter R, et al. Patency of autogenous and polytetrfluoroethylene upper extremity arteriovenous hemodialysis accesses: a systematic review. J Vasc Surg 2003;38:1005–11.
8. Dhingra RK, Young EW, Hulbert-Shearon TE, et al. Type of vascular access and mortality in U.S. hemodialysis patients. Kidney Int 2001;60:1443–51.
9. Murad M, Sidawy A, Elamin M, et al. Timing of referral for vascular access placement: a systematic review. J Vasc Surg 2008;48:31S–3S.
10. Miller PE, Tolwani A, Luscy CP, et al. Predictors of adequacy of arteriovenous fistulas in hemodialysis patients. Kidney Int 1999;56:275–80.
11. Hakaim AG, Nalbandian M, Scott T. Superior maturation and patency of primary brachiocephalic and transposed basilic vein arteriovenous fistulae in patients with diabetes. J Vasc Surg 1998;27:154–7.
12. Hodges T, Fillinger M, Zwolok R, et al. Longitudinal comparison of dialysis access methods: risk factors for failure. J Vasc Surg 1997;26:1009–19.
13. Niyyar V, Wasse H. Vascular mapping: does it help maximize fistulae placement? Adv Chronic Kidney Dis 2009;16(5):316–20.
14. Lauvao L, Ihnat D, Goshiima K, et al. Vein diameter is the major predictor of fistula maturation. J Vasc Surg 2009;49:1499–504.
15. Silva M, Hobson R, Pappas P. A strategy for increasing use of autogenous hemodialysis access procedures: impact of preoperative noninvasive evaluation. J Vasc Surg 1998;27:302–8.
16. Merten GJ, Burgess WP, Gray LV, et al. Prevention of contrast-induced nephropathy with sodium bicarbonate. JAMA 2004;291:2328–31.
17. Keuter X, De Smet A, Kessels A, et al. A randomized multicenter study of the outcome of brachial-basilic arteriovenous fistula and prosthetic brachial-antecubital forearm loop as vascular access for hemodialysis. J Vasc Surg 2008;47:395401.
18. Arroyo M, Sideman M, Spergel L. Primary and staged transposition arteriovenous fistulas. J Vasc Surg 2008;47:1279–83.
19. Greenberg J, May S, Suliman A, et al. The brachial artery-brachial vein fistula: expanding the possibilities for autogenous fistulae. J Vasc Surg 2008;48:1245–50.
20. Geenen I, Nyilas L, Stephen M, et al. Prosthetic lower extremity hemodialysis access grafts have satisfactory patency despite a high incidence of infection. J Vasc Surg 2010;52:1546–50.
21. Cull J, Cull D, Taylor S, et al. Prosthetic thigh arteriovenous access: outcome with SVS/AAVS reporting standards. J Vasc Surg 2004;39:381–6.
22. McCann R. Axillary grafts for difficult hemodialysis access. J Vasc Surg 1996;24:457–62.
23. Dagher FJ, Gerlber RL, Ramos EJ, et al. Basilic vein to brachial artery fistula: a new access for chronic hemodialysis. South Med J 1976;69(11):1438–40.
24. Badero O, Salifu M, Wasse H, et al. Frequency of swing-segment stenosis in referred dialysis patients with angiographically documented lesions. Am J Kidney Dis 2008;51(1):93–8.

25. The Dialysis Access Consortium Study Group. Effect of clopidogrel on early failure or arteriovenous fistulas for hemodialysis. JAMA 2008;299(18):2164–71.
26. Schwab SJ, Oliver MJ, Suhocki P, et al. Hemodialysis arterio- venous access: detection of stenosis and response to treatment by vascular access blood flow. Kidney Int 2001;59:358–62.
27. Besarab A, Sullivan KL, Ross RP, et al. Utility of intra-access pressure monitoring in detecting and correcting venous outlet stenoses prior to thrombosis. Kidney Int 1995;47:1364–73.
28. Lumsden A, MacDonald M, Kikeri D, et al. Prophylactic balloon angioplasty fails to prolong the patency of expanded polytetrafluoroethylene arteriovenous grafts: results of a prospective randomized study. J Vasc Surg 1997;26:382–92.
29. Allon M, Robbin M. Increasing arteriovenous fistulas in hemodialysis patients: problems and solutions. Kidney Int 2002;62:1109–24.
30. Van der Linden J, Lameris TW, van den Meiracker AH, et al. Forearm venous distensibility predicts successful arteriovenous fistula. Am J Kidney Dis 2006;47:1013–9.
31. Wong V, Ward R, Taylor J, et al. Factors associated with early failure of arteriovenous fistulae for haemodialysis access. Eur J Vasc Endovasc Surg 1996;12:207–13.
32. Garcia L, Davila-Santini L, Feng Q, et al. Primary balloon angioplasty plus balloon angioplasty maturation to upgrade small-caliber veins (<3 mm) for arteriovenous fistulas. J Vasc Surg 2010;52:139–44.
33. Beathard G, Arnold P, Jackson J, et al. Aggressive treatment of early fistula failure. Kidney Int 2003;64:1487–94.
34. Beathard G. Gianturco self-expanding stent in the treatment of stenosis of dialysis access grafts. Kidney Int 1993;43:872–7.
35. Bakken A, Protack C, Saad W, et al. Long-term outcomes of primary angioplasty and primary stenting of central venous stenosis in hemodialysis patients. J Vasc Surg 2007;45:776–83.
36. Kakisis J, Avgerinos E, Giannakopoulos T, et al. Balloon angioplasty vs nitinol stent placement in the treatment of venous anastomotic stenosis of hemodialysis grafts after surgical thrombectomy. J Vasc Surg 2012;55:472–8.
37. Padberg F, Calligaro K, Sidawy A. Complications of arteriovenous hemodialysis access: recognition and management. J Vasc Surg 2008;48:55s–80s.
38. Dougherty M, Calligaro K, Schindler N, et al. Endovascular versus surgical treatment for thrombosed hemodialysis grafts: a prospective, randomized study. J Vasc Surg 1999;30:1016–23.
39. Marston W, Criado E, Jaques P, et al. Prospective randomized comparison of surgical versus endovascular management of thrombosed dialysis grafts. J Vasc Surg 1997;26:373–81.
40. Neville RF, Abularrage C, White P, et al. Venous hypertension associated with arteriovenous hemodialysis access. Semin Vasc Surg 2004;17:50–6.
41. Montreuil B, Leblanc M. Vascular and peritoneal access. In: Souba W, editor. ACS surgery: principles and practice. Ontario (Canada): Decker; 2007.
42. Oguzkurt L, Tercan F, Yildirim S, et al. Central venous stenosis in haemodialysis patients without a previous history of catheter placement. Eur J Radiol 2005;55:237–42.
43. Rizvi AZ, Kalra M, Bjarnason H, et al. Benign superior vena cava syndrome: stenting is now the first line of treatment. J Vasc Surg 2008;47:372–80.

44. Ayala J, Smolock C, Colvard B, et al. Efficacy of covered stent placement for central venous occlusive disease in hemodialysis patients. J Vasc Surg 2011; 54:74–9.
45. Puskas JD, Gertler JP. Internal jugular to axillary vein bypass for subclavian vein thrombosis in the setting of brachial arteriovenous fistula. J Vasc Surg 1994;19: 939–42.
46. El-Sabrout A, Duncan JM. Right atrial bypass grafting for central venous obstruction associated with dialysis access: another treatment option. J Vasc Surg 1999;29:472–8.
47. Katzman H, Mclafferty R, Ross J, et al. Initial experience and outcome of a new hemodialysis access device for catheter-dependent patients. J Vasc Surg 2009; 50:600–7.
48. Padberg FT Jr, Lee BC, Curl GR. Hemoaccess site infection. Surg Gynecol Obstet 1992;174:103–8.
49. United States Renal Data System. USRDS 2007 annual data report: atlas of chronic kidney disease and end-stage renal disease in the United States. Bethesda (MD): National Institutes of Health, National Institute of Diabetes and Digestive and Kidney Diseases; 2007.
50. Tokars JI, Miller ER, Stein G. New national surveillance system for hemodialysis associated infections: initial results. Am J Kidney Dis 2002;30:288–95.
51. Cohen G, Haag-Weber M, Horl WH. Immune dysfunction in uremia. Kidney Int Suppl 1997;62:S79–82.
52. Ayus JC, Sheikh-Hamad D. Silent infection in clotted hemodialysis access grafts. J Am Soc Nephrol 1998;9:1314–7.
53. Palder SB, Kirkman RL, Whittemore AD, et al. Vascular access for hemodialysis: patency rates and results of revision. Ann Surg 1985;202:235–9.
54. Ryan SV, Calligaro KD, Scharff J, et al. Management of infected prosthetic dialysis arteriovenous grafts. J Vasc Surg 2004;39:73–8.
55. Vesely T. Use of stent grafts to repair hemodialysis graft-related pseudoaneurysms. J Vasc Interv Radiol 2005;16:1301–7.
56. Morsy AH, Kulbaski M, Chen C, et al. Incidence and characteristics of patients with hand ischemia after a hemodialysis access procedure. J Surg Res 1998;74:8–10.
57. Tordoir JH, Dammers R, van der Sande FM. Upper extremity ischemia and hemodialysis vascular access. Eur J Vasc Endovasc Surg 2004;27:1–5.
58. Schanzer H, Skadany M, Haimov M. Treatment of angioaccess-induced ischemia by revascularization. J Vasc Surg 1992;16:861–6.
59. Guerra A, Raynaud A, Beyssen B, et al. Arterial percutaneous angioplasty in upper limbs with vascular access devices for haemodialysis. Nephrol Dial Transplant 2002;17:843–51.
60. Khan FA, Vesely TM. Arterial problems associated with dysfunctional hemodialysis grafts: evaluation of patients at high risk for arterial disease. J Vasc Interv Radiol 2002;13:1109–14.
61. Rivers SP, Scher LA, Veith FJ. Correction of steal syndrome secondary to hemodialysis access fistulas: a simplified quantitative technique. Surgery 1992;112: 593–7.
62. Schanzer H, Schwartz M, Harrington E, et al. Treatment of ischemia due to "steal" by arteriovenous fistula with distal artery ligation and revascularization. J Vasc Surg 1988;7:770–3.
63. Schanzer H, Eisenberg D. Management of steal syndrome resulting from dialysis access. Semin Vasc Surg 2004;17:45–9.

64. Minion DJ, Moore E, Endean E. Revision using distal inflow: a novel approach to dialysis-associated steal syndrome. Ann Vasc Surg 2005;19:625–8.
65. Zanow J, Kruger U, Scholz H. Proximalization of the arterial inflow: a new technique to treat access-related ischemia. J Vasc Surg 2006;43:1216–21.
66. Scher L, Shah A. Vascular access neuropathic syndrome: ischemic monomelic neuropathy. In: Wilson S, editor. Vascular access principles and practice. 5th edition. Philadelphia: Lippincott Williams & Wilkins; 2010. p. 182–6.

Index

Note: Page numbers of article titles are in **boldface** type.

A

AAA. *See* Abdominal aortic aneurysm (AAA)
AAS. *See* Acute aortic syndrome (AAS)
Abdominal aorta, **877–891**. *See also* Abdominal aortic aneurysm (AAA)
Abdominal aortic aneurysm (AAA), **877–891**
    asymptomatic, 879–886
        diagnosis of, 880–881
        history taking, physical examination, and laboratory workups in, 880
        imaging modalities in, 880–881
        screening for, 879–880
        treatment of
            open repair *vs.* EVAR, 882–886
            prior to aneurysm repair, 882
    causes of, 878
    defined, 878
    impact of rupture, 877
    risk factors for, 878–879
    ruptured
        symptomatic, 886
    site of, 878
ACAS trial. *See* Endarterectomy for Asymptomatic Carotid Artery Stenosis (ACAS) trial
Acute aortic syndrome (AAS)
    workup for, 747–750
Acute limb ischemia
    described, 789–790
    diagnosis of, 790–791
    treatment of
        endovascular percutaneous thrombectomy and thrombolysis in, 791–794
        open surgical thrombectomy with as-needed adjunctive revascularization or
            thrombolytic therapy in, 794–795
        percutaneous *vs.* open surgical reavascularization in, 795
        post revascularization compartment syndrome following, 795–796
        rhabdomyolysis following, 796
        steps in, 790
Age
  AAA related to, 879
Aneurysm(s)
    abdominal aortic, **877–891**. *See also* Abdominal aortic aneurysm (AAA)
    aortic
        workup for, 742–747
    axillary artery, 920
    brachial artery, 920–921

Surg Clin N Am 93 (2013) 1013–1026
http://dx.doi.org/10.1016/S0039-6109(13)00096-0
0039-6109/13/$ – see front matter © 2013 Elsevier Inc. All rights reserved.

surgical.theclinics.com

Aneurysm(s) (*continued*)
  common femoral artery, 911–913. *See* Common femoral artery (CFA) aneurysms
  as hemodialysis access complication
    management of, 1007
  peripheral artery, **911–923**. *See also* Peripheral artery aneurysms
  PFA, 915–916
  popliteal artery, 916–919. *See* Popliteal artery aneurysms
  SFA, 916
Aneurysmal disease
  abdominal aorta, **877–891**
  thoracic aorta, **893–910**
Angiography
  in asymptomatic AAA diagnosis, 881
  CT
    in carotid stenosis diagnosis, 815
  magnetic resonance
    in carotid stenosis diagnosis, 815
Antiplatelet therapies
  in PAD management, 770–771
Aorta
  abdominal, **877–891**
  diseases of
    workup for, 742–750
  thoracic, **893–910**. *See also* Thoracic aorta; Thoracic aortic aneurysms (TAAs)
Aortic aneurysms
  workup for, 742–747
Arterial embolism, 927
Arterial steal syndrome
  as hemodialysis access complication
    management of, 1007–1008
Arterial thrombosis, 928
Arteritis
  radiation, 853–856. *See also* Radiation arteritis
  Takayasu, 835–841. *See also* Takayasu arteritis (TA)
Aspirin
  in PAD management, 770
Atrial reflux
  superficial venous disease and
    treatment of, 974–976. *See also* Superficial venous disease, treatment of, atrial
      reflux–related
Axillary artery aneurysms, 920

B

BCVI. *See* Blunt cerebrovascular injury (BCVI)
Blood pressure control
  in PAD management, 767–769
Blunt cerebrovascular injury (BCVI), 942–945
Blunt TAI. *See* Blunt thoracic aortic injury (TAI)
Blunt thoracic aortic injury (TAI), 945–949

Brachial artery aneurysms, 920–921
Buerger disease, 833–836. *See also* Thromboangiitis obliterans (TAO)

C

CABG. *See* Coronary artery bypass graft (CABG)
CAD. *See* Coronary artery disease (CAD)
Calf muscle pump and valve system
    in superficial venous disease, 965
Carotid artery occlusive disease, **813–832**. *See also* Carotid stenosis
    ACAS trial, 816–817
    CABG for, 818–819
    carotid artery stenting for, 823–829
        considerations regarding, 825–829
        randomized trials, 823–825
    CEA for, 818–819
    cerebral monitoring in, 819–821
    introduction, 813
    NASCET, 817–818
    pathophysiology of, 814–815
    plague location in, 814
    plague pathology in, 814–815
    symptomatic, 817–819
Carotid artery stenting
    for carotid artery occlusive disease, 823–829. *See also* Carotid artery occlusive
        disease, carotid artery stenting for
Carotid endarterectomy (CEA)
    for carotid artery occlusive disease, 818–819
    complications of, 821–823
    eversion, 819
    technical aspects of, 819
Carotid stenosis. *See also* Carotid artery occlusive disease
    asymptomatic, 817
    diagnosis of, 815
Catheter-directed thrombolysis
    in VTE disease management, 990–991
CEA. *See* Carotid endarterectomy (CEA)
CEAP classification
    of superficial venous disease, 967–970
CFA aneurysms. *See* Common femoral artery (CFA) aneurysms
Chronic arterial occlusive disease
    critical limb ischemia secondary to, 790, 796–808. *See also* Critical limb ischemia,
        secondary to chronic arterial occlusive disease
    defined, 796
    epidemiology of, 796–797
Chronic obstructive pulmonary disease (COPD)
    AAA related to, 879
Churg-Strauss syndrome, 849–853
    treatment of, 853
Cilostazol
    in PAD management, 771

Claudication, **779–788**
    background of, 779–780
    diagnosis of, 780–781
    management of
        endovascular, 783–784
        medical, 781–783
        novel treatments in, 785
        surgical, 784–785
Common femoral artery (CFA) aneurysms, 911–913
    described, 911
    diagnosis of, 912
    epidemiology of, 911–912
    natural history of, 912
    patient presentation, 912
    treatment of
        indications for, 912
        results of, 913
        surgical, 912–913
Compartment syndrome
    post revascularization
        following acute limb ischemia management, 795–796
Compressive syndromes, 936
Computed tomography (CT)
    in asymptomatic AAA diagnosis, 880–881
Computed tomography (CT) angiography
    in carotid stenosis diagnosis, 815
Connective tissue disorders, 895
COPD. See Chronic obstructive pulmonary disease (COPD)
Coronary artery bypass graft (CABG)
    for carotid artery occlusive disease, 818–819
Coronary artery disease (CAD)
    AAA related to, 879
Cranial nerve injuries
    CEA and, 822
Critical limb ischemia, **789–812**
    acute limb ischemia, 789–796. See also Acute limb ischemia
    described, 789–790
    introduction, 789–790
    nonreconstructable tibial occlusive disease and, 808
    secondary to chronic arterial occlusive disease, 790, 796–808. See also Chronic
        arterial occlusive disease
        causes of, 797
        diagnosis of, 798–799
        symptoms of, 797–798
        treatment of, 800–808
            endovascular therapy in, 800–802
            hybrid surgical therapy in, 806
            medical, 800
            open surgical therapy in, 802–806
            postrevascularization surveillance in, 807–808
            revascularization goal in, 800

surgical *vs.* endovascular therapy in, 806–807
CT. *See* Computed tomography (CT)

D

Diabetes mellitus
   management of
      in PAD management, 767
   PAD related to, 764
Dialysis Outcomes Quality Initiative (DOQI), 998
DOQI. *See* Dialysis Outcomes Quality Initiative (DOQI)
Dyslipidemia
   AAA related to, 879

E

Embolism
   arterial, 927
Endarterectomy
   carotid
      for carotid artery occlusive disease, 818–819
Endarterectomy for Asymptomatic Carotid Artery Stenosis (ACAS) trial, 816–817
Endoleak(s)
   after EVAR for asymptomatic AAA, 884–885
Endovascular aneurysm repair (EVAR)
   for asymptomatic AAA, 882–886
      endoleaks after, 884–885
   for ruptured AAAs, 886
Endovascular percutaneous thrombectomy and thrombolysis
   in acute limb ischemia management, 791–794
Endovascular therapy
   for critical limb ischemia secondary to chronic arterial occlusive disease, 800–802,
      806–807
   EVAR, 882–886
   percutaneous thrombectomy and thrombolysis, 791–794
Ethnicity
   AAA related to, 879
EVAR. *See* Endovascular aneurysm repair (EVAR)
Eversion CEA, 819

F

False aneurysms, 913–915. *See also* Femoral artery pseudoaneurysms
Femoral artery pseudoaneurysms, 913–915
   diagnosis of, 914
   natural history in, 913–914
   patient presentation in, 913–914
   postcatheterization, 913
   treatment of, 914–915
      indications for, 913–914
      surgical, 914–915

Femoral (*continued*)
    ultrasound-guided compression in, 915
    ultrasound-guided thrombin injection in, 915
Fistula(s)
  nonmaturing
    as hemodialysis access complication
      management of, 1004–1005

G

GCA. *See* Giant cell arteritis (GCA)
Gender
  AAA related to, 879
Giant cell arteritis (GCA), 841–843
  clinical presentation of, 841
  described, 841
  diagnosis of, 841–843
  pathogenesis of, 841
  treatment of, 843
Graft infection
  as hemodialysis access complication
    management of, 1006–1007

H

Hemodialysis access, **997–1012**
  background, 997
  complications of
    management of, 1004–1008
  DOQI, 998
  ideal, 998
  patient evaluation, 998–999
  postoperative surveillance, 1004
  surgical access creation, 999–1002
    forearm options, 1000–1001
    upper arm options, 1001–1002
  technical considerations in, 1002–1004
High ligation and stripping
  in atrial reflux management in superficial venous disease, 976
Hyperlipidemia
  PAD related to, 765
Hyperperfusion syndrome
  CEA and, 821–822
Hypertension
  AAA related to, 879
  PAD related to, 764–765

I

Infection(s)
  graft
    as hemodialysis access complication
      management of, 1006–1007

patch
    CEA and, 822–823
Ischemia(s)
    critical limb, **789–812**. *See also* Critical limb ischemia
    mesenteric, **925–940**. *See also* Mesenteric ischemia
Ischemic monomelic neuropathy
    as hemodialysis access complication
        management of, 1008

K

Kawasaki disease (KD), 847–849
    clinical presentation of, 848
    described, 847
    diagnosis of, 848–849
    epidemiology of, 847–848
    pathogenesis of, 847–848
    treatment of, 849
KD. *See* Kawasaki disease (KD)

L

Lipid lowering
    in PAD management, 769–770

M

Magnetic resonance angiography (MRA)
    in carotid stenosis diagnosis, 815
Magnetic resonance imaging (MRI)
    in asymptomatic AAA diagnosis, 881
MALS. *See* Median arcuate ligament syndrome (MALS)
Median arcuate ligament syndrome (MALS), 936
Mesenteric ischemia, **925–940**
    acute, 927–931
        arterial embolism, 927
        arterial thrombosis, 928
        presentation and evaluation of, 929–930
        treatment of, 930–931
    anatomy related to, 926–927
    chronic, 931–936
        diagnosis of, 932
        presentation of, 931–932
        treatment of, 932–936
    compressive syndromes, 936
    introduction, 925–926
    MALS, 936
    mesenteric venous thrombosis, 929
    noninvasive imaging workup for, 750–753
        acute mesenteric ischemia, 750–752
        chronic mesenteric ischemia, 752–753

Mesenteric (*continued*)
    nonocclusive, 928–929
Mesenteric venous thrombosis, 929
Microphlebectomy
    in tributary reflux management in superficial venous disease, 977
Microscopic polyarteritis (MPA), 849–853
    treatment of, 851–852
MPA. *See* Microscopic polyarteritis (MPA)
MRA. *See* Magnetic resonance angiography (MRA)
MRI. *See* Magnetic resonance imaging (MRI)

N

NASCET. *See* North American Symptomatic Carotid Endarterectomy Trial (NASCET)
Neuropathy
    ischemic monomelic
        as hemodialysis access complication
            management of, 1008
Nonarteriosclerotic vascular disease, **833–875**. *See also specific diseases, e.g.,*
    Thromboangiitis obliterans (TAO)
    radiation arteritis, 853–856
    Raynaud phenomenon, 856–859
    TAO, 833–836
    vasculitides, 836–853
Nonmaturing fistula
    as hemodialysis access complication
        management of, 1004–1005
Nonreconstructable tibial occlusive disease
    critical limb ischemia and, 808
North American Symptomatic Carotid Endarterectomy Trial (NASCET), 817–818

O

Open surgical thrombectomy with as-needed adjunctive revascularization or
    thrombolytic therapy
    in acute limb ischemia management, 794–795
Open thrombectomy
    in VTE disease management, 989–990

P

PAD. *See* Peripheral artery disease (PAD)
PAIs. *See* Peripheral artery injuries (PAIs)
PAN. *See* Polyarteritis nodosa (PAN)
Patch infection
    CEA and, 822–823
Percutaneous revascularization
    open surgical revascularization *vs.*
        in acute limb ischemia management, 795

Perforator reflux
    superficial venous disease and
        treatment of, 978–979
Peripheral artery aneurysms, **911–923**. *See also specific types, e.g.,* Femoral artery
    pseudoaneurysms
    axillary artery aneurysms, 920
    brachial artery aneurysms, 920–921
    CFA aneurysms, 911–913
    femoral artery pseudoaneurysms, 913–915
    PFAs, 915–916
    popliteal artery aneurysms, 916–919
    SFA aneurysms, 916
Peripheral artery disease (PAD), **761–778**
    background of, 761
    causes of, 763
    diagnosis of, 763–764
    epidemiology of, 762
    pathophysiology of, 762
    risk factors for, 764–765
    screening for, 763–764
    treatment of, 765–772
        antiplatelet therapies in, 770–771
        blood pressure control in, 767–769
        diabetes mellitus management in, 767
        exercise therapy in, 771–772
        lipid lowering in, 769–770
        tobacco cessation in, 766–767
Peripheral artery injuries (PAIs), 949–953
Phlebectomy
    powered
        in tributary reflux management in superficial venous disease, 977
Polyarteritis nodosa (PAN), 843–847
    clinical presentation of, 844
    described, 843–844
    diagnosis of, 844–845
    epidemiology of, 844
    pathogenesis of, 844
    treatment of, 845–847
Popliteal artery aneurysms, 916–919
    anatomy related to, 917
    asymptomatic
        natural history of, 918
    clinical presentation of, 917
    described, 916–917
    diagnosis of, 917–918
    management of, 919
    pathogenesis of, 917
    thrombosis related to
        risk factors for, 918–919
Powered phlebectomy
    in tributary reflux management in superficial venous disease, 977

Pseudoaneurysm(s)
    femoral artery, 913–915. *See also* Femoral artery pseudoaneurysms
    as hemodialysis access complication
        management of, 1007
Pulmonary arterial disease (PAD)
    AAA related to, 879

R

Radiation arteritis, 853–856
    clinical presentation of, 854
    described, 853
    diagnosis of, 854
    pathogenesis of, 853–854
    treatment of, 854–856
Raynaud phenomenon, 856–859
    clinical presentation of, 857
    described, 856
    diagnosis of, 858
    epidemiology of, 856–857
    pathogenesis of, 856–857
    treatment of, 858–859
Renal artery stenosis
    noninvasive imaging workup for, 753–756
Reticular veins
    in superficial venous disease, 967
Rhabdomyolysis
    following acute limb ischemia management
        treatment of, 796

S

Saphenous veins and tributaries
    in superficial venous disease, 964–965
Sclerotherapy
    in atrial reflux management in superficial venous disease, 975–976
    in tributary reflux management in superficial venous disease, 977–978
    ultrasound-guided
        in perforator reflux management in superficial venous disease, 978
SFA aneurysms. *See* Peripheral artery aneurysms
Small-vessel vasculitides, 849–853
Smoking
    AAA related to, 878–879
    PAD related to, 764
Stroke
    CEA and, 821
    mortality due to, 813
Subfascial endoscopic perforator surgery
    in perforator reflux management in superficial venous disease, 978–979
Superficial artery (SFA) aneurysms, 916
Superficial venous disease, **963–982**

anatomy related to, 964–967
CEAP classification of, 967–970
epidemiology of, 963–964
evaluation of, 971–974
introduction, 963
pathophysiology of, 964–967
physiology of, 964–967
SVT, 966
telangiectasias and reticular veins, 967
treatment of, 974–979
    atrial reflux–related, 974–976
        conservative therapy in, 974
        high ligation and stripping in, 976
        sclerotherapy in, 975–976
        thermal ablation in, 974–975
    perforator reflux–related, 978–979
    tributary reflux–related, 976–978
        microphlebectomy in, 977
        powered phlebectomy in, 977
        sclerotherapy in, 977–978
Superficial venous thrombophlebitis (SVT), 966
SVT. *See* Superficial venous thrombophlebitis (SVT)

T

TA. *See* Takayasu arteritis (TA)
TAAs. *See* Thoracic aortic aneurysms (TAAs)
Takayasu arteritis (TA), 835–841
    clinical presentation of, 837
    described, 836
    diagnosis of, 837–838
    pathogenesis of, 836
    treatment of, 839–841
TAO. *See* Thromboangiitis obliterans (TAO)
Telangiectasia(s), 967
Thermal ablation
    in atrial reflux management in superficial venous disease, 974–975
    in perforator reflux management in superficial venous disease, 978
Thienopyridines
    in PAD management, 770–771
Thoracic aorta, **893–910**. *See also* Thoracic aortic aneurysms (TAAs)
Thoracic aortic aneurysms (TAAs), **893–910**
    asymptomatic
        evaluation of, 895–897
    connective tissue disorders, 895
    described, 893–894
    evaluation of, 895–898
    incidence of, 894
    natural history of, 894
    pathobiology of, 895
    risk factors for, 894

Thoracic (*continued*)
  symptomatic
    evaluation of, 897–898
    treatment of, 898–907
      medical therapy in, 898–899
      surgical, 899–907
        anatomic considerations in, 899–900
        aortic arch debranching, 903–904
        branched endografts, 906–907
        endovascular, 902–903
        hybrid procedures, 903–905
        open surgery, 900–902
        preoperative risk stratification in, 900
        visceral debranching, 904–906
Thrombectomy
  open
    in VTE disease management, 989–990
Thromboangiitis obliterans (TAO), 833–836
  clinical presentation of, 834
  described, 833
  diagnosis of, 834–835
  pathogenesis of, 833–834
  treatment of, 835–836
Thrombolysis
  catheter-directed
    in VTE disease management, 990–991
Thrombophlebitis
  superficial venous, 966
Thrombosis
  arterial, 928
  venous
    mesenteric, 929
Tibial occlusive disease
  nonreconstructable
    critical limb ischemia and, 808
Tobacco cessation
  management of
    in PAD management, 766–767
Trauma
  vascular, **941–961**. *See also* Vascular trauma
Tributary reflux
  superficial venous disease and
    treatment of, 976–978. *See also* Superficial venous disease, treatment of, tributary
      reflux–related

  U

Ultrasound (US)
  in asymptomatic AAA diagnosis, 880
Ultrasound-guided compression
  in femoral artery pseudoaneurysms management, 915

Ultrasound-guided sclerotherapy
    in perforator reflux management in superficial venous disease, 978
Ultrasound-guided thrombin injection
    in femoral artery pseudoaneurysms management, 915
University of Wisconsin experience
    in VTE disease, 991–992
US. *See* Ultrasound (US)

V

Varicose veins
    in superficial venous disease, 965–966
Vascular disease
    nonarteriosclerotic, **833–875**. *See also specific diseases, e.g.,* Thromboangiitis
        obliterans (TAO)
    noninvasive imaging workup for, **741–760**
        AAS, 747–750
        aortic aneurysms, 742–747
        introduction, 741–750
        mesenteric ischemia, 750–753
        renal artery stenosis, 753–756
Vascular trauma
    extremity-related
        damage control strategies in, 953–954
    injury types, 941–942
    introduction, 941
    modern advances in, **941–961**
        BCVI, 942–945
        blunt TAIs, 945–949
        endovascular approaches, 955–956
        PAIs, 949–953
Vasculitides, 836–853. *See also specific types, e.g.,* Giant cell arteritis
    GCA, 841–843
    KD, 847–849
    MPA, 849–853
    PAN, 843–847
    small-vessel, 849–853
    TA, 835–841
Venous outflow stenosis/occlusion
    as hemodialysis access complication
        management of, 1005–1006
Venous thromboembolic (VTE) disease, **983–995**
    clinical practice guidelines, 991
    clinical presentation of, 984
    diagnosis of, 984–987
    introduction, 983–984
    prevention of, 987–988
    treatment of, 988–991
        nonoperative therapy in, 988–989
        surgical, 989–991
    University of Wisconsin experience, 991–992

Venous thrombosis
    mesenteric, 929
VTE disease. *See* Venous thromboembolic (VTE) disease

W

Wegener granulomatosis, 849–853
    treatment of, 853

Moving?

Make sure your subscription moves with you!

To notify us of your new address, find your **Clinics Account Number** (located on your mailing label above your name), and contact customer service at:

Email: journalscustomerservice-usa@elsevier.com

800-654-2452 (subscribers in the U.S. & Canada)
314-447-8871 (subscribers outside of the U.S. & Canada)

Fax number: 314-447-8029

Elsevier Health Sciences Division
Subscription Customer Service
3251 Riverport Lane
Maryland Heights, MO 63043

*To ensure uninterrupted delivery of your subscription, please notify us at least 4 weeks in advance of move.

Printed and bound by CPI Group (UK) Ltd, Croydon, CR0 4YY

03/10/2024

01040493-0011